STUDIES IN WELSH HISTORY

Editors

RALPH A. GRIFFITHS   CHRIS WILLIAMS
ERYN M. WHITE

———————

25

UNEMPLOYMENT, POVERTY AND HEALTH
IN INTERWAR SOUTH WALES

UNEMPLOYMENT, POVERTY AND HEALTH
IN INTERWAR SOUTH WALES

by

STEVEN THOMPSON

Published on behalf of the
History and Law Committee
of the Board of Celtic Studies

CARDIFF
UNIVERSITY OF WALES PRESS
2006

Published by the University of Wales Press

University of Wales Press
10 Columbus Walk
Brigantine Place
Cardiff
CF10 4UP

www.wales.ac.uk/press

ISBN-10 0-7083-2042-2
ISBN-13 978-0-7083-2042-6

British Library Cataloguing-in-Publication Data
A catalogue record for this book is available from the British Library.

Printed in Great Britain by Antony Rowe Ltd, Wiltshire

EDITORS' FOREWORD

Since the Second World War, Welsh history has attracted considerable scholarly attention and enjoyed a vigorous popularity. Not only have the approaches, both traditional and new, to the study of history in general been successfully applied to Wales's past, but the number of scholars engaged in this enterprise has multiplied during these years. These advances have been especially marked in the University of Wales.

In order to make more widely available the conclusions of recent research, much of it of limited accessibility in postgraduate dissertations and theses, in 1977 the History and Law Committee of the Board of Celtic Studies inaugurated a new series of monographs, *Studies in Welsh History*. It was anticipated that many of the volumes would originate in research conducted in the University of Wales or under the auspices of the Board of Celtic Studies. But the series does not exclude significant contributions made by researchers in other universities and elsewhere. Its primary aim is to serve historical scholarship and to encourage the study of Welsh history. Each volume so far published has fulfilled that aim in ample measure, and it is a pleasure to welcome the most recent addition to the list.

CONTENTS

FIGURES

TABLES

ACKNOWLEDGEMENTS

I have incurred many debts in the completion of this study. I would like to thank the librarians and archivists of the National Library of Wales, Aberystwyth; the Hugh Owen Library of the University of Wales, Aberystwyth; the West Glamorgan Archive Service, Swansea; the Glamorgan Record Office, Cardiff; the Gwent Record Office, Cwmbran; the National Archives, London; the Museum of Welsh Life at St Fagans; and the South Wales Miners' Library, Swansea. I also acknowledge the help of Elisabeth Bennett, the archivist of the South Wales Coalfield Collection at the University of Wales Swansea; the Director and staff of the Centre for Advanced Welsh and Celtic Studies, Aberystwyth; Antony Smith for drawing the maps; and Professor Richard Moore-Colyer. Early in my doctoral research I was fortunate to benefit from the advice of Dr Mari A. Williams, Dr Robert Smith and Dot Jones of the Centre for Advanced Welsh and Celtic Studies. The support of my colleagues in the Department of History and Welsh History at the University of Wales, Aberystwyth has been invaluable. Their friendship and good humour are a constant source of encouragement and ensure that the Department is an enjoyable place in which to work.

I was very fortunate to have Dr Paul O'Leary as my doctoral supervisor. His comments were at all times useful, his suggestions fruitful and his criticisms insightful, constructive and thought-provoking. My doctoral examiners, Dr Richard Coopey and Dr Charles Webster, were generous in their comments and suggestions and I hope that this study meets their expectations. Professors Ralph A. Griffiths and Chris Williams, as editors of this series, offered many observations, suggestions and comments, and I have benefited enormously from their assistance. Leah Jenkins, Sue Charles and Dafydd Jones at the University of Wales Press facilitated the production of this volume and I am grateful to them for their hard work. Gwenno Ffrancon provided constant support and encouragement throughout the time of my research, and nursed me when I broke my arm – twice! Diolch o galon, cariad. Finally, the completion of the doctoral thesis on which this study is based would not have been possible without the support of my parents, David and Janice Thompson. Their commitment to my education, and that of my brother, has been beyond the call of parental duty. I dedicate this book to them with love and respect.

Steven Thompson
August 2006

ABBREVIATIONS

AC	Administrative County
BMA	British Medical Association
CB	County Borough
CC	County Council
MB	Municipal Borough
MRC	Medical Research Council
NAMH	National Association of Medical Herbalists
NHS	National Health Service
NLW	National Library of Wales
PAC	Public Assistance Committee
RD	Rural District
RMOH	Annual Report of the Medical Officer of Health
RSMO	Annual Report of the School Medical Officer
SWMF	South Wales Miners' Federation
UAB	Unemployment Assistance Board
UD	Urban District
WNMA	Welsh National Memorial Association

MAPS

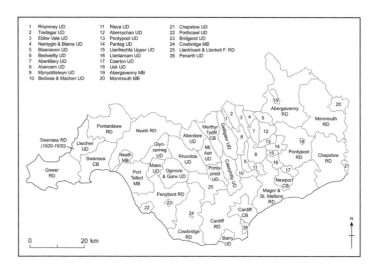

1	Rhymney UD	11	Risca UD	21	Chepstow UD
2	Tredegar UD	12	Abersychan UD	22	Porthcawl UD
3	Ebbw Vale UD	13	Pontypool UD	23	Bridgend UD
4	Nantyglo & Blaina UD	14	Panteg UD	24	Cowbridge MB
5	Blaenavon UD	15	Llanfrechfa Upper UD	25	Llantrisant & Llantwit F. RD
6	Bedwellty UD	16	Llantarnam UD	26	Penarth UD
7	Abertillery UD	17	Caerleon UD		
8	Abercarn UD	18	Usk UD		
9	Mynyddislwyn UD	19	Abergavenny MB		
10	Bedwas & Machen UD	20	Monmouth MB		

Map 1. Local authority administrative districts in south Wales, 1922–34

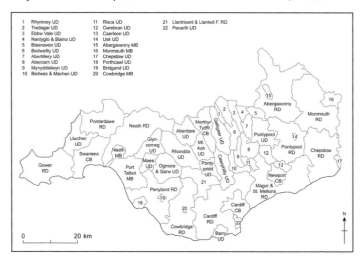

1	Rhymney UD	11	Risca UD	21	Llantrisant & Llantwit F. RD
2	Tredegar UD	12	Cwmbran UD	22	Penarth UD
3	Ebbw Vale UD	13	Caerleon UD		
4	Nantyglo & Blaina UD	14	Usk UD		
5	Blaenavon UD	15	Abergavenny MB		
6	Bedwellty UD	16	Monmouth MB		
7	Abertillery UD	17	Chepstow UD		
8	Abercarn UD	18	Porthcawl UD		
9	Mynyddislwyn UD	19	Bridgend UD		
10	Bedwas & Machen UD	20	Cowbridge MB		

Map 2. Local authority administrative districts in south Wales, 1935–9

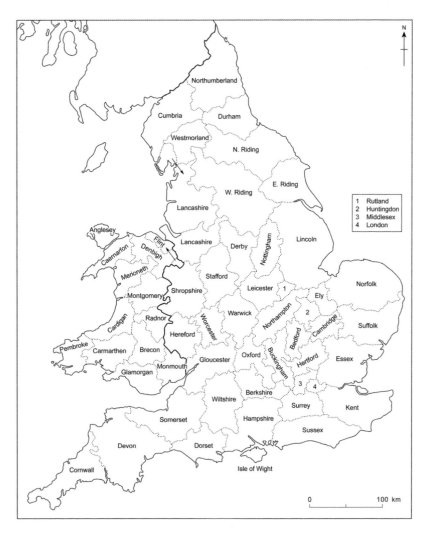

1	Rutland
2	Huntingdon
3	Middlesex
4	London

Map 3. Pre-1974 counties of England and Wales

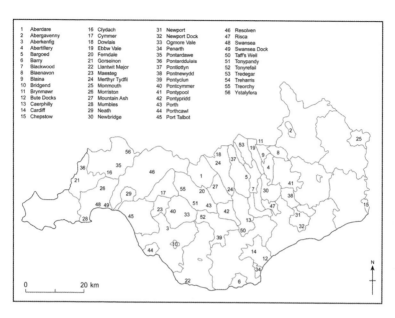

1	Aberdare	16	Clydach	31	Newport	46	Resolven
2	Abergavenny	17	Cymmer	32	Newport Dock	47	Risca
3	Aberkenfig	18	Dowlais	33	Ogmore Vale	48	Swansea
4	Abertillery	19	Ebbw Vale	34	Penarth	49	Swansea Dock
5	Bargoed	20	Ferndale	35	Pontardawe	50	Taff's Well
6	Barry	21	Gorseinon	36	Pontarddulais	51	Tonypandy
7	Blackwood	22	Llantwit Major	37	Pontlottyn	52	Tonyrefail
8	Blaenavon	23	Maesteg	38	Pontnewydd	53	Tredegar
9	Blaina	24	Merthyr Tydfil	39	Pontyclun	54	Treharris
10	Bridgend	25	Monmouth	40	Pontycymmer	55	Treorchy
11	Brynmawr	26	Morriston	41	Pontypool	56	Ystalyfera
12	Bute Docks	27	Mountain Ash	42	Pontypridd		
13	Caerphilly	28	Mumbles	43	Porth		
14	Cardiff	29	Neath	44	Porthcawl		
15	Chepstow	30	Newbridge	45	Port Talbot		

Map 4. Local employment exchanges in south Wales

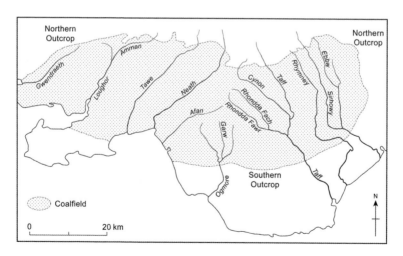

Map 5. Map showing the coalfield and river valleys of south Wales

INTRODUCTION

The economic depression of the interwar period marks a fundamental turning-point in Welsh history, and the history of south
Wales in particular, when decades of breakneck industrialization,
urbanization and immigration came to an end and were followed
by a period scarred by unemployment, poverty and emigration.
The modern history of south Wales or, as some would have it, the
post-modern or post-industrial history of south Wales, began in the
1920s and the region continues to experience the consequences of
that period of economic depression and social deprivation. As
Gwyn Alf Williams commented, 'Whole areas became and have
remained problem areas.'[1] For those people who lived through the
first few decades of the twentieth century, the 'Great Depression' was
equal to the two world wars in terms of the psychological trauma it
inflicted upon the population.[2] 'Never again' was the consensus in
1945 and this referred to the period of unemployment and poverty
that preceded the Second World War rather than the war itself.

Histories of interwar south Wales have almost universally
presented the period as one of economic depression, mass unemployment and widespread poverty.[3] They have posited what
might be termed a 'pessimistic' interpretation which emphasizes the
extensive volume of unemployment and the dire poverty that was
the experience of a large proportion of the population. Histories of
interwar south Wales are, more or less, histories of the unemployed
and the poor. In this historiography, standards of health, and the
broad factors that influenced those standards, such as diet, housing
and unemployment benefits, have been used as indicators of the

---

[1]   Gwyn A. Williams, *When was Wales?* (London, 1985), p. 253.
[2]   For Gwyn A. Williams, the Depression plays a similar role in Welsh history as the
famine in Irish history: Gwyn A. Williams, *The Welsh in their History* (London, 1982), p. 194.
[3]   K. O. Morgan, *Rebirth of a Nation: Wales 1880–1980* (Oxford, 1981), pp. 210–40;
Williams, *When was Wales?*, pp. 252–72; Trevor Herbert and Gareth Elwyn Jones (eds), *Wales
between the Wars* (Cardiff, 1988); John Davies, *A History of Wales* (Harmondsworth, 1994), pp.
509–96; Mari Williams, '"In the wars": Wales 1914–1945', in Gareth Elwyn Jones and Dai
Smith (eds), *The People of Wales* (Llandysul, 1999), pp. 179–206; D. Gareth Evans, *A History of
Wales, 1906–2000* (Cardiff, 2000), pp. 17–31, 46–53.

poverty of the population.[4] In fact, general surveys of the history of Wales have only given consideration to health and medical services at any length in relation to the interwar years, as if this was the only period in which these matters were of any importance, and they have done so in a way that is often economically deterministic.[5] High tuberculosis or maternal mortality rates, for example, although partly attributed to the inefficiency of local authorities and the inadequacy of medical services, have been associated with unemployment and poverty in a relatively simple cause-and-effect manner and have primarily been presented as evidence of the relative poverty of the population and of the tragedy of the Depression in Wales.[6] Popular perceptions have similarly equated ill health and disease with the economic fortunes of the region. Comments such as 'it was a time of disease and high mortality' or 'the smell of death was everywhere' characterize the view of the period found in working-class autobiographies.[7]

Standards of health and levels of mortality and morbidity have been examined almost solely in relation to economic depression and largely in isolation from the wider social, cultural, epidemiological and ecological circumstances of the period. Histories of interwar south Wales underestimate the extent to which the health problems they describe were characteristic of Wales in earlier decades.[8] Wales experienced relatively unfavourable levels of morbidity and mortality during the Victorian and Edwardian periods and has

[4] Morgan, *Rebirth of a Nation*, pp. 233–5; Williams, *When was Wales?*, pp. 264–5; Deian Hopkin, 'Social reactions to economic change', in Herbert and Jones, *Wales between the Wars*, pp. 52–98; Davies, *A History of Wales*, p. 580; Carol White and Sian Rhiannon Williams (eds), *Struggle or Starve: Women's Lives in the South Wales Valleys between the Two World Wars* (Dinas Powys, 1998), pp. 17, 24–5; Chris Williams, *Capitalism, Community and Conflict: The South Wales Coalfield, 1898–1947* (Cardiff, 1998), pp. 73–7; Williams, '"In the wars"', pp. 192–3; R. Merfyn Jones, *Cymru 2000: Hanes Cymru yn yr Ugeinfed Ganrif* (Caerdydd, 1999), pp. 126–8, 140–2; Evans, *History of Wales 1906–2000*, pp. 49–51.

[5] For a notable exception, see Dot Jones, 'Counting the cost of coal: women's lives in the Rhondda, 1881–1911', in Angela V. John (ed.), *Our Mothers' Land: Chapters in Welsh Women's History, 1830–1939* (Cardiff, 1991), pp. 109–33.

[6] Hopkin, 'Social reactions to economic change', p. 60; Deirdre Beddoe, 'Munitionettes, maids and mams: women in Wales, 1914–1939', in John, *Our Mothers' Land*, p. 206; Mari A. Williams, 'Yr ymgyrch i "Achub y Mamau" yng nghymoedd diwydiannol de Cymru, 1918–1939', *Cof Cenedl*, 11 (Llandysul, 1996), p. 121; Williams, *Capitalism, Community and Conflict*, p. 76; Evans, *History of Wales*, pp. 49–51.

[7] Grafton Radcliffe, *Back to Blaengarw* (Blaengarw, 1994), 37; White and Williams, *Struggle or Starve*, p. 129.

[8] A point made in the context of the depressed areas as a whole by Stephen Constantine, *Unemployment in Britain between the Wars* (London, 1980), p. 33.

continued to do so since the Second World War.[9] Therefore, a detailed and systematic consideration of health and mortality in interwar south Wales is long overdue. It is time that the statements and conclusions about the effects of economic depression on standards of health were systematically and empirically tested.

This book examines health, morbidity and mortality in a more holistic way and takes into consideration the 'multiplicity of interactions' that determined health and illness.[10] In 1972 the American medical historian George Rosen advocated an approach to the history of health which integrates biological phenomena, such as health and mortality, with their social and environmental determinants. Pointing out that patterns of health and disease are expressions of the interaction of 'biosocial organisms' with their environment, Rosen argued that:

> health conditions . . . are social phenomena and are to be comprehended within a social context. The social history of health and disease is therefore more than a study of medical problems. It requires as well an understanding of the factors – economic conditions, occupation, income, housing, nutrition, family structure, and others – which create or influence health problems, and of the ways in which they operate.[11]

More recent work in demographic history has posited a more sophisticated conceptualization. Landers, in his study of mortality in London in the 'long eighteenth century', conceptualized the relationship between mortality and its social determinants as a 'vital regime' and defined it 'not as a loosely related collection of vital rates, but as an unbounded network of relationships between the demography of human populations and the structures of their social, economic and political life, as well as their biology and ecology'.[12]

[9] Ieuan Gwynedd Jones, 'The people's health in mid-Victorian Wales', in *idem*, *Mid Victorian Wales: The Observer and the Observed* (Cardiff, 1992), pp. 24–53; Anthony Wohl, *Endangered Lives: Public Health in Victorian Britain* (London, 1983); Anne Hardy, *The Epidemic Streets: Infectious Disease and the Rise of Preventive Medicine, 1856–1900* (Oxford, 1993); James C. Riley, *Sick, Not Dead: The Health of British Workingmen during the Mortality Decline* (Baltimore, 1997); Welsh Office, *Better Health – Better Wales* (London, 1998).

[10] Bill Luckin and Graham Mooney, 'Urban history and historical epidemiology: the case of London, 1860–1920', *Urban History*, 24, 2 (1997), 37.

[11] George Rosen, 'Social variables and health in an urban environment: the case of the Victorian city', *Clio Medica*, 8, 1 (1973), 1.

[12] John Landers, *Death and the Metropolis: Studies in the Demographic History of London, 1670–1830* (Cambridge, 1993), p. 3.

This integration of biological events with social, economic and
cultural determinants has been advocated on many occasions in the
last few decades,[13] and has been achieved in a number of notable
works.[14] These works, however, have been primarily concerned with
the early modern period or the nineteenth century and historians
have yet to address the twentieth century in this way. Studies of
medicine in the twentieth century have been more concerned to
explore the development of health services than to consider the
social factors that determined health and illness.[15] As Samuel
Preston has noted, the decline in mortality that took place in the
developed world in the twentieth century is 'one of mankind's
major achievements' and yet 'we know more about the sources of
change in the relatively quiescent nineteenth century than in the
twentieth'.[16] This study examines the 'multiplicity of interactions'
that determined patterns of mortality in interwar south Wales,
through the use of qualitative and quantitative sources, and demonstrates the interdependence of biological phenomena and their
social, economic and cultural setting.[17] It broadens the hitherto
narrow focus that has characterized studies of health and mortality
in the interwar period and examines the 'vital regime' of interwar
south Wales.

This holistic approach to health requires a 'total history' of
people's lives in interwar south Wales and an approach, as Porter
and Wear have advocated, that does not privilege official docu-
ments at the expense of other sources.[18] This ensures that official or
professional views are complemented by lay attitudes and popular
perceptions. This study is conceived as a social history of health and

---

[13]   E. A. Wrigley, 'The prospects for population history', *Journal of Interdisciplinary History*,
12, 2 (1981), 115; Roy Porter and Andrew Wear, 'Introduction', in *eidem* (eds), *Problems and
Methods in the History of Medicine* (London, 1987), pp. 1–11; Mark S. R. Jenner, review of
Landers, *Death and the Metropolis*, and J. A. I. Chapman (ed.), *Epidemic Disease in London*
(London, 1993), in *Urban History*, 22, 2 (1995), 295–7; Luckin and Mooney, 'Urban history
and historical epidemiology'.

[14]   Richard J. Evans, *Death in Hamburg: Society and Politics in the Cholera Years, 1830–1910*
(Oxford, 1987); Landers, *Death and the Metropolis*; Mary J. Dobson, *Contours of Death and Disease
in Early Modern England* (Cambridge, 1997); Luckin and Mooney 'Urban history and historical
epidemiology'.

[15]   Jane Lewis, 'Providers, "consumers", the state and the delivery of health-care services in
twentieth-century Britain', in Andrew Wear (ed.), *Medicine in Society: Historical Essays* (Cambridge,
1992), p. 317; Virginia Berridge, *Health and Society since 1939* (Cambridge, 1999), p. 1.

[16]   Samuel H. Preston, 'Population studies of mortality', *Population Studies*, 50 (1996), 536.

[17]   Porter and Wear, 'Introduction', p. 8.

[18]   Ibid., p. 5.

medicine 'from below', aiming not only to consider the 'public's view of public health'[19] but also those aspects of life which working men and women believed determined their health and illnesses.[20] For example, it is highly relevant to this approach that many of the working-class women studied by Margery Spring Rice attributed their ill health to the unemployment of their husbands; that respiratory illness in the Swansea valley was blamed on the emissions of a nearby metal-works; that couples purposely limited family size because of concerns about the financial costs of raising children; that a resident of Blaina insisted that every house should have a lavatory – 'It's only healthy'; that working-class families in the Rhondda believed that the way in which they balanced the domestic budget determined their standards of health; that families throughout south Wales aspired to more wholesome standards of housing not just for reasons of comfort or outward respectability but also for the sake of their health; that numerous complaints about environmental pollution were made by members of the public to public health officials; and that efforts were continually made by ordinary people to improve their environment, both inside and outside the home.

This presents a problem. Lay perceptions of the factors that determined health and illness did not necessarily correspond to what actually influenced standards of health. Lay perceptions were partly formed and shaped by experience and, increasingly during the course of the twentieth century, by orthodox biomedicine, but were not always 'rational'. While it is true that orthodox medicine was not as objective or effective as the medical establishment liked to claim, it was also the case that lay knowledge was at times mistaken or even harmful. Moreover, perceptions of the surrounding environment and of the determinants of health led ordinary people to act in a way that had consequences for their lives and for their health. Families made efforts to improve the standard of their diets, housing conditions and immediate public environment, or patronized one type of practitioner instead of another. Cultural factors led people to behave in specific ways which had consequences for their well-being. For example, parents in Cardiff

---

[19]   Michael Sigsworth and Michael Worboys, 'The public's view of public health in mid-Victorian Britain', *Urban History*, 21, 2 (1994), 237–50.
[20]   John V. Pickstone, review of Roy Porter and W. F. Bynum (eds), *Living and Dying in London* (London, 1991), in *Social History of Medicine*, 7, 1 (1994), 147–8.

believed that meat was injurious to the health of children and children's diets in Cardiff lacked protein partly for this reason.

This is not to echo the insistence of many health professionals during these decades that ill health and mortality were to be explained by reference to personal behaviour, without any consideration of the wider social and economic context. Rather, this study sets individual behaviour in the specific context of working-class life and elucidates the internal meaning and logic of lay actions and behaviour.[21] As an example, many public health officials, concerned with the problem of high tuberculosis mortality in interwar Wales, complained of the fatalism of the Welsh population that, it was claimed, derived from their religious convictions and Celtic temperament. While there is evidence to suggest that there did indeed exist a sense of fatalism among the population, it seems that this was a result of close experience of the disease in people's everyday lives and the ineffectiveness of official, therapeutic measures taken against the disease. Only by understanding lay behaviour from within can qualifications of this sort be made.

Apart from this aspect of medical history from below that sheds light on *mentalités*, there is a more prosaic reason for adopting such an approach. By closely examining the everyday realities of people's lives it is possible to obtain a better understanding of the specific ways in which social variables determined standards of health. If the focus of inquiry is altered to examine everyday experiences, a different picture of the past emerges. For example, to describe the extension of water and sewerage provision in interwar south Wales is not to say very much about the mortality risks which faced the population, since connections to individual houses and the qualitative change this involved need to be taken into account too. Similarly, to set out abstract wage indices or unemployment percentages is insufficient to explain high levels of morbidity and mortality since such indices give no indication of qualitative changes in living standards. The practical consequences of poverty were both mitigated and exacerbated by a complex array of factors that determined the quality of life enjoyed by a family and its individual members. For example, only a detailed examination of the sources reveals the fact that workers who experienced short-time

---

[21]   F. Loux, 'Popular culture and knowledge of the body: infancy and the medical anthropologist', in Porter and Wear, *Problems and Methods*, pp. 87–8.

working were worse off than the permanently unemployed, a fact that is not recognized in the traditional historiography and yet it complicates the neat distinction between 'employed' and 'unemployed' and, more importantly, our understanding of the effects of unemployment on health. A micro-level analysis allows a greater understanding of the specific ways in which social factors determined patterns and levels of mortality.

Great advances have been made in recent years in the study of medical history 'from below'. Since the publication of Roy Porter's programmatic article in 1985, an increasing number of scholars have answered his call for the 'patient's view' to be considered and the patient has been moved to the forefront of historical study.[22] Ascertaining the lay attitudes and working-class thought-worlds of interwar south Wales is not easy. There is, for example, an inherent danger in using official sources to interpret the outlook and attitudes of ordinary people since the 'bourgeois sensibilities' of middle-class observers 'rendered them insensitive to the thought-worlds inhabited by members of other social classes'.[23] Fortunately, a number of sources exist in which the opinions and attitudes of working-class people are recorded, while it is also possible to read official sources in a way that suppresses the 'bourgeois sensibilities' of their authors and extracts a specifically working-class or lay rationale for the actions that medical officers condemned.[24]

By taking a view 'from below', the role of human agency in demographic phenomena becomes apparent.[25] To some extent, the emphasis placed on human agency challenges the traditional historiography of interwar south Wales which seems to view working-class people as victims of the powerful forces that acted upon their lives. In this traditional historiography, resistance only manifests itself through overtly political action such as strikes, hunger marches or other forms of political activism; working-class

---

[22] Roy Porter, 'The patient's view. Doing medical history from below', *Theory and Society*, 14 (1985), 175–98; Gert Brieger, 'The historiography of medicine', in W. F. Bynum and R. Porter (eds), *Companion Encyclopedia of the History of Medicine* (London, 1993), vol. 1, pp. 25–6.

[23] Andy Croll, 'Writing the insanitary town: G. T. Clark, slums and sanitary reform', in Brian L. James (ed.), *G. T. Clark: Scholar Ironmaster in the Victorian Age* (Cardiff, 1998), p. 41.

[24] Sigsworth and Worboys, 'Public's view'.

[25] The relationship between human agency and political economy in relation to demography is one that has exercised the attention of anthropologists; see Susan Greenhalgh (ed.), *Situating Fertility: Anthropology and Demographic Inquiry* (Cambridge, 1995), and esp. the chapters by Greenhalgh and Kertzer.

people are otherwise characterized as unresponsive. However, it was also the case that ordinary people acted as conscious decision-makers, active agents in their own history, determined to have at least some control over their lives and their health. Resistance manifested itself in an array of small-scale and subtle everyday acts, attitudes and modes of behaviour. 'Survival strategies' comprise a form of resistance to the circumstances of everyday life.[26]

Issues of morbidity and mortality were contentious during the interwar period and have continued to provide a focus for disagreement ever since, most noticeably in the so-called 'optimistic' and 'pessimistic' interpretations formulated during the 1970s and, more especially, the 1980s.[27] Disagreements centred on the precise effects of unemployment and poverty on the standards of health of the population and whether or not the interwar years should be characterized as a time of marked improvement or significant deterioration in standards of health and levels of mortality.[28] This book is partly conceived as a contribution to that debate and addresses the fundamental issues at stake. It aims to test Anne Crowther's assertion that 'The debate on mortality will be furthered only by careful local studies which relate small-area statistics to the local economy and also to the effectiveness of local policies.'[29] Accordingly, it examines the social history of health in interwar south Wales. This seemingly simple statement requires a great deal of qualification and explanation. In the first place, as historians of 'health' often point out, it is

[26] Laurence Fontaine and Jürgen Schlumbohm, 'Household strategies for survival: an introduction', *International Review of Social History*, 45 (2000), supplement 8, 6.
[27] Derek H. Aldcroft, *The Inter-War Economy: Britain, 1919–1939* (London, 1970), pp. 375–85; John Stevenson and Chris Cook, *The Slump* (London, 1977), pp. 19–21, 38–46, 78–81; Jay Winter, 'Infant mortality, maternal mortality and public health in Britain in the 1930s', *Journal of European Economic History*, 8, 2 (1979), 439–62, and 'The decline of mortality in Britain, 1870–1950', in T. Barker and M. Drake (eds), *Population and Society in Britain, 1850–1950* (London, 1982), pp. 100–20; Charles Webster, 'Healthy or hungry thirties?', *History Workshop Journal*, 13 (1982), 110–29; Jay Winter, 'Unemployment, nutrition and infant mortality in Britain, 1920–50', in *idem* (ed.), *The Working Class in Modern British History* (Cambridge, 1983), pp. 232–55; Charles Webster, 'Health, welfare and unemployment during the depression', *Past and Present*, 109 (1985), 204–29; Margaret Mitchell, 'The effects of unemployment on the social conditions of women and children in the 1930s', *History Workshop Journal*, 19 (1985), 105–27; Ian Gazeley, *Poverty in Britain, 1900–1965* (Basingstoke, 2003), pp. 111–23.
[28] On this debate, see Anne Crowther, *Social Policy in Britain, 1914–1939* (London, 1988), 66–72; Andrew Thorpe, *Britain in the 1930s* (Oxford, 1992), pp. 110–19; Helen Jones, *Health and Society in Twentieth-Century Britain* (London, 1994), pp. 74–6.
[29] Crowther, *Social Policy in Britain*, p. 70.

not health which forms the object of study but ill health, disease and mortality.[30] This study focuses primarily on mortality rather than on 'health' or 'illness' and there are a number of reasons for this. Most importantly, and despite the many methodological problems inherent in the study of mortality, it is easier to examine patterns of mortality than of morbidity. Sickness and illness are subjective states defined by the sufferer, whereas death is definite and irrefutable. No systematic means of recording or measuring sickness incidents existed in interwar south Wales. The notification of certain notifiable diseases was often determined more by the conscientiousness and efficiency of general practitioners and medical officers than by any actual pattern of morbidity.[31]

This study therefore focuses on patterns of mortality in interwar south Wales and their social, economic and cultural determinants. It describes and explains the changing pattern of mortality during the period and evaluates the influence of the interwar economic depression on them. It might be argued that mortality is a rather blunt tool with which to examine the subtle social factors that impacted on people's lives; unemployment and poverty were more likely to influence morbidity than mortality. And yet historians have recognized mortality rates as sensitive indicators of the social and economic well-being of a population.[32] They have been used in the 'standard of living' debate on the effects of the Industrial Revolution,[33] in disagreements about the impact of the First World War on civilian health[34] and, of course, in the controversy over the 'healthy

[30] Derek J. Oddy, 'The health of the people', in Barker and Drake, *Population and Society*, p. 121; Jones, *Health and Society in Twentieth-Century Britain*, p. 1.

[31] On the unreliability of notification, see Monmouthshire CC, RMOH (1924), p. 22; J. M. Mackintosh, *Trends of Opinion about the Public Health, 1901–51* (London, 1953), pp. 80–1; furthermore, it was largely infectious diseases which were classified as notifiable diseases, and cases of other diseases such as respiratory diseases, cancer and heart disease were not enumerated.

[32] Preston, 'Population studies of mortality', 525.

[33] A. J. Taylor (ed.), *The Standard of Living in the Industrial Revolution* (London, 1975); W. A. Armstrong, 'The trend of mortality in Carlisle between the 1780s and the 1840s: a demographic contribution to the standard of living debate', *Economic History Review*, 34, 1 (1981), 94–114; J. G. Williamson, 'Was the Industrial Revolution worth it? Disamenities and death in nineteenth century towns', *Explorations in Economic History*, 19 (1982), 221–45; P. Huck, 'Infant mortality and living standards of English workers during the Industrial Revolution', *Journal of Economic History*, 55, 3 (1995), 528–50; Simon Szreter and Graham Mooney, 'Urbanisation, mortality and the standard of living debate: new estimates of the expectation of life at birth in nineteenth-century British cities', *Economic History Review*, 51, 1 (1997), 84–112.

[34] J. M. Winter, 'The impact of the First World War on civilian health in Britain', *Economic History Review*, 30, 3 (1977), 487–503; idem, *The Great War and the British People*

or hungry thirties'. Infant mortality rates, in particular, have long been considered sensitive indicators of the social and economic well-being of a population.[35]

The first section of this book examines the various social, economic and cultural determinants of mortality. This detailed examination of the material circumstances of working-class life redresses the neglect of these issues that characterizes the 'healthy or hungry thirties' debate. The articles of Webster and Winter do not adequately consider the social determinants of mortality or the material circumstances of working-class life and so are unable to demonstrate fully the relationship between poverty and ill health in interwar Britain. These articles, and much of the work concerned with health in the interwar period, establish the level of unemployment and the poverty of the unemployed and then merely attempt to find the consequences of this poverty in the mortality statistics. As an analysis of the causes of mortality they are inadequate. As Winter recognizes, it is misleading to treat unemployment as an independent variable and infant mortality as a dependent variable, as some studies have done and as Welsh historians have attempted to do using anecdotal evidence. 'To make sense of the immediate consequences of unemployment,' Winter argues, 'it must be seen as part of a network of economic relations, support systems and social attitudes that are deeply embedded in the class structure.'[36] Studies of ill health and mortality in interwar Britain need to examine the material circumstances of everyday life in order to understand the ways in which poverty and unemployment manifested themselves. For example, did unemployment entail a significant decrease in income? Did decreases in income manifest themselves in reduced expenditure on food or did poverty-stricken families move to cheaper rented housing accommodation that was also more insanitary? How did poverty affect the habitability of a house? How long did a person have to be unemployed or exist on a reduced income

(London, 1986); Linda Bryder, 'The First World War: healthy or hungry?', *History Workshop Journal*, 24 (1987), 141–57; J. Winter, 'Public health and the political economy of war: a reply to Linda Bryder', *History Workshop Journal*, 26 (1988), 163–73.

[35] E. G. Stockwell, 'Infant mortality', in Kenneth Kiple (ed.), *The Cambridge World History of Human Disease* (Cambridge, 1993), p. 226.

[36] Winter, 'Unemployment, nutrition and infant mortality', p. 252; this error is committed by N. J. Leiper, 'Health and unemployment in Glamorgan, 1923–1938' (unpubl. University of Wales M.Sc. thesis, 1986), which attempts to correlate time-series unemployment rates for Wales as a whole with the crude death rates for Glamorgan.

before these became issues of concern? What difference did the strategies employed by working-class families make? How important were the actions of local authorities and the central government? A consideration of these sorts of questions is absent from much of the historiography on health and mortality in the interwar period but they are important issues which need to be addressed.

The second section of the book, which examines general mortality and infant mortality, also utilizes descriptive and analytical frameworks. In each case general death rates are disaggregated so as to ascertain subtle patterns and changes in mortality during the interwar period. As Webster pointed out in relation to infant mortality, official, optimistic interpretations were based on a consideration of aggregate death rates, but a radically different perspective is offered by a finer analysis of the mortality data.[37] Patterns and changes revealed by the disaggregation of death rates are explored in more depth and examined in light of the material factors of working-class life outlined in the first section of the book. For example, general histories utilizing anecdotal evidence have suggested the economic and social disadvantages faced by the women of coalmining communities in interwar south Wales, but disaggregating the death rates reveals more precisely the consequences of those disadvantages. Furthermore, these inequalities in mortality experiences can be examined over time so as to show the extent to which the social and economic disadvantages under which women in south Wales laboured changed during the interwar period, but also the degree to which the consequences of unemployment and poverty were disproportionately experienced by women. This is another aspect of the Depression in Wales that is suggested in the general historiography utilizing anecdotal evidence, but it requires more systematic analysis.

The geographical area covered by this study is the counties of Glamorgan and Monmouth. These two counties contained over half the population of Wales by the interwar period and constituted one of the most important industrial regions in Britain. The two counties in their entirety have been chosen so as to utilize the statistics of mortality published in aggregate form in the annual reports of their medical officers of health but also in order to contrast regions within south Wales that were characterized by different

---

[37] Webster, 'Healthy or hungry thirties?', 125.

social, economic and ecological environments. Coalmining communities of the valleys are contrasted with the rural, agricultural areas of eastern Monmouthshire and the large, socially diverse county boroughs on the coast. This comparative dimension provides a number of useful insights and serves to highlight the distinct aspects of the 'vital regime' of each environment.[38]

Elizabeth Andrews wrote of the interwar period that, 'When history comes to be written about this period of mass unemployment it will be dealt with in statistics and percentages. Readers and students of the future will need much imagination and understanding to give the human factor its rightful place.'[39] This is perfectly true. Nevertheless, it is hoped that, though much of this study is based upon quantitative material, the careful engagement with the large number of sources which shed light on people's everyday lives helps to give 'the human factor its rightful place'. It is hoped, for example, that the use of a large number of 'working-class autobiographies' will help to give a feel for the experiences of 'ordinary people'. Despite the use of such material, an effort has been made to make a dispassionate analysis of this emotive period in our history. Understandably, historians have felt a measure of sympathy for the victims of an economic system over which they had no control and, too often, contemporary assertions and judgements on the relationship between poverty, unemployment and health have been accepted uncritically by historians. Welsh historiography has for too long been dependent on a relatively simplistic, one-dimensional view of health in the interwar period and it is necessary to place our understanding of the period on a surer empirical footing.

---

[38]   Descriptions of the nature of the communities of south Wales and the broad history of the interwar period can be found in a number of historical studies; see Arthur H. John and Glanmor Williams (eds), *Glamorgan County History*, vol. 5, *Industrial Glamorgan* (Cardiff, 1980); Prys Morgan (ed.), *Glamorgan County History*, vol. 6, *Glamorgan Society, 1780–1980* (Cardiff, 1988); Morgan, *Rebirth of a Nation*; Williams, *Capitalism, Community and Conflict*; Mari Williams, '"In the wars"'; Herbert and Jones, *Wales between the Wars*.
[39]   Elizabeth Andrews, *A Woman's Work is Never Done* (Ystrad, Rhondda, 1957), p. 27.

I

OBTAINING AN INCOME: WAGES, BENEFITS AND HOUSEHOLD STRATEGIES

His father's toil had been so excessive as to make him stoop like a victim of curvature. That had been just as well, because his father's wages were so low it would have been impossible to count them standing up straight. It had always been necessary to get them very close to the floor to get them in the right perspective.[1]

In any study of interwar Britain, economic depression, unemployment and poverty understandably occupy a central position. Dole queues, soup kitchens, hunger marches, rickety children and hollow-eyed adults have dominated popular perceptions of these 'wasted years'. And yet, as revisionist historians have pointed out, the interwar period was also characterized by impressive economic growth, the development of new light industries and the emergence of new patterns of consumption. While the presence of poverty and hardship is undeniable, it has also been pointed out that the unemployed never constituted more than a minority of the British population during the whole of the period. For those in work the interwar years were a period of rising living standards as real wages increased and as a whole range of consumer durables came within the purchasing power of working-class families.[2] If this central paradox of the interwar years has served to enliven British historiography, it has occasioned much less controversy among Welsh historians. As K. O. Morgan wrote in 1981:

> Some historians of late have tended to paint a more cheerful picture of the thirties than once used to be prevalent . . . in south Wales, this verdict cannot possibly be accepted. The thirties were a time when a whole society was crucified by mass unemployment and near-starvation.[3]

The length and severity of economic depression, the massive volume of unemployment and the dire poverty occasioned by it

---

[1] Gwyn Thomas, *Sorrow for Thy Sons* (London, 1986), p. 67.

[2] Charles L. Mowat, *Britain between the Wars, 1918–40* (London, 1955); Aldcroft, *Inter-War Economy*; John Stevenson and Chris Cook, *Britain in the Depression: Society and Politics, 1929–39* (Essex, 1994 edn).

[3] Morgan, *Rebirth of a Nation*, p. 230; see also Williams, *When was Wales?*, p. 252.

seem to have led Welsh historians to offer a reductionist account of the interwar years which sees a whole society 'crucified'. Histories of interwar south Wales are, more or less, histories of the unemployed and the poor. Certainly there is very little reason to be 'optimistic' about south Wales in the interwar period, but it remains the case that, even in the deepest trough of the Depression in 1932, 55 per cent of the population of Monmouthshire and almost 60 per cent of that of Glamorgan were in employment.[4] For the greater part of the period, approximately 70–80 per cent of the population of south Wales was employed and yet Welsh historians have almost completely overlooked this experience. Perhaps, as Glynn and Oxborrow have observed, historians should not arbitrate between 'optimistic' and 'pessimistic' interpretations but instead present the interwar period in all its complexity and paradoxical nature.[5] The experience of employment was a significant one and an examination of wages and incomes is relevant to a study of the quality of life in interwar south Wales.

Many historians have described the broad nature of changes in wages and incomes in interwar Britain and the general trend in wages can be easily sketched.[6] Large rises in money wages during the First World War meant that by the end of 1920 average salaries in Britain were about double what they had been in 1914. Weekly wage rates had risen 2.7 or 2.8 times for a working week which, in 1919, had been reduced to between 44 and 48 hours from its former range of 48 to 60 hours. There followed a collapse in wages, with a fall in standard wage rates of 8 per cent in the period December 1920 to December 1921 and of 22 per cent in the following twelve months. The average decreases in weekly wages recorded by the Ministry of Labour in 1921 were 17s 6d per week for 7.2 million workers and in 1922 a further 11s for 7.6 million

[4]   Ministry of Labour, *Local Unemployment Index*, 1932; annual average based on 12 monthly averages. A similar observation is made by Davies, *History of Wales*, pp. 559–60; for an insight into the relative incomes of employed and unemployed families in interwar south Wales, see the diagram in Hilda Jennings, *Brynmawr: A Study of a Distressed Area* (London, 1934), p. 162.

[5]   Sean Glynn and John Oxborrow, *Interwar Britain: A Social and Economic History* (London, 1976), p. 13.

[6]   Guy Routh, *Occupation and Pay in Great Britain, 1906–79* (London, 1980), pp. 139–53; Aldcroft, *Inter-War Economy*, pp. 352–4; A. L. Chapman and R. Knight, *Wages and Salaries in the United Kingdom, 1920–1938* (Cambridge, 1953).

workers. Reductions were most severe for coalminers, 1.3 million of whom saw their wages decline on average by £2 per week in 1921 and a further 10s in 1922. Nevertheless, average wage rates in 1924 were still twice those of 1914. Wage rates rested at this level until 1930–1 when a moderate decline occurred until 1934, after which a slow rise took place so that by 1938 wage rates were 5–6 per cent higher than the 1930 level and about double the pre-war level.

Aggregate wage indices and statistics suffer from being abstract averages which conceal as much as they reveal. They conceal significant variations between occupations, industries and regions, and they cover a workforce that varied according to skill, age and sex. Furthermore, these wage indices refer to fully employed workers and do not take into account irregularities of employment such as short-time working, payments in kind, stoppages and even the wilful under-payment by calculating employers. Finally, they take no account of the nature of the family which the wage was intended to support. Its composition in terms of the number and sex of its members, and the proportion of wage earners to dependants, had important implications for the quality of life enjoyed by a family. Therefore, it is important to inquire into the nature of incomes in interwar south Wales beyond the broad outline of real wages.[7]

The pattern of wages in south Wales followed the general outline for Britain as a whole – a sharp decline in the early 1920s, a period of stagnation until about 1933–4, followed by about five years of gradually rising rates in the mid to late 1930s.[8] Workers in the coal industry, working six shifts a week, could earn between about £2 13s and £3 4s a week during the late 1920s and 1930s. Agricultural labourers in Glamorgan could earn a minimum of between £1 12s and £1 18s a week while their counterparts in Monmouthshire on average could earn between £1 11s and £1 15s in the same period. Workers in the engineering, boilermaking and foundry trades in Cardiff and Barry earned typically anything between £2 8s and £3 10s per week depending on their level of skill.

These variations in wages and earnings are, of course, meaningless unless set alongside trends in prices. The assertion by Francis

[7] Aldcroft, *Inter-War Economy*, pp. 351–3.
[8] For a more detailed consideration of wage rates and real incomes in south Wales, see Steven Thompson, 'A social history of health in interwar south Wales' (unpublished University of Wales Ph.D. thesis, 2001), 20–3.

and Smith that the wages bill in the south Wales coal industry fell from £65 million in 1920 to £14 million in 1933 is rather disingenuous.[9] Generally, prices fell gradually during the interwar period.[10] A sharp fall in prices in 1921 meant that, while wage rates fell by 23 per cent, retail prices fell by over 40 per cent. In the following year wages and prices fell equally by about 19 per cent. Prices continued to fall gradually until about 1933–4, after which they rose slowly. The fall in prices, when set against the movement in wages, caused a fairly marked rise in real earnings in Britain as a whole. In south Wales similarly, the standard of living of those in employment was considerably higher in the 1930s, the 'devil's decade', than it had been in the 1920s (see Figure 1.1). Despite the decline in wage rates through the interwar period the even greater fall in prices meant that real incomes rose, albeit gradually.

Rates and indices of wages often have little relation to the reality of working conditions. Economic circumstances, industrial and political factors, and the nature of the labour market need to be considered if an accurate account of incomes is to be obtained. First, the level of skill needed to perform a certain job and the amount of work carried out determined the wages which a worker received at the end of each week. Even within the same industry, workers varied greatly in the skills they possessed and the wages they received. Philip Massey found that in Blaina in the 1930s only one colliery worker in six was a collier. Colliers earned a minimum of 9s 5d a shift and were able to earn anything up to 18s a shift, while repairers earned 9s 9d per shift and helpers and labourers, who made up the majority of the workforce, were only getting 8s 5d per shift. Colliers were therefore the only workers who could earn more than £2 18s 6d a week and those who did so, claimed Massey, were perhaps one in ten of all colliery workers. The weekly earnings of all workers, no matter how high or low they might be, were subject to deductions averaging three or four shillings a week.[11]

The wages of tinplate workers, many of whom worked in west Glamorgan, were similarly based on piece-rates and were also

[9] Hywel Francis and Dai Smith, *The Fed: A History of the South Wales Miners in the Twentieth Century* (London, 1980), p. 33; similarly A. J. Chandler, 'The re-making of a working class: migration from the South Wales Coalfield to the new industry areas of the Midlands c.1920–1940' (unpublished University of Wales Ph.D. thesis, 1989), 51.

[10] On prices see John Burnett, *A History of the Cost of Living* (Harmondsworth, 1969), pp. 309–12; Routh, *Occupation and Pay*, p. 141; Aldcroft, *Inter-War Economy*, pp. 362–5.

[11] Phillip Massey, *Portrait of a Mining Town, Fact*, 8 (November 1937), pp. 29–30.

Figure 1.1. Advertisement for William Harris, grocer, Merthyr Tydfil, 1930

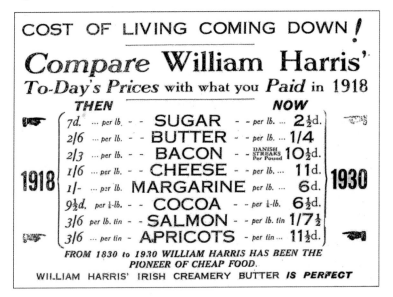

Source: *Merthyr Express* (14 June 1930)

determined by the nature of the task of each worker. A new wage agreement in 1920 meant that workers were paid according to the number of boxes of tinplate they worked. Rollermen were paid 4s 3d per dozen boxes, doublers 3s 5d, furnacemen 3s 2d, behinders 1s 9d, first helpers 3s 0d, second helpers 2s 1d and shearers 1s 4d. In addition, a sliding-scale bonus was paid which was determined by the price of tinplate bar, but, because the price of tinplate fell so low, workers received no additional payments for many years, although they did receive an *ex gratia* bonus, which was paid by the employers in the interest of good industrial relations.[12]

Secondly, the economic conditions of the interwar years and the high levels of unemployment meant that employers enjoyed an advantage in industrial relations. Political activists were victimized and many employers took advantage of their strong position to pay their workers as little as possible.[13] In the coal industry young men of 16 or 17 years of age were preferred to older men since they

[12] W. E. Minchinton, *The British Tinplate Industry: A History* (Oxford, 1957), pp. 220–2.

[13] Cliff Prothero, *Recount* (Ormskirk, 1982), p. 23; see also Matt Perry, *Bread and Work: The Experience of Unemployment, 1918–39* (London, 2000), pp. 67–8.

could be paid less.[14] Another tactic of employers was not to pay wages for the 'small coal' which the colliers cut, despite selling this for a profit.[15] In other instances, workers in the coal industry were dismissed from their jobs for complaining about wilful under-payment by employers.[16]

More widespread was the practice of short-time working. In some industries this was institutionalized as employers and trade unions sought to resolve the problems caused by insufficient demand. In the tinplate industry, for example, there existed a surplus of labour throughout the interwar period which, for various reasons, neither employers nor workers did anything to remedy.[17] Tinplate companies preferred to share the orders they received amongst their mills rather than concentrate production in a smaller number of mills, in readiness for periods of increased demand, and so workers commonly faced periods of short-time working or temporary unemployment. In this instance it is evident that not only was short-time working determined by the variation in demand for a product, but industrial factors were also exerting an influence.[18] The iron, steel and coal industries were similarly characterized by short-time working as efforts were made to maintain an available labour supply for periods of increased demand.

Tinplate companies even exploited the system of unemployment benefit by employing workers for a few days a week, thereby allowing them to claim benefit as well as receive wages for the days on which they were employed.[19] A Political and Economic Planning (PEP) report criticized the tinplate industry for the way in which it was 'wastefully and anti-socially organised' and for 'drawing continuously a hidden subsidy at the expense of other industries through unemployment insurance'. It contrasted the industry with the nickel works at Clydach in the Swansea valley, which was described as a model of 'socially responsible labour policy'.[20]

[14]   See, for example, *Men Without Work: A Report Made for the Pilgrim Trust* (Cambridge, 1938), p. 69.

[15]   B. L. Coombes, *Those Clouded Hills* (London, 1944), p. 10.

[16]   James Hanley, *Grey Children: A Study in Humbug and Misery* (London, 1937), p. 2; see also G. H. Armbruster, 'The social determination of ideologies: being a study of a Welsh mining community' (unpublished University of London Ph.D. thesis, 1940), pp. 273–4.

[17]   Minchinton, *British Tinplate Industry*, pp. 210–14.

[18]   Noel Whiteside and J. A. Gillespie, 'Deconstructing unemployment: developments in Britain in the interwar years', *Economic History Review*, 44, 4 (1991), pp. 665–82.

[19]   Minchinton, *British Tinplate Industry*, p. 213.

[20]   Political and Economic Planning (PEP), *The Problem of South Wales*, *Planning*, 94, 9 (March 1937), 6.

Dockworkers in south Wales were similarly able to exploit the unemployment benefit system.[21] After 1921 insurance benefit contributors were able to claim benefit if they were employed on no more than three days in a six-day period. Before efforts were made in the 1930s to make dock work a closed trade, labour was highly casualized and employees were able to exert some control over their engagements and avoid work that endangered their benefits. 'Three days on the hook and three days in the book' became a common working week. In a survey of 1,000 Newport dockworkers in 1930, for example, it was found that the average weekly wage of £2 18s was supplemented by 8s 7d in unemployment benefit.[22] A slightly different system prevailed in Cardiff among the 1,500 members of the Coal Trimmers' Union. The employers at the docks paid the men's wages not to the individual workmen but to the union, which then distributed the total amount equally among the men. The men worked two weeks on and two weeks off, during which time they also received unemployment benefit. By this method each worker was assured 50s a week whether he worked or not.[23] Dockworkers were able to receive the more generous unemployment benefit rather than assistance or transitional payments because the relatively high wages they received for their work and the regular nature of their employment allowed them to make the necessary contributions.

If employers were in a position to aid their workers with regard to unemployment benefit eligibility they were also able to frustrate their employees' efforts to maintain a steady income. A number of miners in the coal industry during the interwar period remembered how underemployment was common and that colliery managers deliberately set out to deny their workers unemployment benefit. Kenneth Maher of Caerphilly believed that the coal-owners and the government were constantly 'bashing' the miners:

> The favourite trick was to work on Monday and Tuesday, off Wednesday, work Thursday, off Friday, work Saturday, or off Monday, work Tuesday, off Wednesday, work Thursday, off Friday, work Saturday. In this way the men

[21] Gordon Phillips and Noel Whiteside, *Casual Labour: The Unemployment Question in the Port Transport Industry, 1880–1970* (Oxford, 1985), pp. 184–7, 209; for a conflicting view see Sam Davies, '"Three on the hook and three on the book": dock labourers and unemployment insurance between the wars', *Labour History Review*, 59, 3 (1994), 34–43.

[22] Phillips and Whiteside, *Casual Labour*, p. 187.

[23] A. Fenner Brockway, *Hungry England* (London, 1932), pp. 135–6; see also Whiteside and Gillespie, 'Deconstructing unemployment', 667.

could not claim any dole. They were taking home maybe three days' pay –
about £1 or 25/-.[24]

Short-time working was not solely a result of employer exploit-
ation, of course, but was more often the result of the decline in
demand for industrial products and, in particular, coal. All the pits
in Ferndale in the Rhondda Fach were working full-time in 1928,
but coal was not being raised from all the districts and seams, which
meant that, whereas 3,500 to 4,000 men had worked formerly, by
1928 only 2,000 to 2,500 were regularly employed.[25] This large
volume of short-time working meant that large numbers of workers
experienced short spells of unemployment at some point during the
year. The consequences were predictable. Hilda Jennings found that
the average weekly income of the 1,053 Brynmawr miners who had
been employed at some time in the year ending March 1929 was
only 33s 8d, a figure, she noted, well below the legal minimum.
Jennings concluded that the mining industry was not providing a
living for those men still in work and that when stoppages and travelling costs were taken into account miners were in a relatively poor
financial situation.[26]

Similarly, Arthur Lowry, the Ministry of Health investigator
appointed to investigate allegations of inadequate relief made
against the Bedwellty commissioners in 1928, found that a large
proportion of the miners in the district were only receiving the
subsistence wage of 48s 4½d per week despite working full-time.
After deductions and the payment of rent, the families of these men
were forced to meet their food requirements and other needs from
about 30s per week. Workers who only worked three shifts per week
and drew partial benefit, Lowry maintained, were even worse off
and were forced to meet their dietary and other requirements with
much less than 30s per week.[27] Therefore, the weekly wages of
miners working short-time were less than the wages received by the
dockworkers experiencing underemployment who earned over £2

[24]   Nigel Gray, *The Worst of Times: An Oral History of the Great Depression in Britain* (Aldershot,
1985), p. 36; see also Radcliffe, *Back to Blaengarw*, p. 54; B. L. Coombes, *These Poor Hands*
(London, 1939), pp. 215–16; Chandler, 'Re-making of a working class', 88.

[25]   Labour Party Committee of Inquiry, *The Distress in South Wales: Health of Babies and
Mothers Imperilled* (London, 1928), p. 13.

[26] Jennings, *Brynmawr*, p. 159. It must be noted, however, that the year ending March 1929
was a time of excessive short-time working.

[27]   National Archives, London, MH79/304, Correspondence from Arthur Lowry to Sir
Arthur Robinson, 4 December 1928, pp. 1–2.

and even £3 a week. This was partly due to the economic situation in each industry but also to the attitudes of employers and the ability of workers to control their own working arrangements.

The difference between 'temporary' unemployment and 'long' unemployment is an important one. Social commentators and propagandists, writing on south Wales and other distressed areas during the interwar period, focused on the long-term unemployment associated with so-called 'black-spots', with the result that the varied conditions of unemployed people were overlooked. The diverse forms and experiences of unemployment need to be examined if the varied consequences are to be understood.[28] In general terms, a peak in unemployment in 1921 was followed by a short period of relative prosperity in the early 1920s, but by the mid to late 1920s between a quarter and a third of the insured population of Glamorgan and Monmouthshire were unemployed.[29] Rising steadily through the early 1930s, the figure reached a peak of 40.4 per cent in Glamorgan and 42 per cent in Monmouthshire in 1932, after which it declined, albeit gradually, so that in the first eight months of 1939 about a fifth of the 'working' population of south Wales was still unemployed.

However, the unemployment rate of 40 per cent in Glamorgan in 1932 is compatible with situations in which all workers were unemployed for 40 per cent of the year, 40 per cent of the labour force was unemployed for the whole year, or anything between these two extremes.[30] For this reason, aggregate statistics are of only limited value and do not allow an understanding of the consequences of unemployment for living standards. The experience of unemployment was a diverse one. John Hilton, a civil servant of the Ministry of Labour, found on a tour of employment exchanges in the spring of 1929 that the unemployed were characterized by considerable variation in circumstances, experiences and reactions to unemployment:

> Every other person is a special case. Even at Merthyr and Bishop Auckland [in Durham] the unemployed colliery workers, who may be thought of as a

---

[28] Chandler, 'Re-making of a working class', 48–9; on interwar unemployment more generally, see Gazeley, *Poverty in Britain*, pp. 100–28.

[29] See Appendix 1.1. On the reliability of unemployment statistics see W. Garside, *The Measurement of Unemployment: Methods and Sources in Great Britain, 1850–1979* (Oxford, 1980).

[30] Mark Thomas, 'Labour market structure and the nature of unemployment in interwar Britain', in B. Eichengreen and T. J. Hatton (eds), *Interwar Unemployment in International Perspective* (Dordrecht, 1988), p. 98.

group if any body of men can, present the most diverse personal characteristics and circumstances . . . Each man is a category to himself.[31]

Unemployment varied in nature and extent throughout the
interwar period and it is this variation that needs to be examined.
The incidence of unemployment varied greatly in south Wales.[32]
Those 'heads of the valleys' communities, where pits had been
worked out and where the closure of iron and steel works increased
the volume of unemployment and caused a diminution in the
demand for local coal, suffered the highest levels of unemployment.
In an arc of towns stretching from Merthyr in the west to Blaenavon
in the east, and including Dowlais, Brynmawr, Nantyglo and
Blaina, the unemployed often constituted more than half the
'working' population. The experience of the area served by the
Blaina exchange which recorded an unemployment figure of 93 per
cent in 1932 is scarcely imaginable. Elsewhere, communities in the
valleys of the central and eastern coalfield, while not suffering quite
the same high levels of unemployment, did experience considerable
levels of unemployment. Communities stretching from Glyncorrwg
to Pontypool regularly recorded percentages of between 25 per cent
and 50 per cent throughout the 1930s and sometimes higher rates.
To the south and west of these stricken communities relatively
lower levels of unemployment were recorded as the more diverse
nature of their economies and the relatively more buoyant market
for anthracite coal provided greater opportunities for employment.
In the county boroughs of Newport, Cardiff and Swansea, levels of
unemployment were generally lower than in the inland valleys, but
even here they peaked at about a third of the insured population in
the early 1930s.

The geographical incidence of unemployment in south Wales
has long been recognized by Welsh historians. Much less attention
has been given to the structure of unemployment in south Wales.
First, the duration of spells of unemployment needs to be ascer-
tained. A great deal of official attention was focused on 'long
unemployment'.[33] Not only did south Wales experience higher

[31]   NLW, Thomas Jones C.H. papers, J. Hilton, 'Reflections on a tour of certain employment exchanges', 15 June 1929, p. 2.
[32]   Appendix 1.1 sets out unemployment figures for each labour exchange in the period
1927 to 1939. The story these figures convey is a familiar one; see Morgan, *Rebirth of a Nation*,
pp. 210–40; Davies, *History of Wales*, pp. 509–96.
[33]   In official definitions 'long unemployment' referred to periods of unemployment
lasting a year or more.

Long unemp.

levels of unemployment than other areas of Britain, but the unemployed in south Wales were out of work for longer periods of
time. Systematic measurement of this aspect of unemployment was
not carried out until the late 1930s,[34] but even from this period
the relatively worse conditions in Wales were clearly apparent. On
13 December 1937, for example, 31.8 per cent of applicants for
unemployment benefit aged between 16 and 64 in Wales were
unemployed for a year or more. Other regions experienced lesser
degrees of 'long unemployment': London (6.3%), South Eastern
(5.5%), South Western (8.3%), Midlands (13.7%), North Eastern
(13.4%), North Western (19.2%), Northern (30.1%) and Scotland
(24.1%). Similar patterns of regional long-term unemployment
were found up until the outbreak of the Second World War.[35] In
absolute terms, the number of 'long unemployed' in the Wales division varied from almost 49,000 in June 1937 to 30,000 in August
1939 and was therefore also significant in numerical terms.

Detailed figures on the duration of unemployment are only available for the mid to late 1930s and any understanding of this issue
for an earlier period must be based on less complete information.
Various sources suggest that the number of 'temporarily stopped'
workers was highest in the aftermath of the coal lockout of 1926
but declined with the small improvement in the coal trade in
1929.[36] Mark Thomas, in his analysis of unemployment in Britain
as a whole, has found that the turnover of the unemployment
register was very rapid during the 1920s and that the depression of
the early 1930s was marked by a decrease in the rate of absorption
of the unemployed by the labour market and a resultant increase in
the duration of unemployment. After 1932 the labour market gradually returned to a pattern of more rapid turnover so that in the
trough of the depression in the early 1930s unemployment was not
only of greater magnitude but also of longer duration.[37] Although it
is difficult to arrive at any firm conclusions about south Wales, it

[34] Although Crafts found that 21.1% of applicants for benefits in Wales in June 1932
were unemployed for a year or more: N. F. R. Crafts, 'Long-term unemployment in Britain in
the 1930s', *Economic History Review*, 40, 3 (1987), 422.

[35] *Ministry of Labour Gazette* (April 1939), 123; (July 1939), 255; (September 1939), 349; see
also *Men Without Work*, p. 16, for comparable figures; also Crafts, 'Long-term unemployment',
420–2.

[36] Chandler, 'Re-making of a working class', 24–5. Chandler's assertion is based on
National Archives, London, LAB 2/1293, comments of the Divisional Controller. See also
The Times (29 March 1928), 17–18.

[37] Thomas, 'Labour market structure', p. 105.

seems that the peak in unemployment in the early 1930s was characterized by an increase in short-term unemployment (see Table
1.1).

Table 1.1. Numbers of men applying for benefit who had been continuously on
registers for less than 3 months or more than 12 months

On register less than 3 months	
27 June 1932	114,225
19 December 1932	98,024
22 June 1936	69,684
14 December 1936	57,065
On register more than 12 months	
26 June 1933	62,399
18 December 1933	64,822
22 June 1936	63,744
14 December 1936	57,015

Source: Ministry of Labour Gazette (January 1937), 8. These figures again refer to the 'Wales
Division'. The comparison of short-term unemployment to the situation in 1932 and of
long-term unemployment to that of 1933 was because these were the periods in which each
was at its highest.

The increase in unemployment in south Wales in the early 1930s
was due to an increase in the numbers becoming unemployed *and* a
decrease in the labour market's ability to reabsorb unemployed
individuals, rather than to a decline in the labour market rate of
absorption alone, as Thomas found with regard to Britain as a
whole. Unemployment in south Wales during the early 1930s was
primarily characterized by short, rather than long, spells of unemployment. As the figures suggest, while the numbers of
short-term unemployed declined greatly from their peak in 1932[38]
the numbers of 'long unemployed' fell only gradually and still
amounted to about 40,000 by the late 1930s. Although it is possible
to obtain statistics for the duration of unemployment in Wales,
figures for the number of spells of unemployment experienced by a
worker during a twelve-month period, or indeed any period, do not
exist and so an unknown proportion of those in work or registered
as short-term unemployed at any point in time might have experienced numerous spells of unemployment but still be registered as in
employment or as short-term unemployed. Numerous spells of

[38]   See also PEP, *Problem of South Wales*, 3.

unemployment brought with them their own distinct consequences for standards of living.

A further insight to be gained from the evidence is that as the duration of unemployment increased so the likelihood of gaining employment decreased. This may seem obvious since the short-term unemployed were unemployed for short periods precisely because they re-entered the labour market rapidly after becoming unemployed, while the long-term unemployed were without work for so long precisely because they could not obtain work. This seems a tautology but it is not. At any point in time a short-term unemployed person was more likely to gain employment than somebody experiencing long-term unemployment. The Rhondda collier in Beales and Lambert's *Memoirs of the Unemployed* who found himself refused a job because he had been without work for too long was probably typical of a large number of individuals who were victims of the belief that without work a man became 'soft' and 'out of shape'.[39]

This is supported by evidence of the incidence of unemployment according to age. Anecdotal evidence suggests that it was older men who suffered a disproportionate amount of unemployment and for longer periods of time.[40] A survey in Merthyr in 1929 estimated that 60 per cent of the unemployed were over forty years of age.[41] This report also noted that many of these men were physically unfit and were unable to do the work found for them. It is impossible to know whether ill health was a cause or a symptom of unemployment in such cases, whether it was caused by unemployment or merely revealed by it. Mark Thomas found that unemployment rates for older workers were high because older men were as likely to become unemployed as younger men but were less likely to obtain another job subsequently.[42]

---

[39] H. L. Beales and R. S. Lambert (eds), *Memoirs of the Unemployed* (Wakefield, 1973 edn), p. 65; also Massey, *Portrait of a Mining Town*, p. 70.

[40] For statistics on the duration of unemployment according to age, see *Ministry of Labour Gazette* (June 1938), 233; (July 1939), 263; for quarterly statements on the age incidence of unemployment, see *Ministry of Labour Gazette* (1935–9).

[41] NLW, Thomas Jones C.H. papers, John Davies and David E. Evans, 'Report on Merthyr Tydfil', 11 July 1929, p. 5; see also NLW, T. Alban Davies papers, 'The memorandum on the human, cultural and spiritual reactions of the Depression in the special area of south Wales', submitted to the Prime Minister by the United Committee of the Churches in Wales, 22 July 1937, p. 3.

[42] Thomas, 'Labour market structure', pp. 117–19; Thomas also noted that the higher mobility of younger men increased their chances of finding another job.

Long-term unemployment was most often caused by the closure
of pits or iron and steel works whereas temporary unemployment
was caused by places of employment closing for short periods due
to insufficient demand. Francis and Smith calculate that 241 mines
closed in south Wales between 1921 and 1936, and they demonstrate how closures were concentrated in certain periods. Between
January 1927 and April 1928 fifty-six collieries employing 23,370
men closed, while in the eighteen months following January 1929 a
further 138 pits employing 18,300 men closed.[43] Pits in the north of
the coalfield, producing coal for the local iron industry, closed as the
ironworks became redundant or relocated nearer the coast, or as
their coal seams became exhausted. In communities such as Blaina,
Brynmawr, Merthyr, Dowlais and Ebbw Vale the abandonment of
a mine or steel works meant the loss of virtually the only place of
employment in a community.

The report made by Wyndham Portal highlighted the long
unemployment found in the 'Eastern Section' of the coalfield and
demonstrated that of the 80,661 wholly unemployed workers registered at employment exchanges in May 1934, 74 per cent were
unemployed for over a year.[44] In the iron and steel industry this
figure stood at 90 per cent due to the large-scale closure of plants
such as those at Blaenavon, Ebbw Vale and Dowlais. The closure of
iron and steel works at Ebbw Vale in 1929 and at Dowlais in 1930
meant that 2,000 men had had no regular work in the intervening
years.[45] Thus in Ebbw Vale, 87 per cent of the unemployed had not
worked for over a year by May 1934 and 83 per cent of the unemployed at Merthyr were similarly disadvantaged.[46]

In the Rhondda valleys, on the other hand, collieries did not
close but were often temporarily stopped,[47] while in the Garw
valley, which produced coal for export, the levels of employment
and unemployment fluctuated with variations in international
demand and the size of stockpiles at the ports. Furthermore, since
the collieries of the Garw valley were owned by different combines,
there was no coordination of production between the different

---

[43]   Francis and Smith, *The Fed*, pp. 33, 97, 176.
[44]   Ministry of Labour, *Reports of the Investigation into the Industrial Conditions in certain Depressed
Areas, III: South Wales and Monmouthshire* [Cmd. 4728], 1933–4, xiii, p. 135.
[45]   Ibid.
[46]   Ibid., p. 136.
[47]   Ibid., p. 130; see also Labour Party Committee of Inquiry, *Distress in South Wales*, p. 12.

collieries which meant that they were all working or shut as demand fluctuated. Fluctuations in the demand for coal registered themselves more directly on the unemployment figures for that area.[48] Clearly, the local circumstances of the coal industry determined the nature of the labour market in each area and the experiences of employment and unemployment.

Apart from these various measurements of unemployment, there were a great many workers who had been unemployed for a long time but who were, at the time of the measurement of unemployment, in temporary employment. There were workers, for example, who had suffered severe hardship for a long time, and perhaps were still doing so, but who had found temporary employment and were not registered as unemployed. H. W. Singer gave the theoretical example of a Merthyr collier counted among the short-term unemployed in February 1939 who had been unemployed since before the lockout of 1926, but 'who happened to have the privilege of being employed as an auxiliary postman in the last week just before Christmas, when even people in Merthyr Tydfil send and get letters and parcels'.[49]

While it is not possible to ascertain the number of spells of unemployment suffered by the unemployed, it is possible to gain some idea of the amount of unemployment they experienced. This can be done using the returns of benefit and assistance payments made at local employment exchanges in March and June 1936. These returns were occasional surveys of the number of payments made to the unemployed and they distinguished between unemployment insurance benefit, unemployment assistance and transitional payments. To be eligible for unemployment benefit a worker was required to have paid thirty contributions in the previous two years, but if the worker had exhausted this benefit without paying sufficient contributions he or she received unemployment assistance or transitional payments. Therefore, this source indicates what proportion of the unemployed at each exchange had paid thirty contributions in the preceding two years.[50]

The first return, made on 23 March 1936 and published in

---

[48] Chandler, 'Re-making of a working class', pp. 81–4.

[49] H. W. Singer, *Unemployment and the Unemployed* (London, 1940), pp. 3–4.

[50] The payment of 30 contributions did not necessarily mean that a worker had worked at least 30 weeks in the last two years, only that he or she had obtained at least some work in 30 separate weeks and had paid that many contributions.

Table 1.2. Percentages of unemployed insured persons (aged 16–64) applying for insurance benefit, unemployment assistance (UAB) or other relief in Britain, 23 March 1936.

Region	Estimated no. of insured persons	No. of unemployed	% of unemployed claiming		
			insurance benefit	allowances (UAB)	other
London	2,466,310	183,211	68.6	20.5	10.9
South East	1,074,190	84,287	68.9	18.5	12.9
South West	928,900	95,751	63.6	27.7	8.7
Midlands	1,952,260	179,535	56.5	36.5	7.0
North East	2,075,230	352,826	41.1	49.4	9.5
North West	2,156,420	372,055	47.8	41.1	11.1
Scotland	1,355,510	266,728	39.9	45.4	14.7
Wales	618,180	198,778	38.7	54.3	7.0
Great Britain	12,627,000	1,733,171	49.2	40.4	10.4

Source: Planning, 75 (19 May 1936), 9.

summary form in an issue of *Planning*, demonstrates the position of Wales relative to the other areas of Britain as can be seen in Table 1.2. Evidently, Wales had the lowest proportion of unemployed persons eligible for benefit, reflecting the greater incidence of long-term unemployment. A second return, published by the Ministry of Labour, offers a much more detailed breakdown of unemployment payments and serves to demonstrate the structure of unemployment in south Wales. Figure 1.2 represents the percentage of unemployed at each exchange who had gained sufficient work in the previous two years to pay the required thirty contributions. In Pontlottyn, for example, 20 per cent of the unemployed had gained sufficient work in the last two years to be eligible for benefit while 80 per cent had not and were dependent on means-tested assistance and transitional payments.

This more detailed return allows figures to be calculated for south Wales alone and, as might be expected, the proportion of unemployed claiming benefit was lower than in Wales as a whole in the previous March. Of the 133,800 unemployed registered at the fifty-six employment exchanges (including Brynmawr) in south Wales, only 47,916 (35.8 per cent) were claiming benefit.[51]

---

[51] This does not include those ineligible for benefit and refused assistance.

Figure 1.2. Percentage of unemployed persons at each local employment exchange claiming unemployment benefit as opposed to unemployment assistance or transitional payments, 26 June 1936

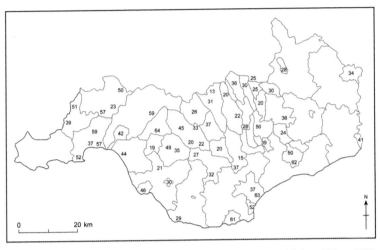

Source: Return of the number of payments made at local offices of the Ministry of Labour, 26 June 1936 [Cmd. 5240], 1935–6, xvii, p. 1011; for key to the map, see Map 4, p. xvii; each percentage figure is located on the employment exchange to which it refers.

Therefore, almost two-thirds of the unemployed of south Wales in June 1936 received means-tested assistance or transitional payments.

The high percentages at the ports of Newport, Cardiff, Barry, Port Talbot and Swansea are immediately obvious, demonstrating the casual nature of the labour employed there and the systems of work-sharing which allowed dockworkers to maintain their contribution payments and receive benefit.[52] Similarly, high percentages are evident in west Glamorgan where tinplate works and anthracite pits offered greater opportunities for employment during the course of a year. Likewise, large numbers of the unemployed at Glyncorrwg, Ogmore Vale, Pontycymmer, Treharris and Newbridge were able to maintain sufficient payments to retain eligibility for benefit. Elsewhere the unemployed were not so fortunate. The very low figures in the 'heads of the valleys' area reflected the high levels of long-term unemployment experienced there. In Dowlais, for example, only 13 per cent of the unemployed had been able to gain

---

[52]   See Map 4, p. xvii.

sufficient employment in the previous two years to be eligible for unemployment benefit and as many as 87 per cent were dependent on the less generous unemployment assistance payments or transitional payments.

The incidence and structure of unemployment are only important, as far as this chapter is concerned, for the implications they had for the incomes of the unemployed. If unemployment had an impact on standards of health it was primarily because of the way in which it influenced a family's income. Therefore, an examination of the various welfare systems intended to relieve unemployment and poverty is necessary to determine the mechanisms by which the unemployed obtained an income. Furthermore, an estimate of the benefits and allowances obtained by the unemployed needs to be made in order to establish the standards of living of the unemployed, and so that these standards can be set alongside the quality of life enjoyed by those in employment.

First, the unemployed could obtain support from the Unemployment Insurance scheme.[53] Introduced by a Liberal government in 1911, the National Insurance Act allowed for 7s unemployment benefit to be paid to the unemployed up to a maximum number of fifteen weeks in any fifty-two-week period. Workers in certain occupations[54] contributed $2\frac{1}{2}$d every week out of their wages, employers matched the employee's contribution and the state made a contribution equal to one-third of the joint contribution of the employers and the 'insured' worker. While the basic principles of the system remained unaltered in the following decade, the scheme was extended, most notably in 1920, to include all manual workers and non-manual workers earning less than £250 per annum, with the exception of agricultural workers and domestic servants. As a result, the Act covered approximately twelve million workers by 1920. Moreover, alterations were made to the rates of benefits and contributions, the number of 'waiting days' of unemployment during which benefit could not be claimed, and the number of contributions needed before benefit was paid. Men received 15s per week and women 12s.

---

[53] See D. C. Marsh, *National Insurance and Assistance in Great Britain* (London, 1950), pp. 39–47; B. B. Gilbert, *British Social Policy, 1914–39* (London, 1970), pp. 51–97, 162–92; Alan Deacon, 'Systems of interwar unemployment relief', in Sean Glynn and Alan Booth (eds), *The Road to Full Employment* (London, 1987), pp. 31–42; Pat Thane, *Foundations of the Welfare State* (London, 1996), pp. 87–8, 137–9, 162–73.

[54] The trades initially selected in 1911 as insurable were the building and construction industries, ship-building and engineering. 2,250,000 workers were initially insured.

Fears of revolution and a desire to reward ex-servicemen, on the one hand, and pressure from the City, economic dislocation and a concern to discourage voluntary unemployment, on the other, led the government to make many changes to the unemployment insurance scheme in the immediate post-war years. These conflicting pressures resulted in a number of changes which alternately extended and restricted central government's financial support for the unemployed. In 1921 dependants' allowances of 5s a week for a dependent wife and 1s for each dependent child were introduced and these were later increased. Furthermore, although unemployment insurance had been intended to provide for short periods of unemployment, the depression of the immediate post-war years left many of the unemployed without work for much longer periods. In response to this, extended or 'uncovenanted' benefit was introduced in 1921 whereby claimants who had exhausted their right to standard benefit were granted benefit for an extended period of eight to ten weeks after the 'covenanted' fifteen weeks. This extended benefit was, from February 1922, subject to a means test for certain groups of workers while later in that same year a clause was introduced to discourage 'malingerers' by making all claimants prove that they were 'genuinely seeking work'.[55]

In all, there were more than twenty Acts in the decade before 1931 amending the system of unemployment insurance. These amendments were intended as responses to the economic difficulties of the 1920s and were primarily concerned with the rates of benefits and contributions, the policing of the administration of the scheme through the 'genuinely seeking work' clause and the means test, and the terms of entitlement for claimants. In theory, benefit was paid almost indefinitely during the 1920s, regardless of the number of weeks on benefit or of the number of contributions made. From 1925 to August 1931 the minimum number of contributions was eight in the previous two years or thirty at any time, and by the late 1920s large numbers of claimants had not worked for long periods. The unemployment insurance system had moved a long way from the actuarial system which its creators had envisaged. However, in practice the means test and the 'genuinely seeking work' clause served to lessen the amounts received by unemployed families or to disallow their claims altogether.

[55]   See Alan Deacon and Jonathan Bradshaw, *Reserved for the Poor: The Means Test in British Social Policy* (Oxford, 1983).

After the resignation of the Labour government in August 1931 over its difficulties in resolving the problems that beset the unemployment insurance system, the Conservative-dominated National government, which was determined to restrict expenditure, cut benefits by 10 per cent and restricted them to those who had paid thirty contributions in the last two years, thus disallowing 800,000 of the 2,800,000 people who were at that moment drawing benefit. Claimants disallowed benefits now had to apply for transitional payments, which were to be paid at the same rates as insurance benefits but were to be means-tested by the Public Assistance Committees (PACs) of the local authorities. Transitional payments were, therefore, to be assessed in the same way as poor relief, the administration of which the PACs had recently assumed from the Boards of Guardians. While insurance benefits were paid on the basis of entitlement, the transitional payments were granted according to criteria of need.

While the means test applied to transitional payments did decrease household payments in a large number of cases, many PACs successfully limited its effects. Glamorgan County PAC, for example, disregarded nearly all the income of other members of the household.[56] This defiance on the part of locally elected bodies convinced the government of the need to take the administration of unemployment relief out of the control of the local authorities. With this intention, Part II of the Unemployment Act of 1934 created the Unemployment Assistance Board (UAB). The UAB was to administer non-contributory benefits for the uninsured unemployed and attempted to introduce uniform scales of assistance and to standardize the terms of entitlement so that unemployed persons received assistance commensurate with their needs rather than according to the political complexion of the local PAC. Upon discovering that assistance payments would, in many cases, be reduced by the new uniform scales, massive numbers of people took to the streets in one of the most notable instances of direct popular protest in the interwar period and forced the government into an embarrassing climb-down.[57]

[56] Deacon, 'Systems of interwar unemployment relief', p. 38; see also Chris Williams, 'Labour and the challenge of local government, 1919–1939', in Duncan Tanner, Chris Williams and Deian Hopkin (eds), *The Labour Party in Wales, 1900–2000* (Cardiff, 2000), pp. 156–7.

[57] See Neil Evans, '"South Wales has been roused as never before": marching against the means test, 1934–1936', in David W. Howell and Kenneth O. Morgan (eds), *Crime, Protest and Police in Modern British Society: Essays in Memory of David J. V. Jones* (Cardiff, 1999), pp. 176–206.

The 'standstill order', passed in response to the opposition, required the UAB to assess all claims twice: first according to its own scales and then according to the scales the PACs had used. The claimant received whichever payment was greater. Although the 'standstill order' remained in place for only eighteen months, with the new regulations gradually being implemented thereafter, the administration of unemployment assistance was carried out more sympathetically in the remaining years of the 1930s. Assistance officers were encouraged to make generous use of their discretionary powers by granting additional payments and disregarding larger proportions of a claimant's savings and the earnings of other members of the household. Nevertheless, the hated means test continued to determine the living standards of large numbers of families.

Therefore, the standard of living of the unemployed was bound up with the administrative changes made to the unemployment insurance system. A family of four received less than 30s in the late 1920s and early 1930s, much less than those in work, which meant that after rent had been paid and other forms of non-food expenditure met there was only a small sum left to meet dietary requirements. In favourable circumstances, unemployment benefit allowed families to ward off hunger and survive from one day to the next. If the money was spent with the greatest care, if the family was not too large and if no money whatsoever was spent on 'wasteful' luxuries such as leisure or entertainment then unemployment benefit allowed a family to function without too many adverse consequences for standards of health. But this was, as Stephen Constantine has described it, a standard of existence rather than a standard of living and one only achieved through the most careful budgeting.[58]

However, many families were large in size, some had exhausted their right to benefit, while others found their assistance decreased by the workings of the means test. If unemployment was prolonged, families increasingly found that they were forced to divert money from food expenditure to other forms of expenditure. Unemployment benefits and assistance provided a low safety net for the unemployed and their families which could provide for their needs in favourable circumstances but often did not.[59] Too many families slipped through the gaps in welfare provision and found their health threatened by the poverty they experienced.

---

[58] Constantine, *Unemployment in Britain between the Wars*, p. 27.
[59] Ibid., p. 30.

Indices for insurance benefits have been calculated[60] and the difference in real benefits between the early 1920s and 1930s is immediately apparent, demonstrating not only that benefit levels increased quite substantially in the early 1920s but also that food prices fell during the interwar period. The increases in dependants' allowances over the period substantially improved the quality of life of unemployed families relative to their position in the early 1920s. While the dependant's allowance for children (2s per child up to October 1935 and 3s thereafter)[61] bore no relation to the cost of raising a child, it nevertheless recognized the existence of children in a way that wage payments did not.

Many historians have argued that by the late 1930s Britain possessed an unemployment benefit system that was more generous than comparable systems in other developed countries and that, at the very least, it allowed a family to ward off starvation and to survive.[62] In this context, the comment made by John Hilton in 1929 that the 4,000 unemployed men at Merthyr, who had been supported by unemployment payments for the previous five years, were 'still alive and moderately flourishing' is intriguing.[63] This comment cannot be dismissed as the justification of a government official defending the unemployment system that he administered. Not intended for publication, his report is a remarkably sympathetic appraisal of the unemployment situation, displaying a common sense absent from other, more public, statements. In an evaluation of the workings of the 'genuinely seeking work' clause, for example, Hilton found that the vast majority of the unemployed in the depressed areas were not tramping the streets, searching for work day after day, week after week, as they claimed to investigation committees and Courts of Referees. Such a search, which the clause was designed to provoke, would be pointless, Hilton concluded, and he was in complete sympathy with those who subverted its implementation by false assertions to relief officers. Hilton advised that the clause be abolished.[64] Elsewhere, Hilton criticized the belief

[60]   See Thompson, 'Social history of health', 387–8.
[61]   Ministry of Labour, *Twenty-Second Abstract of Labour Statistics*, pp. 68–71.
[62]   See A. Green and M. MacKinnon, 'Unemployment and relief in Canada', in Eichengreen and Hatton, *Interwar Unemployment in International Perspective*, p. 388; Stevenson and Cook, *Britain in the Depression*, p. 71; Deacon, 'Systems of interwar unemployment relief', p. 41; Constantine, *Unemployment in Britain between the Wars*, p. 30; Gary S. Cross, *Time and Money: The Making of Consumer Culture* (London, 1993), pp. 135–6.
[63]   Hilton, 'Reflections on a tour of certain employment exchanges', p. 22.
[64]   Ibid., pp. 3–7.

that the unemployed were 'work-shy' and that benefit encouraged unemployment. If a 'work-shy' member of the unemployed refused a job, he reasoned, it left that job available to the vast majority of the unemployed who were not work-shy.

Therefore, the sympathetic and perceptive nature of Hilton's report means that his comment that the unemployed of Merthyr were 'moderately flourishing' needs to be given at least some consideration. As was demonstrated by Figure 1.2, the proportions of unemployed at each exchange receiving benefit and assistance varied geographically. It might be thought that larger proportions of the unemployed in the more depressed communities (such as the heads of the valleys communities) were receiving less assistance and fewer transitional payments than those receiving benefit elsewhere. However, the local administration of the means test in those depressed areas worked to raise the levels of assistance so that they approximated to the level of unemployment insurance benefits. This can be seen in microcosm in the Merthyr County Borough and its three exchanges of Dowlais, Merthyr and Treharris. The percentages of the unemployed receiving benefit in Dowlais, Merthyr and Treharris, as illustrated in Figure 1.2, reflected the varying economic conditions in each area. Dowlais, with its worked-out and redundant ironworks, was characterized by a high proportion of long unemployment whereas Treharris showed a large proportion of unemployed receiving benefit, reflecting the fact that underemployment rather than unemployment was more the norm there. Fenner Brockway, on his visit to Merthyr, was told that while the number of disallowances and reductions of benefit were small for the borough as a whole, 'In the central part of the borough the reductions in benefit have been more, at the lower end of the valley they have been considerable.' The PAC refused to establish a scale and preferred to judge each case on its merits. It took the view that at Dowlais the ordinary benefit rates were 'not too much to keep hunger from the home'.[65]

Thus, in this case, the actions of the PAC placed all the unemployed on an approximately equal footing, generally making transitional and assistance payments equal to those of benefit payments. Reductions were presumably made in cases of recent unemployment where a family still had some resources on which to

[65]   Fenner Brockway, *Hungry England*, p. 165; see also Jennings, *Brynmawr*, pp. 155–6, 170.

fall back. It was thus preferable to be unemployed in an area where a Labour majority sympathetic to the plight of the unemployed controlled the local authority.[66] While the unemployed in the large seaport towns of Swansea, Cardiff and Newport were more likely to have gained sufficient work to make them eligible for the supposedly more generous benefit payments, the long-term unemployed of the more depressed communities were more likely to obtain assistance and transitional payments equal to, or approaching, the level of benefit payments owing to the more sympathetic attitude of the authorities.

In south Wales as a whole, transitional payments and assistance were generally more generous than elsewhere in Britain.[67] In Merthyr, for example, 98.9 per cent of all applicants for transitional payments in the period 25 January to 3 September 1932 received the maximum rate (that is, equal to that of unemployment benefit). Of the 3,042 applicants, only 17 were granted payments less than the maximum and only 16 were allowed no payment at all. Similarly, the Glamorgan County PAC made maximum payments in 93 per cent of its cases in the same period.[68] During the furore surrounding the Unemployment Assistance Act of 1935 many councillors boasted that the means test had never been operative in their districts as local committees had circumvented its workings.[69]

While in relative terms the unemployed of south Wales were more favourably placed than their counterparts in other parts of England and Wales, in absolute terms the sums they received were still very low. Furthermore, despite the relative generosity of public welfare authorities in south Wales, there remained a large number of families whose income from public sources was exceedingly low. A notebook kept during the 1930s by Phillip Abraham, a member of the National Unemployed Workers' Movement who advised unemployed people in Nantyglo on their applications for public assistance, illustrates the low level at which many families lived. In

---

[66] For a similar situation in regard to Poor Law Guardians in the 1920s, see Williams, 'Labour and the challenge of local government', pp. 154–6.

[67] On regional differences in the benefit and transitional payments made to the unemployed, see Webster, 'Health, welfare and unemployment during the Depression', 206–11.

[68] *Final Report of the Royal Commission on Unemployment Insurance*, p. 62. The very low percentages of unemployed receiving neither benefit nor assistance in Wales, as evidenced by Table 1.2, supports this point.

[69] Evans, '"South Wales has been roused as never before"', p. 181.

November 1934, Abraham wrote to the relieving officer on behalf of a family of three adults and three children who were receiving 25s per week, while in December he wrote on behalf of a family of three adults, a man, his wife and their adult son, who were receiving 19s per week.[70] Thus, many families existed on very low levels of income in interwar south Wales and the welfare systems established by the central state did not allow an adequate standard of life.

Nevertheless, the long unemployed in interwar south Wales, especially in the more depressed communities, which also happened to be those with a Labour majority on local councils, were assured of a more-or-less regular income. As savings were used up and as homes were stripped of any furniture or belongings of any value, the long unemployed were promised a regular income from one week to the next. This is not to argue that the sum they received was sufficient to ensure an adequate standard of life, only that any peaks or troughs in their weekly income experienced while in employment were flattened out. This can be contrasted with the fate of the short-term unemployed and those who experienced intermittent spells of employment. Members of unemployed households who gained a job would initially require better food and clothing, and more heating, lighting and cleaning materials, and would thus further depress the standards of the other members of their households. These initial costs could swallow up any increase in income, and when the duration of employment was short, a family could find itself worse off because one of its members had been fortunate enough to obtain work. This was because in many instances the amount received in wages was little better, if at all, than unemployment benefit or public assistance.

Herein lies the danger in comparing unemployed with employed standards of life. The division between employed and unemployed was not always a clear-cut distinction – unemployment could be experienced for relatively short periods or for years at a time. Neither was the distinction obvious in an economic sense: with wages so closely approximating incomes from public sources the demands on each family's resources rendered the economic distinctions between those in work and those without employment almost meaningless. For example, in the report made to the Pilgrim Trust

[70] South Wales Coalfield Collection, Pocket book containing notes by Phillip Abraham on financial circumstances of named families on relief in Nantyglo, November 1934 to February 1935, pp. 5, 60.

an analysis of seventy-five records of wages obtained in Tonypandy demonstrated how very close were the amounts earned in wages to rates of unemployment benefit paid in the area. It was found that:

> In 16 of the 17 cases of men with wives and two or more children there was very little advantage in working rather than living on unemployment allowances, the difference being less than 15s. a week, without taking into account deductions from wages and the additional expenses of working. In 10 out of 11 cases of men with three or four children there was probably no advantage at all in working – the gross difference in earnings and allowances being less than 10s. a week. In 6 cases out of 7 of men with more than four children there was probably a definite advantage, from the point of domestic economy, in not working, for the gross difference between 'stop' wages and allowances in these cases was less than 5s. a week.[71]

Significant here are Andy Chandler's findings that those communities characterized by short-term unemployment tended to experience higher rates of emigration than did communities with higher proportions of long unemployed. In an analysis of four employment exchange areas, Chandler found that the emigration rates were inversely proportional to the overall levels of unemployment. Thus, between 1921 and 1938 Brynmawr lost 22 per cent of its population, Merthyr 28 per cent, Pontypridd 30 per cent and the Garw valley 35 per cent.[72] An investigation into Welsh migrants to Oxford concluded that the long-term unemployed were half as mobile or half as likely to move as the rest of the unemployed. Chandler concluded that in many cases 'migration was a relatively immediate response to unemployment'.[73] Expressed another way, if the unemployed were going to migrate then they were more likely to do so after only a short spell of unemployment.

Part of the reason for this might have been the costs incurred by the short-term unemployed and which the long-term unemployed did not face. Many commentators in the interwar period made the point that many in employment were worse off than the un-

---

[71] *Men Without Work*, p. 204; see also the comments in B. Eichegreen and T. J. Hatton, 'Interwar unemployment in international perspective: an overview', in *Interwar Unemployment in International Perspective*, p. 43.

[72] Chandler uses the unemployment figures for the exchanges of Brynmawr, Pontypridd, Pontycymmer and Merthyr, Dowlais and Treharris and population figures obtained from Jennings, *Brynmawr*, p. 53; *Second Industrial Survey of South Wales*, p. 165.

[73] Andy Chandler, '"The black death on wheels": unemployment and migration – the experience of inter-war south Wales', in Tim Williams (ed.), *Papers in Modern Welsh History*, 1 (Cardiff, 1982), 8.

employed.[74] For example, a Treasury memorandum on the Coalfields Distress Fund in November 1929 noted that in all mining areas the statement was being made that 'The unemployed man is better off than the man in work', and commented that 'The prevalence of this belief is quite remarkable'.[75] As was pointed out on many occasions, an unemployed man did not face National Health and Unemployment Insurance contributions, trade union subscriptions, donations to working men's clubs, libraries, pithead baths, nursing associations, hospitals, aged miners' homes and the upkeep of tools, boots and clothing or the extra food expenditure that heavy manual work required. Hilda Jennings estimated in 1929 that stoppages typically amounted to between 3s and 4s a week.[76] In addition to this extra expenditure, working men in many cases faced travelling costs. The Second Industrial Survey of South Wales found that of 120,000 employed miners, 44,000 lived beyond walking distance of their workplace and their weekly fares averaged just over 2s 3d which, in many cases, amounted to 10 or 20 per cent of their earnings.[77] Therefore, the difference between the incomes of the employed and the unemployed was so small in many cases that, the Treasury memorandum claimed, if the unemployed man did not pay his rent he was better off than many employed men and definitely better off than those men working short-time.[78]

In addition to wages, benefits and dole payments, the age and family structure of the population had a bearing on incomes in interwar south Wales. These had profound implications for wage earners as well as for the unemployed and have long been recognized as important determinants of the standard of life.[79] Traditionally, south Wales, in common with other mining regions, was characterized by a high birth rate and correspondingly large

[74]   *Men Without Work*, pp. 201–12; *The Times* (29 March 1929), 17; this was something that was recognized by government investigations; see National Archives, London, MH79/336, J. Pearse, J. A. Glover, A. P. Hughes and T. W. Wade, 'Inquiry into the present conditions as regards the effects of continued unemployment on health in certain distressed areas', 3 July 1934, p. 11; National Archives, London, MH79/339, T. W. Wade, 'Dietary of persons in receipt of public assistance', 1 October 1935, p. 4.

[75]   NLW, Thomas Jones C.H. papers, 'The Coalfield Distress Fund', Treasury memorandum for the Cabinet (November 1929), p. 3.

[76]   Jennings, *Brynmawr*, p. 159; this is supported by Massey, *Portrait of a Mining Town*, pp. 63–4.

[77]   Quoted in PEP, *Problem of South Wales*, 11; Jennings, *Brynmawr*, p. 159, estimated that the fares of Brynmawr miners approximated 3s. a week.

[78]   'The Coalfield Distress Fund', p. 3.

[79]   Stevenson, *British Society, 1914–45*, pp. 143–81.

families compared with other parts of Britain. This continued to be the case during the interwar period, but south Wales also shared in the decline in birth rates and family size experienced throughout Britain from the end of the nineteenth century. From a level of about 29 live births per 1,000 population in 1920, the birth rate fell by almost 50 per cent in interwar south Wales to reach roughly 15 or 16 births by the late 1930s.[80] This fall in the birth rate, together with the effects of migration of individual members of families, caused a corresponding fall in family size (see Table 1.3).

Table 1.3. Persons per family in south Wales and England and Wales, 1911–51

Census year	Glamorgan (including county boroughs)	Monmouthshire (including county boroughs)	England and Wales
1911	4.89	4.90	4.36
1921	4.62	4.56	4.14
1931	4.01	3.99	3.72
1951	3.37	3.41	–

Source: Census of England and Wales, 1921, 1931, 1951.

Smaller families meant that the weekly income was divided between fewer persons; income per family member would have increased during the interwar years even had incomes remained the same merely because of the fall in family size. As Glynn and Booth argue, the fact that real GDP improved to a greater extent than real wages points to the importance of changing age structure and family size for standards of living and this also applies to unemployment payments.[81] Wages or benefits had to support smaller families during the interwar period.

The fall in family size experienced in interwar south Wales improved the quality of life of working-class families relative to their position in the Edwardian period or the nineteenth century. Against this needs to be set the fact that families were still larger in south Wales than elsewhere in England and Wales. More importantly, the proportion of dependants to earners was much higher in south Wales than elsewhere. An issue of *Planning*, the journal of Political and Economic Planning (PEP), published in 1935, contrasted the demographic structure of the Rhondda with that of

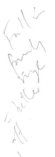

[80]   Glamorgan CC, RMOH (1920–39); Monmouthshire CC, RMOH (1920–39).
[81]   Glynn and Booth, *Modern Britain*, p. 26.

another depressed community, Oldham.[82] Both communities, according to the census of 1931, had a population of about 140,000 inhabitants and while there were 13,500 unemployed in the Rhondda in 1935 there were some 18,500 without employment in Oldham. The situation appeared to be worse in Oldham but, as was pointed out, there were 63,000 workers in employment in Oldham as against only 42,000 in the Rhondda, a difference of over 20,000 wage earners. Total earnings would have to have been about a third lower in Oldham to place it on the same economic level as the Rhondda but the total was, in fact, higher in Oldham. South Wales, *Planning* concluded, was suffering from a 'strikingly large number of dependent children and a strikingly small number of workers in each family compared with the national average'.[83]

H. W. Singer attributed this low proportion of wage earners to dependants to the policy of transference that drained depressed areas such as south Wales of their population of working age.[84] Singer asserted that, of the 15–20-year-old population of the Rhondda valley in 1921, no less than 40 per cent had left by 1931 and he estimated that 65–70 per cent had left by 1938. This had an adverse effect on the age-structure of the population. Taking the population aged between 15 and 55 as the 'breadwinners', and those below and above these ages as dependent on the breadwinner, or on public welfare systems, Singer asserted that whereas in 1921 four breadwinners maintained one other person, by 1941 it could be estimated that five breadwinners were forced to maintain three dependants. While five people had existed on the earnings of four workers in 1921, eight people were forced to exist on the earnings of five workers in 1941.[85] Therefore, according to the report in *Planning*, while the average number of workers per family in England and Wales was 1.63, the figure stood at only 1.22 for the Rhondda.[86]

However, the formal, 'official' forms of employment were not the only sources of income. When faced by inadequate income working-class families, whether employed or unemployed, increased

82 *Planning*, 59 (8 Oct. 1935), 4–7.
83 Ibid., 5; see also Massey, *Portrait of a Mining Town*, p. 66.
84 Singer, *Unemployment and the Unemployed*, pp. 32–3.
85 The Royal Commission on Unemployment Insurance (p. 63) also recognized that the number of wage-earners per family was comparatively high in an area like Lancashire but was low in the mining valleys of south Wales.
86 *Planning*, 59, 7.

their weekly income by a variety of means. Various strategies were utilized in order to allow a better standard of life than was allowed by a wage or unemployment payment. The first strategy adopted by families was for any women in the family to obtain paid employment.[87] This varied from 'official' employment, such as domestic service, catering, shopwork and clerical work, to 'unofficial' employment within the 'neighbourhood economy' such as childminding, cleaning, paperhanging, taking in washing or sewing, or taking in lodgers.[88] Working-class women had resorted to these means of supplementing the family income previously but were forced to do so to a greater extent because of the unemployment of the interwar period. As Wyndham Portal's report of 1934 noted, 'In prosperous times, women folk in the mining valleys normally remained in the home doing domestic tasks, but owing to the acute depression many are now compelled to earn a living.'[89] Children were similarly forced to find some form of employment or means of earning an income and many entered the labour market at fourteen years of age, often ending hopes of continuing their education and pursuing a career in the 'professions'.[90]

Furthermore, working-class families resorted to various means of 'penny capitalism' to supplement the weekly income.[91] Men grew food on allotments, picked coal, kept chickens or pigs, cobbled shoes or did all manner of 'odd jobs' for a small payment.[92] Women set up parlour shops, sold faggots and peas, and nettle beer, or made items of clothing, while children collected jam-jars, rag-and-bone,

---

[87] See White and Williams, *Struggle or Starve*, pp. 13–14, 173–4, 201–11; Beales and Lambert, *Memoirs of the Unemployed*, p. 140.

[88] See Elizabeth Roberts 'Women's strategies, 1890–1940', in Jane Lewis (ed.), *Labour and Love: Women's Experience of Home and Family, 1850–1940* (Oxford, 1989), pp. 223–47; Elizabeth Roberts, *A Woman's Place: An Oral History of Working-Class Women, 1890–1940* (Oxford, 1984), pp. 136–42.

[89] Ministry of Labour, *Reports into Certain Depressed Areas*, p. 140. See also Armbruster, 'Social determination of ideologies', 158, and Barry Eichengreen, 'Unemployment in interwar Britain: new evidence from London', *Journal of Interdisciplinary History*, 17, 2 (1986), 335–58.

[90] For examples, see Rachael Ann Webb, *From Caerau to the Southern Cross* (Port Talbot, 1987), pp. 84–6; White and Williams, *Struggle or Starve*, pp. 161–74; Jennings, *Brynmawr*, p. 109.

[91] For a definition of 'penny capitalism', see John Benson, *The Penny Capitalists: A Study of Nineteenth-Century Working-Class Entrepreneurs* (Dublin, 1983), p. 5; see also *Entrepreneurism in Canada: A History of 'Penny Capitalists'* (Lampeter, 1990), esp. pp. 83–92.

[92] Jennings, *Brynmawr*, p. 187; Hilton, 'Reflections on a tour of certain employment exchanges', p. 15; White and Williams, *Struggle or Starve*, pp. 60–1.

whinberries, blackberries, manure for gardens or else carried out some small task or ran errands for a small payment.[93] The extent of penny capitalism, and its importance in the budgets of working-class families, is impossible to ascertain. Elizabeth Roberts's study of three towns in Lancashire found that, despite considerable differences in the industrial and economic structures of the towns, in each case 40–4 per cent of families engaged in some form of penny capitalism at some time between 1890 and 1914.[94] This is, of course, a considerable period of time and the extent to which penny capitalism figured in the weekly budgets of these families is unclear. John Benson's study of what he labels the 'submerged economy'[95] suggests that it constituted the chief means of income for 10 per cent of all working-class families and the partial support of 40 per cent at the start of the twentieth century.[96] The significance of these estimates when applied to standards of life in interwar south Wales is hard to determine. It seems that large proportions of the population would have considered such strategies as a remedy for their low incomes but, at the same time, the impoverishment of the population lessened the amount of money in circulation.

As David Vincent has argued, these survival strategies, originating in the previous century and in the Edwardian period, were inconsistent with the requirements of the public welfare systems of the interwar period.[97] Means-tested payments were reduced if other members of a family earned something or if an unemployed man carried out 'odd jobs' to supplement his meagre allowance. John Hilton was scathing in his criticism of this aspect of the unemployment system, claiming it repressed enterprise.[98] Therefore, while working-class families could still implement strategies for supplementing their income, as they had done before the interwar period, the unemployed were constrained to some extent by the nature of the means test. It was possible, of course, to conceal

[93] Jean John, *Grey Trees: Childhood Memories of Llwydcoed* (Bristol, 1996), p. 133; Harold Finch, *Memoirs of a Bedwellty MP* (Newport, 1972), p. 62; Webb, *From Caerau to the Southern Cross*, p. 59; Simon Eckley and Don Bearcroft (eds), *Voices of Abertillery, Aberbeeg and Llanhilleth* (Stroud, 1996), pp. 29–30; White and Williams, *Struggle or Starve*, pp. 114–16.

[94] Elizabeth Roberts, 'Working-class standards of living in Barrow and Lancaster, 1890–1914', *Economic History Review*, 30, 2 (1977), 306–21.

[95] Benson, *Entrepreneurism in Canada*, p. 1.

[96] Benson, *Penny Capitalists*, p. 134.

[97] David Vincent, *Poor Citizens: The State and the Poor in Twentieth Century Britain* (Harlow, 1991), pp. 73–9.

[98] Hilton, 'Reflections of a tour of certain employment exchanges', pp. 13, 15.

additional sources of income[99] but the efforts of means test officers to uncover deception and the tip-offs of jealous neighbours usually put paid to such efforts.[100]

It is evident that a number of conflicting forces determined the incomes of families in interwar south Wales. Trends in wages, prices and family sizes meant that considerable improvements took place in the living standards of families fortunate enough to obtain secure employment. But, as has been demonstrated, the considerable volume of unemployment and the extensive incidence of short-time working meant that for much of the interwar years large proportions of the population of south Wales were not able to enjoy fully the benefits which these changes brought. Due to the difficulties of reconciling these conflicting forces, it is impossible to determine the proportion of families that benefited from these changes and experienced improvements in their quality of life. And yet, the unemployed of the interwar period were more fortunate than their Victorian and Edwardian equivalents as the much more extensive, and relatively more generous, welfare systems and, in particular, the unemployment insurance system allowed a higher standard of living than had been experienced previously. The introduction of dependants' allowances and the influence of falling food prices served to emphasize this process. This does not necessarily amount to an 'optimistic' interpretation of the interwar years. Rather, the poverty that existed was of a different nature to that experienced previously and was more a lack of access to consumer durables and commodities than the life- and health-threatening indigence of the nineteenth century.[101] However, as Aneurin Bevan noted, 'It is no answer to say that things are better than they were. People live in the present, not in the past. Discontent arises from a knowledge of the possible, as contrasted with the actual.'[102] The living standards of the Welsh working class were worse than those of their counterparts elsewhere in Britain during the interwar period.

---

[99] Finch, *Memoirs of a Bedwellty MP*, p. 62; White and Williams, *Struggle or Starve*, pp. 129, 173, 166–7; Armbruster, 'Social determination of ideologies', 300, stated that this was prevalent among the unemployed.

[100] White and Williams, *Struggle or Starve*, pp. 166–7, 186–7.

[101] Jennings, *Brynmawr*, pp. 142–3.

[102] Aneurin Bevan, *In Place of Fear* (London, 1961), p. 22.

II

'THE GARMENT HAS TO BE CUT ACCORDING TO THE CLOTH': BALANCING THE BUDGET IN WORKING-CLASS HOUSEHOLDS

> The garment has to be cut according to the cloth, and any mishandling in the spending of a shilling reacts on the sum to be spent on other commodities, and some item has to be curtailed or denied altogether to make it up.
>
> (A Rhondda householder)[1]

In any assessment of the extent to which poverty caused ill health and premature death, it is not enough merely to describe the income obtained from various sources. Lack of money alone did not, and does not, cause ill health and mortality. As E. Ivon Davies, the medical officer of Barry, observed:

> Poverty with its attendant hardships – poor food, bad housing, overcrowding, overwork and worry – diminishes resistance to . . . disease; while prosperity which buys good food, rest, change of air and scene, choice of occupation and diversion decreases the chance of infection, increases the resistance and avoids contact with the infection.[2]

Davies was writing in regard to tuberculosis but his comments can also be applied to health and mortality more generally. The degree to which these 'attendant hardships' influenced an individual's quality of life was determined not only by the income a family obtained but also by the manner in which a family utilized this income.[3] As William Rosser Jones, in recounting his experiences of unemployment in Mardy, explained: 'You know your income, but it's the method of distribution that counts.'[4] Historians have hitherto been satisfied to explain that families existing on low incomes experienced inadequate diets, sub-standard housing, overcrowding, limited access to medical care and so on, without examining the

---

[1]   Quoted in E. Ll. Harry and J. R. E. Phillips, 'Expenditure of unemployed and employed households', *Welsh Journal of Agriculture*, 14 (1938), 103.

[2]   Barry UD, RMOH (1938), p. 6.

[3]   The analysis in this chapter largely refers to families and gives little attention to single men. This reflects the prominence given to families in the sources and the almost complete neglect of single men.

[4]   SWML, AUD/180, Interview of William Rosser Jones, 4 July 1973.

relationship between insufficient income and its consequences. This, however, is inadequate. Each week, families were forced to make decisions as to the most effective way of apportioning their income to meet the various costs they faced. Different families prioritized their requirements in vastly different ways. Each family had its own ideas about the importance of meeting the requirements of housing, food, clothing, leisure and so on, and managed their finances accordingly. They were forced to choose between these essentials, and the ways in which they did so are relevant to a study of the determinants of ill health and mortality.

In fact, it is not possible to evaluate the influence of poverty and unemployment on health and mortality by a consideration of incomes and needs alone. The material consequences of poverty were complicated by the many strategies employed by poor families and individuals to maximize their purchasing power. These strategies partly explain why it is so difficult to find a conclusive correlation between unemployment and mortality in interwar Britain. They complicated the relationship between an inadequate income and ill health. It might also be argued that such strategies insulated families from the full effects of the interwar economic depression and acted as 'shock absorbers'[5] against the worst effects of the poverty engendered by unemployment and low income.

In examining the economies of working-class families, historians have described the various sources of income, have assessed the levels of income obtained from these sources, and have evaluated the importance of housewives' strategies to deploy the family income and to 'make a little go a long way'.[6] David Vincent, for example, has written that the essence of the housewife's task was 'constantly deciding what basic requirement had to be sacrificed for the attainment of another' and he has also stated that the more destitute the family, the greater the number of luxuries in the budget. 'During a given week, almost any purchase could be substituted or postponed. Clothing, virtually all household items except

---

[5]   This phrase is used to describe 'penny capitalism' by S. Berger, 'The uses of the traditional sector in Italy', in F. Bechhofer and B. Elliott (eds), *The Petite Bourgeoisie: Comparative Studies of the Uneasy Stratum* (London, 1981), pp. 71–89.

[6]   See for example Jane Lewis (ed.), *Labour and Love: Women's Experience of Home and Family, 1850–1940* (Oxford, 1989 edn), pp. 223–43; Deirdre Beddoe, *Back to Home and Duty: Women between the Wars, 1918–1939* (London, 1989), pp. 99–101; Vincent, *Poor Citizens*, 5–19; Deirdre Beddoe, *Out of the Shadows: A History of Women in Twentieth-Century Wales* (Cardiff, 2000), p. 89.

coal, and most forms of food and drink except bread, potatoes, tea and margarine, could be dispensed with.[7] In other words, items which might be considered essential by other families were sacrificed for luxuries by poorer families in order to provide some light relief from the tedium of everyday life.

Similarly, Susan Porter Benson has written that 'The historian . . . needs to look inside the working-class family in order to understand the dynamics of allocating scarce resources; the more vexed the choices, the more complex and intriguing the processes by which they are made.'[8] And yet the priorities, preferences and needs which determined these choices and decisions are not examined. These decisions are extremely important in identifying the aspirations, desires and values of working-class families and are therefore deserving of consideration. They are also important to a consideration of the social determinants of mortality since the choice of an adequate diet on the one hand, or wholesome housing conditions on the other, which many families were forced to make, had important consequences for the life-chances of individuals within a family.

While working-class families utilized a wide range of strategies in their daily efforts to 'make ends meet', there existed a more general tradition or habit of careful budgeting. Experience of low wages and hardship inculcated into working-class families a frugality which continued during more prosperous times and which was summed up in the proverb 'Cut your coat according to your cloth'.[9] This was even more apposite during the economic crises of the interwar period. The American sociologist G. H. Armbruster believed that the experience of inadequate incomes had had a limiting effect on the aspirations of the people of south Wales and had forced them to limit their weekly expectations. A circumscribed income had forced people to allot each penny of their income in advance of spending it.[10]

The degree of success with which families were able to satisfy their needs with the incomes they received was determined, to some

---

[7]   Vincent, *Poor Citizens*, pp. 94, 9.

[8]   Susan Porter Benson, 'Gender, generation, and consumption in the United States: working-class families in the interwar period', in Susan Strasser, Charles McGovern and Matthias Judt (eds), *Getting and Spending: European and American Consumer Societies in the Twentieth Century* (Cambridge, 1998), p. 224.

[9]   See for example John Ackerman, *Up the Lamb* (Bridgend, 1998), pp. 117–18, 115.

[10] Armbruster, 'Social determination of ideologies', 159–60, 162.

extent at least, by a woman's ability to budget and to 'make a shilling do half a crown's work'.[11] It is not necessary to accept middle-class criticisms that working-class women were lacking in basic budgeting skills to acknowledge that women varied in the skill with which they allocated a limited income to the various items of expenditure. The smaller the income a family received, the greater the effort that was made in spending it. David Vincent has written how the poorer the household, the more sophisticated the financial wheeling and dealing. Each day required new plans and calculations.[12] Wastage meant further impoverishment for low-income families and therefore the wife's role as 'key strategist' in the battle to 'make ends meet' was vital.[13] The Pilgrim Trust report claimed that households in the Rhondda were 'generally well-managed, clean and tidy'.[14] Nevertheless, women differed in their abilities to manage the household budget. As the Save the Children Fund report of 1933 commented: 'A family which has been accustomed to an income of £5 per week must suffer more when reduced to £2 than a family which had lived on a £3 scale'.[15] Faced with an inadequate income, it was those women who had learnt the complicated calculations and strategies necessary for survival who coped most ably.

In addition to this general attitude of thriftiness, working-class women utilized numerous strategies in their weekly efforts to balance the budget. In times of economic difficulty, strategies were adopted to decrease food expenditure, for example, from buying less of a product, to buying cheaper alternatives, or to shopping on a Saturday night or purchasing defective stock such as bacon trimmings or broken biscuits.[16] At this level of existence, the differences that such strategies made were marginal in real terms if significant in proportional terms and, as Joanna Bourke has pointed out,

---

[11] J. M. Keane, 'The impact of unemployment: a study of the effects of unemployment in a working-class district of Cardiff in the depression years, 1930–35' (unpubl. University of Wales M.Sc. (Econ.) thesis, 1983), 52.

[12] Vincent, *Poor Citizens*, p. 92.

[13] Ibid., p. 94; this was a point made by interwar investigations: see *Men Without Work*, p. 105; Margery Spring Rice, *Working Class Wives: Their Health and Conditions* (Harmondsworth, 1939), p. 165.

[14] *Men Without Work*, p. 129.

[15] Save the Children Fund, *Unemployment and the Child* (London, 1933), pp. 37–8.

[16] The nature of food expenditure will be examined in more detail in Chapter 3. For examples of these strategies see Keane, 'Impact of unemployment', 46–7.

Figure 2.1. Advertisement for William Harris, grocer, Merthyr Tydfil, 1929

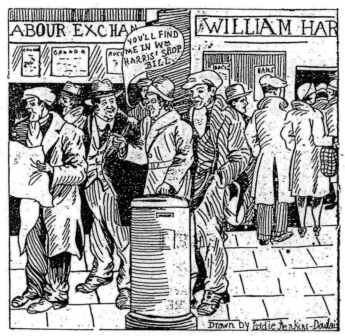

Source: Merthyr Express (6 April 1929), 11.

working-class people did not behave as profit maximizers but instead worked the system to their minimum disadvantage.[17] For example, the mother of Reginald Morgan of Cefn Fforest walked many miles to Bargoed to save a few pennies in the shops there. In the same way, Philip Massey noted how people were buying in small quantities from different shops in an effort to save on the comparative costs of the same commodity in each shop.[18]

Similarly, various strategies were employed in the purchase of clothing. It was virtually impossible for many families to purchase an expensive item of clothing in one payment and so a variety of means to buy clothing had evolved. 'Packmen' or 'Scotch drapers' had long been prevalent in the south Wales valleys by the interwar years and although they charged 'exorbitant and extortionate prices' they were patronized because they granted credit and accepted small weekly payments.[19] 'Club' methods, provident cheques, mail order and club systems run by local shops were utilized by the families which Philip Massey encountered in his investigations in the Nantyglo and Blaina area. As Massey commented, 'These methods are not liked by many as it is recognised that you don't get such good value for money, but it is difficult to pay the necessary cash down, even for men in work.'[20] Increasingly during the interwar period, hire purchase methods of credit were employed to obtain clothes, furniture, wireless sets and a whole range of commodities. However, not all families utilized credit to purchase clothes – some viewed it as an uneconomic way of spending money that demonstrated the financial difficulties of a family.[21] Therefore, while these strategies enabled families to purchase clothing it was recognized that they were not ideal methods and that there were costs involved.

Forms of credit purchasing such as hire purchase were relatively acceptable forms of borrowing. Other methods were much less 'respectable' but were often employed to ease the budgeting difficulties of working-class families. Pawnshops, for example, were a

---

[17] Joanna Bourke, *Working-Class Cultures in Britain, 1890–1960: Gender, Class and Ethnicity* (London, 1994), pp. 65–6.

[18] E. Morgan, *Mad Morgan: Child of the Forest, Man of the Mines. The Autobiography of Reginald Victor Morgan* (Bradford, 1995), p. 42; Massey, *Portrait of a Mining Town*, p. 59.

[19] Ackerman, *Up the Lamb*, p. 97.

[20] Massey, *Portrait of a Mining Town*, p. 59; see also Keane, 'Impact of unemployment', 49.

[21] Edith S. Davies, *The Innocent Years: The Story of my Childhood in Ynysybwl* (Creigiau, 1995), 79.

stigmatizing means of obtaining money but they nevertheless played an important role in the budgeting strategies of the urban poor.[22] Families made use of the credit available from pawnshops in different ways – 'For some the pawnshop was the last resort and for others it became a way of life' commented Bill Twamley of Cardiff.[23] Items of value assumed great significance as they could either be sold, pawned or else loaned for a small fee to a neighbour or friend who could then pawn the item as their own property.[24] Precious items or articles of clothing, indeed anything of value, were bought during more prosperous periods in readiness for leaner times – a sort of 'thrift in reverse'.[25] And yet, the use of pawnshops depended on families having items of value, and such was the poverty in some areas, and the gradual denuding of homes by poverty and means test officers, that pawnshops also suffered the effects of the trade depression. Philip Massey found that there were no pawnshops left in Nantyglo and Blaina by the mid 1930s.[26] Furthermore, pledging items at a pawnbroker's store was an expensive means of credit if used regularly. An interest rate of $^1/_2$d on each 2s was charged no matter how long an item had been in pawn and was also charged on items of less than 2s in value. The smaller the loan, the higher the rate of interest.[27]

In assessing the living standards of the interwar period and the strategies utilized by families in response to low incomes, historians have failed to consider the importance of the savings of working-class families. Historians have emphasized how families purchased

[22]   On the place of pawning in the domestic economies of the working class, see Melanie Tebbutt, *Making Ends Meet: Pawnbroking and Working-Class Credit* (London, 1984); Johnson, 'Credit and thrift and the British working class, 1870–1939', in Winter, *The Working Class in Modern British History*, pp. 154–7; in south Wales, see Anne Eyles and Con O'Sullivan, *In the Shadow of the Steelworks: Reminiscences of a Splott Childhood in the 1930s* (Cardiff, 1992), 13–14, and *In the Shadow of the Steelworks*, vol. 2 (Cardiff, 1992), p. 5; *Kelly's Directory of Monmouthshire and South Wales* (1920), pp. 320, 1393, lists 137 pawnbrokers' shops in Glamorgan and Monmouthshire.

[23]   Bill Twamley, *Cardiff and Me – Sixty Years Ago: Growing up in the Twenties and Thirties* (Cardiff, 1984), p. 80.

[24]   For a fascinating instance of this and an insight into pawning, see R. L. Lee, *The Town that Died* (London, 1975), pp. 108–9; see also Gray, *Worst of Times*, p. 34.

[25]   Gareth Stedman Jones, *Outcast London* (London, 1971), p. 49; Lee, *The Town that Died*, pp. 54–5; P. Johnson described this phenomenon as 'real asset accumulation': Johnson, *Spending and Saving*, p. 196; see also Tebbutt, *Making Ends Meet*; Johnson, 'Credit and thrift', 157; Maggie Pryce Jones, *Kingfisher of Hope* (Llandysul, 1993), pp. 41, 47; Webb, *From Caerau to the Southern Cross*, p. 18.

[26]   Massey, *Portrait of a Mining Town*, p. 68.

[27]   Tebbutt, *Making Ends Meet*, p. 9.

articles of value during times of regular employment so as to utilize their resale or pawning value but have largely neglected the accumulation and liquidation of savings accounts as a budgeting strategy.[28] Hilda Jennings believed that 'considerable savings' were accumulated during the years of relatively high wages before the interwar period but the precise amount and nature of working-class saving is difficult to ascertain.[29] Some families and individuals saved informally. Maggie Pryce Jones of Trelewis remembered how the lodger in her house hoarded sovereigns in his Bible and that these were rapidly used up during her mother's illness.[30] Others paid a friend or neighbour to look after their money[31] or, as will be demonstrated below, conceived of housing as a form of saving. Such methods of saving are impossible to quantify but it is evident that they were adopted.

Similarly, the evidence relating to formal means of saving is scant and fragmentary, and it is difficult to disaggregate the savers of south Wales from national statistics. One informative source is the records of the co-operative societies in south Wales. The Labour Party Committee of Inquiry of 1928 was in no doubt of the societies' importance in helping families to cope with the financial difficulties of unemployment and low wages, stating that the Nantyglo and Blaina district was 'living on its savings' during the late 1920s.[32] It pointed out that the share capital of the Blaina society fell from £250,000 in 1920 to £80,000 at the beginning of 1928, demonstrating the extent to which members had drawn upon this source during the industrial crises of the 1920s.[33]

Statistics relating to savings accounts held in the co-operative societies in south Wales suggest that savings were high in the early 1920s and late 1930s as members were more able to put something aside.[34] The amounts per member invested with the societies were small and presumably could only support a family for a short length

---

[28]   Johnson, *Saving and Spending*, generally considers saving and its implications for times of need but does not examine this tendency in the interwar years at any length.

[29]   Jennings, *Brynmawr*, p. 152.

[30]   Pryce Jones, *Kingfisher of Hope*, p. 62.

[31]   Jennings, *Brynmawr*, p. 163.

[32]   Labour Party Committee of Inquiry, *Distress in South Wales*, p. 6.

[33]   Ibid. The report also gave the examples of Cymmer and Abergwynfi societies whose share capital fell from £19,000 to £7,000 and from £14,000 to £4,000 respectively in the period 1920 to 1927 (p. 15); see also *The Times* (28 March 1928), 17; Armbruster, 'Social determination of ideologies', 268; and Prothero, *Recount*, p. 19.

[34]   *Co-operative Congress Annual Reports*, 1921–1940.

of time. That those who needed them most possessed these savings seems unlikely. Even during times of prosperity a large proportion of the working class, and especially members of larger families, was unable to save. Of those who did save, it seems likely that they were able to utilize their savings in 1921 and, to a lesser extent, in 1926 but had exhausted them by the late 1920s and 1930s. At the same time, however, a survey carried out in the Rhondda in July 1936 found that some saving was being carried out in 'employed households' during the 1930s but that this saving was 'socially undesirable' because householders went without necessities so as to put money aside for future periods of unemployment.[35] Therefore, despite the relatively low incomes of families in the interwar period, efforts were made to put money aside to cope with crises such as unemployment or illness or to cope with the unexpected demands on the budget that sometimes arose. This was, of course, a finite resource that could only be of use over a very short period, but it did figure in the budgeting strategies of working-class families.

Historians have already examined most of the strategies mentioned above but there existed a further range of factors specific to south Wales which have received much less systematic attention and yet which played a significant role in the living standards of families in the interwar period. These factors were all associated with the payment of rent for housing accommodation in interwar south Wales. Rent was one of the largest single expenditures that working-class families made and it seems that rents were rising in relation to wages during the 1920s.[36] Any means by which this outlay could be lessened, or even avoided, had considerable implications for the other requirements of daily life.

First, the high level of working-class owner-occupation of housing in south Wales had implications for the quality of life enjoyed by families.[37] The extent to which this was true varied from town to town and even from one street to another. Generally though, south Wales, in common with the Lancashire cotton towns, shipbuilding towns such as Jarrow and, to a lesser extent, the

[35] E. Ll. Harry and J. R. E. Phillips, 'Household budgets in the Rhondda Valley', *Welsh Journal of Agriculture*, 13 (1937), 85–6.

[36] Glamorgan CC, RMOH (1929), p. 29.

[37] See Steven Thompson, '"Conservative bloom on Socialism's compost heap": working-class home ownership in south Wales, *c.*1890–1939', in R. R. Davies and Geraint H. Jenkins (eds), *From Medieval to Modern Wales: Historical Essays in Honour of Kenneth O. Morgan and Ralph A. Griffiths* (Cardiff, 2004), pp. 246–63.

Yorkshire wool districts and some isolated suburbs of south-east London, was characterized by a high level of working-class owner-occupation.[38] H. Stanley Jevons estimated in 1914 that the level of owner-occupation in the mining communities of south Wales ranged from 15 per cent to 60 per cent (the latter being the figure for Mardy and Ferndale in the Rhondda Fach valley).[39] Even in Nantyglo and Blaina, an area characterized by severe economic depression during the interwar period, there existed high levels of owner-occupation. A housing survey made in 1920 found that 29 per cent of the houses in the urban district were owner-occupied and this had increased to 33 per cent by 1934.[40] The level of working-class owner-occupation was even higher in the western anthracite district. It was estimated that at least 40 per cent of the workmen residing in the Pontardawe Rural District owned the houses they inhabited, while in the Llanelli Rural District the proportion was in excess of 80 per cent.[41] Therefore, the level of owner-occupation varied from one town to the next but was generally high for a working-class region.

The ownership of houses was a highly significant economic strategy of working-class families in south Wales and one that had important consequences in the interwar period. While many families had paid off their mortgages and owned their houses outright by the interwar years,[42] others were still paying mortgages, though even these were sometimes preferable to rent payments.[43] In times of economic difficulty owner-occupiers were able to sell or mortgage their houses to provide a badly needed source of income. It was noted in the late 1920s, for example, that a large proportion of the houses formerly owned by miners had either been sold or had been heavily mortgaged.[44] A respondent to G. H. Armbruster noted how, due to the economic difficulties forced by the industrial

---

[38]   M. Swenarton and S. Taylor, 'The scale and nature of the growth of owner-occupation in Britain between the wars', *Economic History Review*, 38, 3 (1985), 378.

[39]   Quoted ibid., 379.

[40]   Gwent Record Office, Nantyglo and Blaina UDC, Sanitary Inspector's Report Book (calculated from the summaries of Housing Surveys printed at back of Report Book).

[41]   Ministry of Health, *Report of the South Wales Regional Survey Committee* (1921), pp. 15–16.

[42]   Houses built by building clubs were usually bought through short-term mortgages of about 10–20 years.

[43]   Elizabeth Roberts, 'Working-class standards of living in Barrow and Lancaster, 1890–1914', *Economic History Review*, 2nd ser., 30, 2 (1977), 318, notes that mortgages were cheaper than rents in Preston in the early twentieth century; see also C. G. Pooley and S. Irish, 'Access to housing on Merseyside, 1919–39', *Transactions of the Institute of British Geographers*, 12 (1987), 182.

[44]   Labour Party Committee of Inquiry, *Distress in South Wales*, p. 6.

strife of the 1920s, house-owners were forced 'to sell the house and eat it'.[45] This remarkable phrase – 'to sell the house and eat it' – neatly encapsulates the consumption of housing as an economic commodity to be realized if economic circumstance dictated.

This assertion needs to be qualified, however, by a recognition of the difficulties house-owners in the more depressed communities encountered in their attempts to sell houses or obtain a mortgage during the interwar years. The market in house property ebbed just at the moment when owner-occupiers needed money. Cottage property was said to be almost worthless in Mardy where in 1928 one house was sold for a mere £50 while in the Glyncorrwg Urban District many cottages were abandoned and one collier was only able to obtain a mortgage of £25 on the house he owned.[46] As was commented, 'houses in these districts are a drug in the market, and both private owners and public authorities find their property almost valueless'.[47] This was in the most depressed districts, however, during the depths of the Depression and it seems likely that some return could be gained on property in other parts of south Wales and at other times during the interwar period.

It was the issue of rent, however, that placed owner-occupiers in a relatively favourable position. With rents of working-class housing in south Wales varying between 5s and about 15s,[48] families that owned their own homes made a significant saving by not having to pay rent. Providing the house had been paid for, owner-occupiers did not face rent payments and retained a much greater proportion of their income to spend on food and other necessities.

Another significant factor in regard to rent was the widespread practice of sub-letting that was so prevalent in south Wales. Some historians have already pointed out that many families supplemented their income by taking in a lodger and that this was characteristic of working-class communities throughout Britain.[49] The lodger-uncle who contributed to the family finances in return for board and lodge is a familiar figure in the memories of people

---

[45]   Armbruster, 'Social determination of ideologies', 273.
[46]   Labour Party Committee of Inquiry, *Distress in South Wales*, pp. 14, 15; Jennings, *Brynmawr*, p. 92.
[47]   Labour Party Committee of Inquiry, *Distress in South Wales*, 16.
[48]   Jennings, *Brynmawr*, p. 157, stated that average rents in Brynmawr ranged from 5s to 12s 6d. Rents in Cardiff would have been higher again.
[49]   Lewis, *Labour and Love*, p. 228; Vincent, *Poor Citizens*, p. 90; Benson, *Penny Capitalists*, p. 77.

who grew up in the interwar period.[50] A more significant phenomenon was the practice of sub-letting a portion of a house to another family. This phenomenon of multi-occupation varied in intensity throughout Britain but was marked in south Wales. The 1921 census revealed that 29 per cent of families in Glamorgan and 28 per cent of those in Monmouthshire were living at a density of two or more families per dwelling and this figure probably increased during the early 1920s.[51] New houses built during the 1920s and emigration from south Wales, most noticeably in the late 1920s, meant that by the time of the census of 1931, 28 per cent of families in Glamorgan and 23 per cent in Monmouthshire still shared a house.[52]

These high levels of multi-occupation enabled valuable savings to be made in the weekly outlay in rent. The tenant received a weekly contribution to his income from the sub-tenant, which could be put towards the rent he owed the landlord or to the other needs of his family. At the same time, the sub-tenant paid less in rent than if he had rented a whole house direct from a landlord. Sub-letting was clearly, in many cases, a sign of a family's poverty and the shortage of affordable accommodation but it also represented the efforts of other families to minimize their outlay on rent payments and increase their expenditure on other items.

An investigation made in 1928 by Oliver Harris, the treasurer of the South Wales Miners' Federation, provided a few examples of the economic relationship between tenant and sub-tenant. In a house rented for 12s per week in Cefn Fforest near Blackwood, sub-tenants contributed 6s per week, while in two houses in Abertillery bearing rentals of 9s 7d and 10s per week apartments were being let at 5s per week.[53] Therefore, while it is clear that multi-occupation was partly caused by housing shortage, the most important rationale was economic.[54]

---

[50]   White and Williams, *Struggle or Starve*, p. 67; Walter Haydn Davies, *The Right Place – The Right Time: Memories of Boyhood Days in a Welsh Mining Community* (Llandybie, 1972), pp. 66–7.

[51]   Census of England and Wales, 1921, Glamorgan p. xiii; Monmouthshire p. xii; Rhondda UD, RMOH (1920), pp. 86–7.

[52]   Census 1931, Glamorgan p. xi; Monmouthshire p. xii.

[53]   Oliver Harris, *Poor Law Administration: A Report on the Investigation into Poor Law Relief Cases in the Bedwellty Union* (*c.*January 1929), pp. 1, 4.

[54]   For examples see Abersychan UD, RMOH (1932), p. 22; Gelligaer UD, RMOH (1930), p. 15; Glamorgan CC, RMOH (1926), p. 27; (1931), p. 40; see also Jennings, *Brynmawr*, p. 91; Rhondda UD, RMOH (1930), pp. 100–1.

One last significant feature concerning the place of rent in the household budgets of working-class families is the varied attitudes to the payment of rent. Families differed greatly in their attitudes towards their contractual agreements with their landlords. Many families made rent the first charge on their income and then allocated the remaining money to the other expenses which they faced. There existed a strong desire on the part of many families always to pay the rent and thereby gain a reputation as 'tidy tenants'.[55] The family of Reginald Morgan of Cefn Fforest, Blackwood, was one such family. 'A roof over your head is your main concern' and 'The rent first, before anything else' were favourite aphorisms of his grandfather.[56]

This diligence in the payment of rent had important consequences for the remaining expenses a family had to cover. Hilda Jennings in her study of Brynmawr commented that 'The more independent families keep their rent paid whatever sacrifices it costs them' and contrasted these families with the 'Very many others [who] pay it only when the landlord brings pressure to bear.'[57] That the sacrifice Jennings described often meant expenditure on food is borne out by the findings of Fenner Brockway in his study, *Hungry England*. 'Again and again', he stated, 'I have found during this enquiry that it is in the homes which are seemingly above destitution level that the greatest privation is suffered.'[58] Brockway related the story of a family of four living in Merthyr who were paying 10s 6d a week in rent out of their weekly income of 24s 9d. The effort to pay this rent and to maintain high standards in the home meant that this family was existing on 'bread and margarine . . . meal after meal, day after day'.[59] Other investigators found that families were prepared to pay rents out of proportion to their incomes so as to occupy local authority houses of a better quality than privately rented accommodation.[60] Therefore, some families considered a

[55]   Davies, *The Right Place – The Right Time*, p. 66.
[56]   Morgan, *Mad Morgan*, p. 34.
[57]   Jennings, *Brynmawr*, p. 157.
[58]   Fenner Brockway, *Hungry England*, p. 160.
[59]   Ibid., p. 162.
[60]   Port Talbot MB, RMOH (1936), p. 63; this point is similar to the well-known findings of M'Gonigle and Kirby that former residents of slum housing in Stockton-on-Tees were forced to spend less on food when they were rehoused in local authority housing in the 1930s as a result of the higher rents; G. C. M. M'Gonigle and J. Kirby, *Poverty and Public Health* (London, 1936), pp. 108–29.

clear rent book or the attainment and possession of a new local authority house to be important enough to endure an inadequate diet. It is impossible to ascertain what proportion of the population this extended to, but it is clear that certain families prioritized rent payments over food expenditure with detrimental effects on their health.

However, there were also large numbers of tenants who, for various reasons, did not pay rent to a landlord. First, no rent was paid by the tenants of some of the most insanitary property in south Wales. A large number of leases reverted to the ground landlord in the interwar period but, in some cases, these ground landlords were not interested in collecting rent from their tenants.[61] Furthermore, tenants of houses scheduled for clearance in many cases refused to pay the rent. Landlords were reluctant to carry out repairs to such houses and had written off any hope of receiving a return on them. In the mid to late 1930s landlords of houses scheduled for clearance in the slum clearance campaigns found that their tenants stopped paying rent as soon as the clearance order was made.[62]

Apart from these tenants who, for various reasons, did not have a rent obligation, there was a much larger class of tenants who purposely sought to avoid their contractual obligation and defaulted on their rent. There existed a small hard core of tenants who seem to have withheld their rent, or have been unable to pay it, for long periods of time. In Blaenavon in 1934, it was apparently 'not uncommon' to find in houses bearing rents of seven to ten shillings per week, arrears of £70 to £100 and more.[63] Such arrears could conceivably consist of anything up to five and a half years of unpaid rent. Some tenants of the Ebbw Vale Urban District Council apparently owed as much as £130 in unpaid rent.[64] A large proportion of the rent arrears that accumulated in the interwar period was a result of the lockout of 1926. It seems that the majority of locked-out miners did not pay rent for the duration of the lockout.[65] The amount of arrears occasioned by the lockout was

---

[61] For example, see NLW, Welsh Board of Health collection, Box 58Q, R. Bruce Low, Untitled report on the Sanitary Administration of the Nantyglo and Blaina UD, 17 January 1929, p. 1.

[62] See for example *Merthyr Express* (10 June 1939), 7.

[63] Blaenavon UD, RMOH (1934), p. 37.

[64] *Western Mail* (26 Sept. 1931), 8.

[65] Steven Thompson, '"That beautiful summer of severe austerity": health, diet and the working-class domestic economy in south Wales in 1926', *Welsh History Review*, 21, 3 (2003), 552–74.

staggering and by the time of the report made to the Pilgrim Trust in the late 1930s there were still families whose arrears from the lockout amounted to £50 or £60.[66] The lockout of 1926 was the most notable example of tenants defaulting on their rent during a period of crisis, but other strikes and lockouts, such as in 1921, also caused arrears to rise. It was a generally accepted principle that rent would not be paid during these times of difficulty, as earlier strikes had demonstrated.[67]

More generally, families allowed themselves to go into arrears with their rent in order to make ends meet during personal, small-scale crises such as illness, unemployment or short-time working. More common than the small number of tenants who purposely set out to withhold rent payments for as long as possible were those families who, in the words of the report made to the Pilgrim Trust, 'default on the rent to meet any sudden expense'.[68] W. Darby, a member of the Ebbw Vale Urban District Council, summed up succinctly the 'choices' facing a tenant with a limited income when he stated:

> If an unemployed man had to pay his rent this week, and his child wanted a pair of boots, that man asked who could stand it best, the authority or himself? Owing to his being out of work for a long time, that man bought a pair boots for his child, and let the rent go.[69]

Increases in arrears owed to Merthyr County Borough Council from one month to the next were explained with reference to the Dowlais works being stopped for a number of weeks or to the fact that the pits at Treharris were working short-time.[70] Alternatively, more prosaic reasons were given for an increase in arrears. The housing committee found that it was usual for arrears to increase during holiday periods, such as at Christmas or Easter.[71] Such a choice was probably easier for local authority tenants to make but the same factors governed the actions of tenants of private land-lords. Bill Twamley of Cardiff remembered the 'ever present problem of priority in the use of available cash':

[66] *Men Without Work*, p. 125.
[67] For other examples, see *South Wales Daily News* (3 June 1898), 3; *Merthyr Express* (11 March 1911), 5.
[68] *Men Without Work*, p. 125.
[69] *Merthyr Express* (9 June 1934), 17; see also Jennings, *Brynmawr*, p. 167.
[70] *Merthyr Express* (6 September 1930), 13; (7 July 1934), 11.
[71] For examples see *Merthyr Express* (10 May 1924), 9; (12 July 1930), 13; (9 May 1931), 12; (7 January 1933), 12.

> It came at times to the point of the rent being paid, the rates being paid or
> the food bill in the Direct Trading Company, well the kids had to eat so that
> solved the problem and Mr. Wass the landlord could rant and rave for his
> rent, but too late the money was gone.[72]

As a result of this non-payment of rent, tenants of local authorities accumulated massive arrears. Near the end of 1928, 486, or 61 per cent, of Merthyr County Borough's tenants were in arrears and the proportion had not changed appreciably by March 1934.[73] In nearby Ebbw Vale, the arrears of the council's 492 houses amounted to £6,733 (approximately £13 13s per tenant) by June 1935, while in neighbouring Nantyglo and Blaina they stood at a staggering £20,031 on 214 houses (over £93 per tenant).[74] In the Rhondda, arrears had increased from £2,368 in March 1927 to £3,413 a year later and stood at about £4,500 in September 1928. At this last date, 222 of the council's 234 tenants were in arrears with their rent, while over half of these (117) owed more than £10.[75] Even relatively prosperous towns such as Cardiff and Swansea faced severe difficulties in regard to arrears. In February 1928, 1,570 of Cardiff's 3,179 tenants were in arrears, although 1,083 (nearly 70 per cent) of these owed less than £2.[76] In Swansea, 601 out of 1279 tenants were in arrears in December 1924.[77]

Martin Daunton has demonstrated how tenant–landlord relations existed within a general context of existing building styles and the legal system, and were determined by the house-building cycle on the one hand and trends in real wages on the other. They 'rested upon a complicated interplay of forces'.[78] Therefore, although interwar south Wales was characterized by a trough in the house-building cycle, large-scale emigration and widespread poverty, not to mention the rent controls imposed during the war, meant that

---

[72] Twamley, *Cardiff and Me*, p. 77.
[73] *Merthyr Express* (10 November 1928), 12; (10 March 1934), 13. The proportion of tenants in arrears by March 1934 was 63%.
[74] *Merthyr Express* (1 June 1935), 17.
[75] *Western Mail* (14 February 1929), 10; the average arrears per tenant in arrears was over £20 5s.
[76] *Western Mail* (21 March 1928), 10.
[77] West Glamorgan Record Office, Swansea CB, Housing of the Working Classes Committee minutes, 29 Jan. 1925.
[78] Martin J. Daunton, *House and Home in the Victorian City: Working-Class Housing, 1850–1914* (London, 1983), pp. 99–100, 131, 155; on this question of changing tenant–landlord relations, see also J. H. Treble, *Urban Poverty in Britain, 1830–1914* (London, 1979), pp. 136–7.

landlords were not able to impose high rents and were forced to acquiesce in the accumulation of rent arrears. In the years leading up to the First World War, allegations of rack-renting and exploit-ation were continually being made against landlords in south Wales and it is significant that such allegations were not made during the interwar period.[79] The balance of power between landlords and tenants had been transformed in the meantime. Furthermore, it was during the interwar period that local authorities became land-lords to a significant degree and they were either not willing or not able to be as ruthless in their treatment of rent defaulters as private landlords had been.

An investigation made in 1928 by officials of the Ministry of Health hints at the large proportion of tenants who did not pay the full rent due to their landlord.[80] As the investigation was still ongoing, Arthur B. Lowry, the chief general inspector of the Ministry of Health, reported his general preliminary impressions to Sir Arthur Robinson, the Minister of Health. Lowry was of the opinion that families dependent on poor law relief were no worse off than families where the man was in work 'since in the majority of cases they can and do refrain from paying any rent'.[81] Lowry elaborated upon this point a month later in another investigation which he undertook in south Wales for the Ministry of Health. He explained that a 'considerable number' of unemployed miners in the Bedwellty Union, and indeed elsewhere in the coalfield, were able to avoid the payment of rent.

This second investigation was in response to a report written by Oliver Harris, the treasurer of the South Wales Miners' Federation, on the relief administered by the commissioners appointed to replace the Bedwellty Board of Guardians.[82] Lowry criticized Harris's statements as to the financial situation of the thirty-four families which Harris surveyed,[83] and complained that he had

[79] For examples, see Edgar L. Chappell, *Gwalia's Homes: 50 Points for Housing Reform* (Ystalyfera, 1911), pp. 9–10, 15, 24.
[80] National Archives, London, MH 79/304, 'Public assistance, distress in mining areas, winter 1928–9'.
[81] National Archives, London, MH 79/304, Correspondence from Arthur Lowry to Sir Arthur Robinson, 4 December 1928, p. 2.
[82] Harris, *Poor Law Administration*.
[83] In fact, Harris does make reference to cases where the full rent was not paid or where sub-letting families paid the tenant, but Lowry seems to have believed that non-payment of rent was a bigger factor than Harris admitted. There is no way of ascertaining which was the more accurate interpretation.

ignored any income except that legally belonging to the family and that, secondly, he assumed that all rent due was paid. Lowry conducted his own investigation into the households surveyed by Harris and found that, of thirty-one households for which he was able to obtain information, seven shared their houses with near relations. It was not unreasonable, Lowry argued, to assume that the sub-letting relations were making some sort of financial contribution to the household. Of the remaining twenty-four families, seven paid no rent whatsoever, while others paid less than the amount due to the landlord. Lowry was firmly of the opinion that this non-payment of rent, and the payment of lesser amounts than were due, had an important effect on the financial situation of the families involved. He calculated that the average income per head in the twenty-four families which did not have relations residing with them was 3s 9$^1/_2$d because of the unpaid rent, rather than the 2s 9d per week stated by Harris.[84]

Therefore, from this admittedly small sample of thirty-one households, about a fifth of the families had relations staying with them who probably contributed to the household budget, another fifth paid no rent and a further unspecified proportion paid the landlord a lesser amount than was due. The increase in money available for other expenditures in the family budget was, if Lowry's calculations are to be believed, large in proportional terms if small in real terms. Nevertheless, the sum of 3s 9$^1/_2$d in food expenditure was still below the 4s per person per week of John Boyd Orr's group I, which existed on a diet wholly inadequate for perfect health in all the constituents considered (protein, fat, calories, calcium, phosphorous, iron and Vitamins A and C).[85]

It must be stressed that conditions specific to south Wales created unique relationships between landlord and tenant that were not necessarily replicated in other depressed areas and which had unique consequences for the standard of life experienced by the population of south Wales. Few working-class districts possessed comparable levels of owner-occupation to those of south Wales or experienced the high levels of multi-occupation witnessed in the region. It might also be argued that the specific tenant–landlord relations of south Wales created unique attitudes towards the

[84]   National Archives, London, MH 79/304, A. B. Lowry, 'Bedwellty Union: complaints of inadequate relief', 15 January 1929.

[85]   John Boyd Orr, *Food, Health and Income* (London, 1936), pp. 33–6.

payment of rent. Fenner Brockway, in his *Hungry England*, constantly reiterated the point that the people of the north-east of England made great efforts to pay the rent and consequently arrears were at a minimum.[86] 'To pay the rent is a religion among the women', Brockway noted.[87] He did not make this comment about south Wales. The significance of these comments can be recognized when the diet of an unemployed family in south Wales which Brockway described is considered. He commented that this diet: 'allows much more variety in food than some of the budgets which I have obtained in other districts; almost for the first time I see fruit included in the budget of an unemployed family.'[88] This was not an isolated comment. Philip Massey, while comparing John Boyd Orr's income groups with the expenditure on food by families in Nantyglo and Blaina in the mid 1930s, noted how expenditure on food was higher in south Wales than was anticipated by Orr's classification and he attributed this to the fact that rents in the district were low.[89] G. H. Armbruster, similarly using Orr's classification but this time comparing it with the budgets of miners in the Blaenavon–Pontypool area in the late 1930s, also noted the relatively high expenditure on food and attributed it to the fact that rents were comparatively low, commenting that 'more money is available for other essentials'.[90] Lastly, the survey into household budgets in the Rhondda also noted the high expenditure on food and, in fact, pointed out that this 'relatively poor group . . . showed a tendency to consume some articles of food in a way much more characteristic of wealthy than of poor communities'.[91]

Therefore, from these comments comes the suggestion that the diet of the working class and unemployed of south Wales was better than that enjoyed in other depressed areas. This might have been due to the forms of housing tenure that existed. The higher prevalence of

---

[86]   This is refuted to some extent by R. Ryder, 'Council house building in County Durham, 1900–39: the local implementation of national policy', in Martin J. Daunton (ed.), *Councillors and Tenants: Local Authority Housing in English Cities, 1919–1939* (Leicester, 1984), pp. 86–90, but the general impression given by Ryder's figures suggests that arrears were indeed higher in south Wales.

[87]   Fenner Brockway, *Hungry England*, pp. 105–8, 124.

[88]   Ibid., pp. 167–8.

[89]   Massey, *Portrait of a Mining Town*, p. 66; *The Times* (29 March 1928), 17, on the other hand, commented on the 'high rents' that were charged for housing in the valleys of south Wales.

[90]   Armbruster, 'Social determination of ideologies', 303.

[91]   Harry and Phillips, 'Household budgets in the Rhondda Valley', 83.

working-class owner-occupation, the greater degree of sub-letting, and the unique relationship between landlord and tenant that allowed the greater accumulation of arrears, might have meant that more money was available to families in south Wales in their attempts to meet their dietary requirements. Such increases, however, probably did not raise the level of food expenditure to a level that promoted good health or even prevented ill health, but merely lessened the disadvantages under which poor families laboured.[92]

In addition to rent arrears, it is evident that other debts were accumulated by poor families in the interwar period and yet debt has not been systematically studied by historians of the working-class domestic economy or by historians of the interwar years. Historians have examined the wages and benefits that families received and the prices of commodities that they could and did purchase, but they have failed to consider the commodities that were not paid for, the products that families went into debt to obtain. Debt undoubtedly signified poverty but it also represented the purchase of commodities or services that were not paid for or that were paid for when a family could afford the cost. Therefore, the greater the amount of debt that could be built up, the better the standard of life that could be enjoyed by poorer families.

Sources for the nature and extent of debt in interwar south Wales are disparate and scarce but at least some suggestions can be made. First, to take an example, the 1,700 families which made up the community of Brynmawr owed £130,000 in rates, rents and charges to the Urban District Council by 1929. Also, a further £50,000 in poor relief had been given on loan and £45,000 was owed to traders and shopkeepers.[93] These levels of debt could conceivably represent debts of over £132 per family. A large proportion of this total amount owed was a consequence of the lockouts of 1921 and 1926. Co-operative societies and private shopkeepers gave credit to locked-out miners and their families in 1921 and, to a lesser extent, in 1926.[94] The credit granted by the Dowlais

[92]   There were, of course, many comments that, in fact, the diets of the unemployed and the poor of south Wales were inadequate.

[93]   NLW, Thomas Jones C.H. papers, National Council of Social Service, Coalfields Distress Report, c.1929–30.

[94]   Peter Gurney, *Co-operative Culture and the Politics of Consumption in England, 1870–1930* (Manchester, 1996), pp. 220, 226–8; W. Hazell, *The Gleaming Vision, being the History of the Ynysybwl Co-operative Society Ltd., 1889–1954*, p. 61; Jennings, *Brynmawr*, pp. 105–6, commented on the 'tradition by which the unemployed workers fell back on the family tradesmen in times of industrial depression'.

Co-operative Society rose from £3,017 in 1920 to £30,518 the following year while in the Western Division of the Co-operative Union in the same period, the average amount of credit per member rose from 16s 5d to £3 15s 5d.[95]

The effect was to increase massively the debts owed to shop-keepers. In the Blaina and Nantyglo area, one shopkeeper who gave credit freely in 1921 had debts of £2,000 owing to him in the space of six months, while some families owed £40, and even £60, to a single shopkeeper.[96] Some grocers in Brynmawr had unpaid bills of £5,000 by the early 1930s.[97] The co-operative societies found that their debtors hoped to pay off their debts through the dividend which they accrued but that this was not a very effective way of clearing debts.[98] As a result of the huge debts built up in the 1920s and the difficulties experienced in clearing those debts, shopkeepers and co-operative societies limited the amount of credit they granted in the late 1920s and 1930s. By the 1930s, therefore, the larger shopkeepers in the more depressed communities allowed some credit to attract business, but only on a short-term basis, while smaller shops confined themselves to cash trading.[99]

If this question of credit is examined from the other point of view, that of the consumer, then it can be seen that credit did play an important part in the balancing of the domestic budget. Armbruster found that 'In the lowest of income groups there is no opportunity to save and expenditure is to the full limit of the income or goes beyond it.'[100] Examining the weekly budget of a family whose husband was in employment, Armbruster found that the family had spent 6d more than it had earned. The family, like most families in the district, was paying one week's grocery bill with the following week's wages and was therefore always in arrears. But because the following week's wages or benefit did not always amount to the previous week's bills, debts built up.[101] Studies of the budgets of families in the Rhondda by the Department of

---

[95] Johnson, 'Credit and thrift', pp. 153–4 (the Western Division included Herefordshire and Gloucestershire as well as societies in Breconshire and Carmarthenshire).

[96] Massey, *Portrait of a Mining Town*, pp. 23–4.

[97] Jennings, *Brynmawr*, p. 153.

[98] *57th Annual Co-operative Congress Report*, Southport (1925), p. 227.

[99] Massey, *Portrait of a Mining Town*, pp. 23–4, 59.

[100] Armbruster, 'Social determination of ideologies', 297.

[101] Ibid., 160, 298. In the case of this particular family quarterly dividends of 1s in each £1 spent at the local co-operative store partly made up the difference.

Agricultural Economics at the University College of Wales, Aberystwyth, further supported the observation that low-income families utilized credit in their weekly efforts to balance the budget. In a study of forty-six households in July 1936 it was found that expenditure exceeded income in about half of the households surveyed and that 'considerable ingenuity' was being exercised in making the budget balance.[102]

However, credit was not an unmixed blessing for working-class families and its costs need to be taken into account. Families were generally anxious to clear any debts they accumulated and often commenced repayments immediately upon an improvement in their situation. In real terms, credit often depressed a family's income over a period of time and the servicing of a debt when circumstances improved served to further depress living standards.[103] The costs of credit varied with each store. In many stores interest was charged indirectly by the selling of inferior products at inflated prices to debt-ridden customers.[104] The credit extended by co-operative societies, on the other hand, was without cost and did not incur interest payments, and members were more likely to be treated sympathetically than by private traders. However, it must be remembered that while some storekeepers were bankrupted by the large volumes of credit they allowed in 1921 and 1926,[105] still others were forced to write off the large debts of many customers which they had no chance of receiving, and in this way some families were able to avoid repayment.[106]

The cost of servicing rent arrears varied a great deal. No interest had to be paid on rent arrears but they still had to be repaid in better times. Private landlords generally managed their property on purely economic terms although in the heightened sensitivity of the interwar period actions such as eviction, distraint or action for the recovery of arrears would have been unwise. It was noted that

---

[102] Harry and Phillips, 'Household budgets in the Rhondda Valley', 85, 92–3.

[103] However, note Beales and Lambert, *Memoirs of the Unemployed*, p. 141.

[104] Johnson, 'Credit and thrift', p. 154; see also White and Williams, *Struggle or Starve*, p. 117.

[105] Jennings, *Brynmawr*, p. 153. Jennings found that in Brynmawr thirteen tradesmen had filed for bankruptcy while another eight had closed down (p. 106).

[106] *57th Annual Co-operative Congress Report*, Southport (1925), p. 227; Massey, *Portrait of a Mining Town*, pp. 23–4; at the same time Jennings, *Brynmawr*, p. 153, noted that some grocers had sold off their debts to 'enterprising persons who have had less compunction in demanding repayment from the workers'.

'the eviction of [a] family . . . for non-payment of rent in an industrial area is almost unthinkable'.[107] The balance of power in tenant–landlord relations had shifted considerably in favour of the tenant and many tenants were able to accrue arrears to an extent that was impossible in Victorian or Edwardian south Wales. Furthermore, 'small' landlords were unable to enforce repayment while others used legal means but to little avail. What seems to have been more usual was that the various types of landlord would allow their tenants to build up arrears during instances such as the lockout of 1926 and expect them, or take action to force them, to clear arrears after returning to work.[108] The colliery companies deducted the rent due from their workers directly from their pay packets and thereby denied families the opportunity to manage their own finances. Such a deduction was an onerous burden and served to reduce living standards substantially, especially during periods of short-time working.[109]

Local authorities did not have this degree of control over their tenants but still expected arrears to be repaid after a strike. Local authorities did obtain court judgments to enforce the clearing of arrears but councillors in many districts, such as the Rhondda, seem to have viewed the rent due from tenants as a subsidy from the council on which families could draw in times of need, and allowed arrears to be carried indefinitely. Some Labour-led local authorities in south Wales saw it as their duty to ameliorate the harsh conditions faced by the inhabitants of their areas by investing money in local authority services and by granting relatively 'generous' levels of relief to the unemployed.[110] Rent arrears can in some ways be seen as another instance of the ways in which local authorities aided the people they served.[111]

---

[107] 'The Coalfields Distress Fund', p. 3.

[108] South Wales Miners' Library, AUD/201, Interview of Henry Lewis, 4 December 1972; see also AUD/180, Interview of William Rosser Jones.

[109] National Archives, London, MH79/312, 'Public assistance, out-relief – Rhondda administration' (1936), Report by D. J. Roberts, p. 4; see also *Merthyr Express* (30 April 1927), 16.

[110] Morgan, *Rebirth of a Nation*, pp. 292–3; Evans, '"South Wales has been roused as never before"', pp. 180–1; Sian Rhiannon Williams, 'The Bedwellty Board of Guardians and the Default Act of 1927', *Llafur*, 4, 2 (1979), 65–77.

[111] Jennings, *Brynmawr*, p. 95; more generally on local authorities see Chris Williams, 'Labour and the challenge of local government, 1919–1939', in Tanner, Williams and Hopkin, *The Labour Party in Wales*, pp. 140–65.

Furthermore, unemployed families were more able to carry debts than those families in employment. A Treasury memorandum on the Coalfields Distress Fund noted in 1929 that the unemployed did not incur the costs of 'arrears of rent or other debts contracted in previous periods of unemployment or stoppages of work' that the employed did.[112] This was most obviously the case in regard to colliery housing where rent was deducted from the wages, but was also true more generally. This difference between employed and unemployed families is supported by the assertion of Rhys Davies, the writer from Clydach Vale, whose mother, responsible for looking after their grocery's ledger of debts, would file a suit for recovery of debt upon hearing that a family which owed money had improved its financial situation. Debts were carried until an improvement in a family's economic circumstances.[113] Some debts were easier to clear than others. The 'South Wales Miner' whose memoirs were published in Beales and Lambert's collection, *Memoirs of the Unemployed*, remembered how he had cleared the £20 debt he had built up at the co-operative store in the 1926 lockout by allowing the dividend on purchases to accumulate but had been unable to clear his rent arrears – 'we have as much as we can do to pay the current rent'.[114]

Many of the budgeting strategies of unemployed families were revealed in greater detail by an investigation carried out by the Department of Agricultural Economics at the University College of Wales, Aberystwyth in 1936. The investigation revealed the monthly pattern of expenditure of twenty-one Rhondda households in which the head was unemployed and seventeen households where the head was employed (see Table 2.1). It is evident that when faced by a decreased income a family reduced its expenditure on clothing and footwear and 'made do' by darning clothes and cobbling shoes in the hope that they could soon return to their former level of income. The expenditure of unemployed households on clothing was only 35 per cent of that of employed households and it is not surprising that many observers believed that it was in the clothing and footwear of the unemployed that

[112] 'Coalfields Distress Fund', p. 3; see also *The Times* (29 March 1928), 17; National Archives, London, MH79/339, T. W. Wade, 'Dietary of Persons in Receipt of Public Assistance', 1 October 1935, p. 4.

[113] Rhys Davies, *Print of a Hare's Foot* (Bridgend, 1998 edn), pp. 21, 23.

[114] Beales and Lambert, *Memoirs of the Unemployed*, pp. 66–7.

Table 2.1. Monthly expenditure of 'employed' and 'unemployed' Rhondda families on various necessities, July 1936

Item of expenditure	Head unemployed with no supplementary earners		Head employed		Amount spent by unemployed as % of amount employed
	Amount spent on product	% of total expenditure	Amount spent on product	% of total expenditure	
Food	77s	49.2	138s 6d	42.1	55.3
Rent and rates	27s 10d	17.8	47s	14.3	59.2
Fuel and lighting	12s 3d	7.8	24s 4d	7.4	50.3
Clothing	11s 9d	7.5	33s 3d	10.1	35.3
Insurance	8s	5.1	11s 6d	3.5	69.6
Personal	5s 6d	3.5	22s	6.7	25.0
Soap and laundry	3s 5d	2.2	7s 7d	2.3	45.1
Thrift clubs	2s 10s	1.8	5s 3d	1.6	54.0
Books, library, subs, etc.	2s	1.3	5s 7d	1.7	35.8
Medical and chemist	2s	1.3	9s 10d	3.0	20.3
Other	3s 11d	2.5	24s	7.3	16.3
Total	**£7 16s 7d**	**100**	**£16 8s 11d**	**100**	**49.7**

Source: Harry and Phillips, 'Household budgets in the Rhondda valley', calculated from table II, p. 86, and table III, p. 88.

poverty was most evident.[115] Similarly, household goods and utensils were considered non-essential items of expenditure and the purchase of items such as furniture, floor coverings, bedclothes, towels, cutlery and crockery was curtailed in order to maximize the expenditure on more essential items such as food.[116] Means-tested unemployment assistance and poor relief tended to exacerbate the dispersal of household assets so that unemployed households were soon stripped of most pieces of furniture.[117]

Expenditure on clothing or household goods could not be put off indefinitely. The pressure of social acceptability, not to mention sheer necessity, meant that at some point, usually after an extended period of unemployment or existence on a low income, clothes and shoes could be mended no more and the pressure to spend money on household goods became too great.[118] A critical point was reached at which expenditure on 'non-essential' items could be put off no longer and expenditure on food correspondingly suffered.

This serves as a useful reminder that expenditure was not solely directed at securing the necessities of life but that social expectations also influenced patterns of consumption. Hilda Jennings argued that during short periods of unemployment the tendency was to dispense with all such luxuries, but that when unemployment became prolonged and there was 'no apparent hope of improvement' then 'some means of escape from the prevailing drabness and apathy' became necessary.[119] Even then expenditure was very low. The investigation in the Rhondda valleys found that the unemployed had merely a quarter of the money for 'personal' expenditure that employed families possessed.

Jennings also stated that betting and gambling were on the increase and it was this form of expenditure that most provoked

---

[115] National Archives, London, MH 57/3, J. E. Underwood, 'Report on conditions of health, nutrition, clothing and boots of school children in the south Wales colliery districts', *c.*1930, p. 14.

[116] Keane, 'Impact of unemployment', pp. 50–1.

[117] A columnist in *The Labour Woman* (1 May 1924), 78, made similar observations.

[118] National Archives, London, MH 55/691, Dr Eicholz, Dr Underwood and Birch Jones, 'Physical condition in Welsh mining areas, Board of Education Report' (1928), p. 29.

[119] Jennings, *Brynmawr*, pp. 158–9. However, it is evident from other studies that expenditure on the consumption of leisure decreased as a result of the Depression; see Gareth Williams, 'From grand slam to great slump: economy, society and rugby football in Wales during the Depression', in *1905 and All That: Essays on Rugby Football, Sport and Welsh Society* (Llandysul, 1991), pp. 175–200; Martin Johnes, *Soccer and Society: South Wales, 1900–1939* (Cardiff, 2002), pp. 64–75.

the ire of middle-class critics. A report made by E. P. Cathcart and A. M. T. Murray into the adequacy of diets in Glasgow, Cardiff, Reading and St Andrews, gleefully reported in the *Western Mail*, suggested that cheap, unhealthy food was being purchased by many families so as to allow bets to be laid on horse or dog races.[120] It seems likely that these instances of gambling were attempts to bring some 'colour and excitement in[to] the empty and monotonous existence of the unemployed'.[121] As Ross McKibbin has shown, the possibility of staking a shilling to win £5 or more was too good an opportunity for many people to miss.[122]

One last area of working-class expenditure that was considered wasteful by conservative writers was life insurance. The intense dislike of 'pauper funerals', the cost of funerals and the high likelihood of death in large, poor families meant that a life insurance policy for the purpose of covering the expenses of death was a high priority for most working-class families. According to Table 2.1 the proportion of income devoted to this expenditure by the poorer families was high in comparison to other items of expenditure and amounted to 70 per cent of the expenditure of employed households. Evidently, insurance was considered an important item of expenditure and efforts were made to maintain the weekly policy payments whatever the consequences. The Pilgrim Trust investigators, seemingly astounded by the depth of working-class feeling in favour of burial insurance, described the desire to maintain weekly insurance payments, rather patronizingly, as 'something akin to superstition'.[123] Even (or perhaps especially) among the poorest sections of the population, the effort to maintain regular payments was made and unemployment did not change this.

Most families seem to have taken out policies for each member of the family. The unemployed Rhondda family described as typical by Miles Davies, consisting of man, wife and three children, paid policies of 6d a week for the husband, 6d for the wife and 1d for each child.[124] Reggie Lee of Merthyr remembered how 'Gran, had

---

[120] *Western Mail* (27 January 1937), 5; another good example of such criticism can be found in *Merthyr Express* (3 March 1923), 13.

[121] Jennings, *Brynmawr*, p. 158.

[122] Ross McKibbin, 'Working-class gambling in Britain, 1880–1939', in *idem*, *The Ideologies of Class: Social Relations in Britain, 1880–1950* (Oxford, 1991), pp. 101–38; for an example from south Wales, see Fenner Brockway, *Hungry England*, p. 155.

[123] *Men Without Work*, p. 183.

[124] Miles Davies, 'The Rhondda Valley', *Geographical Magazine*, 2, 5 (1936), 380.

a lot of insurance books, covering all the family'.[125] The criticism that this was an inefficient means of saving did have some grounds, in that policies were being surrendered at a reduced value while others were allowed to lapse because of the poverty engendered by the Depression.[126] Certainly the poorer a family the less efficient a system of life insurance it could afford. While this ignores the social importance and pressure felt to have a 'respectable' funeral, it remains the case that this was an important item of expenditure in the family budget and one that was maintained even in times of financial difficulty.

In addition to these forms of social spending intended to relieve the gloom of unemployment or poverty or to meet certain specific needs, there were also forms of consumption which were intended to assert an individual's identity or respectability. Budgeting strategies were not determined by economic considerations alone but were also intended to cultivate and preserve social and cultural capital.[127] As Paul Johnson has argued, virtually all people use their power to consume to define their social position within their community.[128] Individuals defined themselves and asserted their status by their 'conspicuous consumption' of certain products, commodities and resources. Pecuniary strength was demonstrated to peers in the local community according to a well-defined and easily recognizable system of value that attached worth to specific forms of expenditure.[129] These social considerations, however, were often inconsistent with attempts to improve living standards since they diverted valuable resources from food expenditure or rent payments.

The most obvious way in which working-class families demon-

---

[125] Lee, *The Town that Died*, p. 83.

[126] National Archives, London, MH 55/691, R. J. Davies, F. W. Pethwick-Lawrence and H. Evans, 'The Distress in South Wales', 8 March 1928, p. 8.

[127] Fontaine and Schlumbohm, 'Household strategies for survival', 12, 14.

[128] Paul A. Johnson, 'Conspicuous consumption and working-class culture in late-Victorian and Edwardian Britain', *Transactions of the Royal Historical Society*, 38 (1988), 29; more generally, see Peter Burke, '*Res et verba*: conspicuous consumption in the early modern world', in John Brewer and Roy Porter (eds), *Consumption and the World of Goods* (London, 1993), p. 149; see also Mary Douglas and Baron Isherwood, *The World of Goods: Towards an Anthropology of Consumption* (Harmondsworth, 1980 edn.).

[129] At the same time, purchases considered 'feckless' were frowned upon and common sense in the management of the household budget conferred status upon a housewife; see Rosemary Crook, '"Tidy Women": women in the Rhondda between the wars', *Oral History*, 10, 2 (1982), 40–6.

strated pecuniary strength was through the consumption of housing but other means could also be used. Walls were whitewashed with lime, curtains decorated windows, and doorsteps whitened and brass polished.[130] Even food could be used as a means to convey social status. Luxury items such as eggs, vegetables or tinned fruits could only be afforded by the more affluent and were likely to be used to mark a special occasion. Conversely, certain foods were considered inferior and their consumption demonstrated a family's poverty. In Merthyr, 'Buying foreign meat showed that you were really poor' and was therefore something to be hidden from public knowledge.[131]

Other forms of expenditure similarly conferred status on an individual or family. The almost universal habit of keeping clothes as 'Sunday best' was even more prevalent in south Wales than elsewhere in Britain.[132] It is also notable that pawnbrokers were at their busiest on a Monday morning when money was scarce and on a Friday night 'to get the old man's suit out for the weekend'.[133] The American sociologist G. H. Armbruster found that dress was extremely important to many of the unemployed and that it constituted an expression of self.[134] 'Keeping up appearances' assumed greater significance for an unemployed man than for a man in work because an unemployed man no longer had 'a good wage' to proclaim his respectability.[135] The wives of unemployed men faced even greater difficulties. Many derived satisfaction from having their children dressed as well as possible but often did so at their own expense. Many women failed to attend Social Service Clubs, or chapels on a Sunday, owing to their self-consciousness at their appearance, and only ventured out of the house to do the shopping.[136] Other observers similarly noted the importance of 'keeping up appearances' for the unemployed.[137] This desire to

[130] Museum of Welsh Life Sound Archive, Tapes 7089 and 7090, Janet Davies, recorded 26 July and 2 August 1984.

[131] Lee, *The Town that Died*, p. 5.

[132] *Men Without Work*, p. 308.

[133] Eyles and O'Sullivan, *In the Shadow of the Steelworks*, p. 13.

[134] Armbruster, 'Social determination of ideologies', 68–78; see also Jennings, *Brynmawr*, p. 158; Davies, *Innocent Years*, p. 79.

[135] Armbruster, 'Social determination of ideologies', 75.

[136] Ibid., 77; Armbruster also gave examples of the tiny minority of women who neglected their children's diet so as to have money to spend on clothing and the household (77–8); see also Davies, *Innocent Years*, p. 79; Jennings, *Brynmawr*, p. 158.

[137] Cyril E. Gwyther, *The Valley shall be Exalted* (London, 1949), p. 16; H. V. Morton, *In Search of Wales* (London, 1945 edn), p. 260; Miles Davies, 'The Rhondda Valley', 380.

maintain appearances placed the unemployed in a difficult position as means-test officers tended to lessen unemployment payments when confronted by a well-dressed family and a well-maintained home.[138] In this way, the unemployment assistance system clashed against the values of working-class families and engendered a great deal of bitterness in the process.

The need felt to compete with peers and to establish status within the local community led many families to divert finances from more necessary forms of expenditure and into forms of 'conspicuous consumption'. Critics, ignorant of the culture that made such purchases necessary, condemned what they saw as wasteful spending and misplaced pride. And yet the expression of status in this way was important enough to sacrifice necessities and some-times to acquiesce in a lowered standard of living. One social survey drew a distinction between those of the unemployed wearing old clothes, 'in itself a good sign', and the 'flashily' dressed young men of south Wales who were 'not often the best'.[139] At the very low level at which many families existed, a small reduction in the food bill was worth making if it meant that some statement could be made about the family's social worth.[140]

A family's income was undoubtedly the most important factor in determining the life-chances of that family. And yet the way in which income was utilized in the form of expenditure also had important consequences. Balancing the budget was a creative and dynamic process that was often carried out differently from one week to the next and which, for many families, presented contin-uous difficulties to be overcome. Moreover, families differed in their requirements. Items of expenditure were prioritized according to the attitudes, preferences and ideas of the man of the family and attained by the calculated strategies of his wife. This is not to argue that the family formed a single, cohesive unit of consumption, for this was evidently not the case. Each individual within the family

---

[138] Armbruster, 'Social determination of ideologies', 67.

[139] *Men Without Work*, p. 185.

[140] Johnson, 'Conspicuous consumption and working-class culture', 40. The strength of the desire to 'keep up appearances' perhaps goes some way to explaining the motivation behind strike-breaking; see also Armbruster, 'Social determination of ideologies', 64–5; White and Williams, *Struggle or Starve*, p. 122.

made demands on the family's resources and experienced varying degrees of success in having those demands met. Nevertheless, the family remained the basic unit of consumption and the ways in which it consumed various products and resources had significant consequences for its experience of everyday life. Needs other than the satisfaction of hunger and nutrition meant that the money available for the purchase of food was reduced.

When faced with the sudden decrease in income that unemployment entailed, working-class women utilized many more strategies to make ends meet than have hitherto been recognized. In the first place, a number of changes were made in the way that the household budget was managed. Expenditure on 'luxuries' such as entertainment, clothing and personal items was discontinued and expenditure concentrated in essential areas such as food. Cheaper alternatives to the food usually consumed were purchased and a general thriftiness was observed. These strategies were probably sufficient to allow a family to survive a short period of unemployment relatively unscathed and with minimum effect on standards of health, but as the spell of unemployment lengthened so other strategies had to be employed. People entered the 'submerged economy' and attempted to make up the shortfall in their income by selling their own services or goods. Savings, whether in the form of savings accounts, houses, goods or co-operative share capital, were realized in order to provide the necessary money for a family to feed itself.

Furthermore, if a family's conception of respectability did not prevent it, credit could be utilized and debts accumulated so as to put the available money to better use. In many cases, the debts that could be accumulated were finite but, in many other cases, massive debts were allowed to accrue. At the low level of existence of poverty-stricken families, relatively small sums of additional money could make a significant difference. The utilization of savings and credit in this way has been completely overlooked by historians of interwar south Wales and yet they seem to have been significant survival strategies. The Labour Party Committee of Inquiry of 1928 stated that life was being sustained in the Nantyglo and Blaina area by six sources of income and support, and it placed savings and indebtedness as the first two sources.[141]

[141] Labour Party Committee of Inquiry, *Distress in South Wales*, pp. 6–7, 16; the four other sources were jobs outside the area, relatives from other areas sending money and clothes, welfare payments and private charity.

These strategies acted as 'shock absorbers' against the effects of
unemployment. By lessening the financial obligations of a household and by realizing alternative forms of money, these strategies
went some way to mitigating the financial effects of unemployment
and poverty. In many cases they served to increase the burden on
the budget after regaining employment but this was not always the
case. For these reasons, the sudden and often significant decrease in
income that unemployment occasioned was not matched by a
corresponding change in the material standards of life. A change
from employment to unemployment did not necessarily involve a
dramatic transformation in the quality of diet or the standard of
housing of a family. The effects of unemployment only registered
themselves over a much longer time-period. As savings, goods and
other sources of money were used up, as the opportunities to obtain
credit or default on the rent diminished, and as the pressure grew to
make expenditure on worn-out clothing, footwear and household
equipment, so the amount of money available for expenditure on
food decreased and so unemployment came to have an effect on
health and levels of mortality.[142]

---

[142] Massey, *Portrait of a Mining Town*, p. 69; see also Jennings, *Brynmawr*, p. 138.

III

'FAIR CLEMMED': DIET AND NUTRITION

A great deal is spoken and written about diet. The general assumption is that the problem is one of widespread interest. Academically this is undoubtedly true; practically it is not. The only question asked by the majority of people is whether there is enough to eat.[1]

Our priority was food, not eating it, but how to get it. We were always scheming and dealing and trying to find ways of cooking what little we had to our best advantage. For instance, we used a lot of flour in our food because it was filling. We put it in our broth to thicken it, and in eggs so as they would go further. Sometimes, if we didn't have bread on Thursdays my mother would mix flour and water together and add a pinch of salt and cook it on an enamel plate in the oven. Then we would have it with dripping. It tasted all right, not like real bread perhaps, but it was edible. Yes, we made some odd recipes in those days . . . We put anything edible into our pot, anything and everything.

(Beatrice Wood, Dowlais)[2]

Diet and nutritional standards became issues of political importance in the interwar period. Developments in the science of nutrition coincided with a period of prolonged industrial depression to provoke furious controversies over the adequacy of the diet of the population and the effects of inadequate diet on physical well-being. Diet and nutritional status were politicized in various ways: definitions of poverty formulated during the period (and, of course, before and since) included dietary adequacy as a criterion; critics of the government utilized descriptions of the diets of the unemployed and their families to criticize central government welfare provision and unemployment policies; and the government responded by drawing up wholesome diets that could supposedly be purchased on very low incomes while attributing malnutrition to ignorance and fecklessness. In short, diet became a sensitive political issue.[3]

---

[1] E. P. Cathcart and A. M. T. Murray, *An Inquiry into the Diet of Families in Cardiff and Reading*, MRC Special Report Series, 165 (1932), p. 18.

[2] White and Williams, *Struggle or Starve*, p. 127.

[3] Madeleine Mayhew, 'The 1930s nutrition controversy', *Journal of Contemporary History*, 23, 3 (1988), 445–64; Gazeley, *Poverty in Britain*, p. 726.

The bitter controversies that raged at that time have continued as historians have fought over the apparent dichotomy between rising nutritional and dietary standards in Britain as a whole set against the obvious deficiencies of diets of families living in the depressed areas.[4] It might be thought that, owing to the relatively high levels of unemployment in south Wales, this dichotomy is irrelevant, but it is not. Rather, the general trend of improving nutritional standards and the continuation, and even intensification, of pockets of malnutrition and inadequate diet can be observed even in depressed areas such as south Wales, and even at the level of individual communities. For despite the massive volume of unemployment and poverty that characterized interwar south Wales, a regular income could mean an adequate diet and even, as the period progressed, an increasing supply of nutritious food. As will be demonstrated, the considerable fall in food prices that occurred in the interwar period had significant consequences for both those in work and the unemployed.

This aspect of the history of diet in interwar south Wales needs to be recognized. While dietary averages of the population of a region are important, so too are variations within the population. Using qualitative as well as quantitative data, this chapter describes the food consumed by different sections of the population at different times during the 1920s and 1930s. Since the purpose of the chapter is to inform a study of standards of health, nutritional analyses of the diets are made wherever possible and evidence of the nutritional status of various sections of the population considered. In this way, an empirical evaluation of the standards of diet that prevailed during the interwar period is made in an attempt to replace the more impressionistic accounts that have hitherto characterized Welsh historiography.

Anecdotal evidence suggests that the diets of the unemployed were inferior to those enjoyed by families with wage earners. Hilda Jennings, in her study of Brynmawr published in 1934, described the diets of unemployed families as 'scanty and unnutritious':

---

[4]   Winter, 'Infant mortality, maternal mortality and public health in Britain in the 1930s'; Webster, 'Healthy or hungry thirties?'; Winter, 'Unemployment, nutrition and infant mortality in Britain'; Webster, 'Health, welfare and unemployment during the Depression'; Mitchell, 'Effects of unemployment on women and children'; John Burnett, *Plenty and Want: A Social History of Diet in England* (London, 1989), pp. 268–87; Thorpe, *Britain in the 1930s*, pp. 110–19; Perry, *Bread and Work*, pp. 69–74.

At breakfast, tea, and at supper, if taken, it consists mainly of bread and butter and tea. Dinner is the only meal at which meat is eaten, and in most cases this is only freshly cooked on Sundays. Vegetables, also, except where men have allotments are often regarded as Sunday fare. On other days, the remains of the Sunday dinner, bacon, bread and cheese, sausages and faggots, form the menu.[5]

Allen Hutt compared the diets of two families in Glynneath, each of which consisted of a man, wife and one child. The man of the first family was unemployed, received 25s 3d in unemployment benefit a week and subsisted on a diet which consisted of bread, butter, potatoes, bacon, tea and 'minute' quantities of meat, fresh milk (only one pint a week), vegetables, cheese and lard. The husband of the second family, an employed miner, earned almost £3 a week and was able to provide his family with 60 per cent more bread, 30 per cent more butter, twice as much milk, meat and vegetables, three times as many potatoes, six times as much cheese, twice as much lard, and in addition had fish, eggs, fruit, currants, rice and jam which the unemployed family was never able to afford.[6] Hutt opined:

On the straitness of the unemployed man's budget further comment is hardly necessary; what should be stressed here is that the employed miner is only able to spend on vital foodstuffs sums that by any proper standard are derisory. Thus the [employed] family considered above only spend 3s. a week on meat, 1s. on vegetables (apart from potatoes), 1s. on fruit and 6d. on fresh milk (two pints). And the anthracite miners are the aristocrats of the Welsh mining valleys![7]

Similarly, the authors of the report made to the Pilgrim Trust found that in the 'better type of unemployed home at least' bread tended to be the staple diet. 'So in a family of seven in Wales, in which the children were aged from 11 to 21, the record notes: "Saw five large loaves of bread; evidently it is the main diet."'[8] Further anecdotal evidence confirmed this impression that the unemployed existed on completely inadequate diets.[9]

---

[5]   Jennings, *Brynmawr*, p. 156.
[6]   Allen Hutt, *The Condition of the Working Class in Britain* (London, 1933), pp. 29–30.
[7]   Ibid., p. 30.
[8]   *Men Without Work*, p. 135.
[9]   Save the Children Fund, *Unemployment and the Child*, appendix IV, 'Some selected family budgets', pp. 116–18; Fenner Brockway, *Hungry England*, pp. 167–8.

The verdicts passed on the diets of the unemployed by writers such as Hutt, Fenner Brockway and Wal Hannington were often dismissed as highly polemical, politically inspired attacks on government policy. But even government-appointed investigations commented on the qualitatively inferior diet of the unemployed. The findings of an investigation published in 1929 confirmed that unemployed households subsisted on bread, margarine, potatoes, sugar, jam, tea, bacon and little else. Meat was seldom eaten and fresh milk could only be obtained when provided free by clinics.[10] In their confidential discussions, government ministers were even more concerned at the poor dietary standards of the unemployed. At a conference in July 1934 at which the Minister of Health, the President of the Board of Education and the Minister of Labour discussed various investigations that had been made into the diets of the unemployed in the distressed areas of Durham and Tyneside, Lancashire and south Wales, the Minister of Health stated that the reports, and especially that referring to south Wales, were a cause for 'grave disquiet'. The conditions found in south Wales were said to be 'particularly disturbing' and the nutritional status of children and young persons, particularly boys aged between 14 and 18, especially worrying.[11]

While this anecdotal evidence provides a valuable, albeit impressionistic, account of the diets of the unemployed, it needs to be placed in context by quantifiable source material. Contemporaries were broadly agreed that the unemployed experienced inferior diets in comparison with the rest of the population, but the extent of the difference in standards needs to be assessed. Various studies made in the mid to late 1930s by E. Harry and J. R. E. Phillips of the Department of Agricultural Economics at the University College of Wales, Aberystwyth, attempted to compare the household budgets of various 'unemployed' and 'employed' families. These hitherto neglected studies serve as a useful source for the consideration of unemployment and its effects on dietary standards. A study of forty-six households in the Rhondda in 1936 revealed clearly the differences between households of different types. Total expenditure on food for the month of July varied from 17s 5½d per person

[10] Ministry of Health, *Report on Investigation in the Coalfield of South Wales and Monmouthshire*, 1929 [Cmd. 3272], 1928–9, viii, p. 6.

[11] National Archives, London, MH79/337, 'Malnutrition among the unemployed: discussion with President of the Board of Trade and Minister of Labour', 12 July 1934, pp. 1–2.

in 'unemployed' households to £1 6s 6 ³/₄d in those households where the head was employed, a difference of over 9s per person per month.[12]

A further study carried out by Harry and Phillips compared the expenditure of 'employed' and 'unemployed' households in the Rhondda over the course of the year between July 1936 and June 1937. Four 'employed' households spent £1 15s 1d per head per month compared with 16s 9¹/₂d by the 'unemployed' households, a difference of almost £1 per head per month.[13] The difference was greater than that found in the survey of July 1936 and suggests that dietary inequality between the employed and the unemployed was more marked after long periods of unemployment. As the investigators commented, families that suffered short periods of unemployment tended to maintain their food expenditure near to the level of when they were employed.[14] On experiencing unemployment, families initially reduced their expenditure on non-food items, such as boots, clothing, household furniture and utensils, and entertainment, in the hope that the spell of unemployment would not last long. As the period without work lengthened, so families were less able to bear the hardships that reduced expenditure on these items entailed and were forced to sacrifice their food expenditure to compensate. Therefore, the differences in the standard of diet experienced by the employed and the unemployed were most keenly felt over long periods of time.

Table 3.1 shows how the expenditure of the households surveyed in July 1936 was distributed among various food products. The greatest differences in expenditure were on meat, eggs and 'milk-stuffs', but vegetables and fruit also showed marked variation. Therefore, employed families were able to buy much larger quantities of the so-called 'protective foods' than were the unemployed. At the same time, some 'unemployed' households spent more on bulky and cheap foodstuffs than did those households whose members were employed. These foodstuffs included cereals and other breakfast foods, butter, cheese and margarine, and it was from these that 'the unemployed households supplied bodily needs'.[15]

[12] Harry and Phillips, 'Household budgets in the Rhondda Valley', 87.
[13] Ibid., 'Expenditure of unemployed and employed households', 95.
[14] Ibid., 94.
[15] Harry and Phillips, 'Household budgets in the Rhondda Valley', 87–8; these patterns of expenditure were confirmed by the study carried out by Harry and Phillips in the period July 1936 to June 1937; Harry and Phillips, 'Expenditure of unemployed and employed households', 96.

Table 3.1. Per capita expenditure on different foodstuffs in 'employed' and 'unemployed' Rhondda households, July 1936

	Head unemployed without supplementary earners	Head in employment	All families surveyed
No. of households	21	17	46
No. of persons	90	72	207
Average income per person	£1 16s 6d	£3 17s 9d	£2 14s 2d
Meat, suet, fish, eggs	5s 10½d	7s 10¾d	6s 3d
Cereals and breakfast foods	2s 11d	3s 8¾d	3s 7d
Butter, margarine and cheese	3s 4½d	4s 4½d	3s 11½d
Milkstuffs	1s 4¾d	2s 6d	1s 9¼d
Fruit	7¾d	1s 11¼d	1s 1¾d
Vegetables	1s 8¾d	2s 2¾d	1s 10½d
Preserves	1s 3¼d	2s 1½d	1s 8½d
Beverages	1s 0d	1s 6½d	1s 3½d
Home-produced food and meals from home	1d	2¾d	4½d
Total food expenditure	17s 5½d	£1 6s 6¾d	£1 1s 11¼d

Source: Adapted from Harry and Phillips, 'Household budgets in the Rhondda Valley', table III, p. 88.

Therefore, certain strategies can be observed in the way in which families dealt with the hardship that unemployment occasioned. Following a fall in a family's income, its consumption of different foodstuffs did not fall uniformly but tended instead to decline in the relatively expensive 'protective' foods and to rise in the cheaper, bulky products in order to satisfy hunger.

This strategy is also hinted at in a study of Cardiff diets carried out by the nutritional scientist E. P. Cathcart. The diets of fifty-six Cardiff families were compared with those of seven unemployed families within the sample. Although the diets of these unemployed families contained less fat and, to a smaller extent, less protein, they nevertheless contained more carbohydrate than the average diet in the sample. By substituting cheaper carbohydrate-loaded foodstuffs for the more nutritious products they could no longer afford, un-employed families were able to obtain a diet which, at least in terms

Calorific value, roughly equal, protein + fat.

of the calorific value, was almost comparable to that of employed families.[16]

The studies of Harry and Phillips reveal another strategy utilised by working-class women to provide enough food for their families. In times of economic stress, Harry claimed, an attempt was made to 'make do' by lowering quantities as well as the quality of products purchased. Those on low incomes attempted to satisfy the same food requirements on a reduced income:

> The attempt takes two forms – first some redistribution of the total purchasing power allocated to foods as between the different classes of foods, and second a change from a better to a lower quality, and from higher to lower price commodities, within some of the classes like 'meatstuffs' and 'milkstuffs'. The redistribution causes reductions in quantities and proportions at some points and increases at others.[17]

A further notable indicator of the poverty endemic in the Rhondda which was brought out by Harry's investigations is the way in which large quantities of meat and fish, and indeed other foodstuffs not included in the study, were purchased at auctions.[18] These auctions were held once or twice a week in different parts of the valley on different days of the week. The quality of the food sold varied widely but, it was stated, large households with small incomes welcomed this means of obtaining food. Since relatively large quantities were offered for sale at these auctions, smaller households were unable to afford the higher prices for these larger amounts and so households often 'clubbed' together to buy meat. In this way, poorer families were also able to achieve economies of scale. Poorer families were usually only able to buy in small quantities, and prices for such small amounts were often relatively higher per unit of product purchased than for larger quantities.[19]

[16] Cathcart and Murray, *Diet of Families in Cardiff and Reading*, table II, p. 7; table XIa, p. 16.

[17] Harry and Phillips, 'Household budgets in the Rhondda', 90–1; this substitution of cheaper products for those previously purchased means that the nutritional adequacy of diets cannot be accurately assessed using expenditure patterns, since cheaper alternatives might have been purchased without in any way lessening the nutritional adequacy of a diet. This demonstrates the methodological flaws inherent in any attempt to assess dietary standards based on expenditure patterns.

[18] E. Ll. Harry, 'Meat consumption in the Rhondda Valley', *Welsh Journal of Agriculture*, 12 (1936), 70 and 81; for examples see Eyles and O'Sullivan, *In the Shadows of the Steelworks*, p. 46; Fenner Brockway, *Hungry England*, pp. 163–4.

[19] Massey, *Portrait of a Mining Town*, p. 25.

The study carried out by Harry and Phillips also revealed the relatively small improvement, at least in the short term, in the living standards of households which moved from unemployment to employment. Members of 'unemployed' households who gained a job initially required better food and clothing, and more heating, lighting and cleaning materials, and thereby further depressed the standards of other members of their households. These initial costs swallowed up any increase in income and when the duration of employment was short a family found itself worse off because one of its members had been lucky enough to obtain employment. This was so because in many instances the amount received in wages was little better than unemployment benefit or public assistance.

The level of income was clearly the most important factor in determining the quality of diet experienced by a family. However, while differences *between* families were highly significant, the divisions *within* families also conditioned experiences and determined standards of living and so the social relations within families also need to be taken into account. While it is helpful to use households or families as the unit of analysis, it needs to be remembered that resources were not allocated equally among members of those units. Households can be conceptualized as a 'forum for centrifugal and centripetal forces' where individual members competed to satisfy their needs.[20] Most importantly, gender relations influenced the allocation of food resources within families. This worked in a number of ways. In the first place, there was a cultural ideal that the earning capacity of the family needed to be maintained and that this was best achieved by maximizing the food consumption of the (usually male) breadwinner or breadwinners.[21] Secondly, the nature of the coal industry meant that women played a supporting role in the home and there was a tendency for working-class wives to place the needs of their husbands before their own needs.[22] The heavy workload of a collier's wife meant that she was forced to take meals as best she could. A respondent to J. M. Keane suggested that he never saw his mother sit down and eat a meal throughout his childhood.[23]

Thirdly, the pressures placed on a family by unemployment served to exacerbate this gendered allocation of resources within a family. Many contemporary investigators noted how it was women

[20] Fontaine and Schlumbohm, 'Household strategies for survival', 5–6.
[21] White and Williams, *Struggle or Starve*, pp. 128, 133, 134.
[22] As an example see, Hanley, *Grey Children*, p. 19.
[23] Keane, 'Impact of unemployment', 46.

who bore the brunt of the deterioration in dietary standards that unemployment occasioned.[24] Responsible for the management of the household budget, many working-class women sacrificed their own food consumption so as to ensure that their husbands and children received sufficient nutrition. The sacrifices made by mothers and, to a lesser extent, fathers meant that children were to some extent sheltered from the worst effects of poverty. Maggie Pryce Jones of Trelewis, remembering the allocation of food resources in her family, stated rhetorically that it was 'The best for Dad, the next best for the children; for her, I suspect now, nothing'.[25]

The report of the Tuberculosis Physician for the Swansea area noted in 1921 that the diets of girls suffered during economic hardship. He commented: 'I fear we shall reap the whirlwind in the case of the young women of 17 onwards who required full nourishment and went short', suggesting that it was not merely that women were responsible for the household budget and so sacrificed their own food consumption to ease the weekly burden but that the allocation of food resources within families was specifically organized according to gender.[26] Nevertheless, while children below a certain age were protected from the worst effects of poverty by the sacrifices of their parents and especially their mothers, girls similarly experienced shortages in their food intake when they reached a certain age.

This was borne out by the findings of the Rhondda school medical officer and his staff during the mid to late 1930s when medical inspection was extended to children attending secondary and continuation schools in the district. They found that girls attending these schools were 'physically inferior' to the boys and asserted that this was due to a number of factors, most importantly to diets deficient in 'the constituents which serve to maintain phys-

[24] Jennings, *Brynmawr*, p. 157; Eli Ginzberg, *A World Without Work* (London, 1942), p. 37; *Men Without Work*, pp. 112, 133; Gelligaer UD, RMOH (1926), pp. 38–9. Government investigators came to the same conclusions: National Archives, London, MH55/629, Ministry of Health, J. Pearse, T. W. Wade, O. Evans and J. E. Underwood, 'Report of an inquiry into conditions affecting health through unemployment in South Wales and Monmouthshire', 23 October 1936, pp. 10–11, 49–50; MH55/691, Board of Education, Dr Eicholz, Dr Underwood and B. Jones, 'Physical condition in Welsh mining districts', 1928, pp. 9, 29–30; Ministry of Health, *Report on Investigation in the Coalfield of South Wales and Monmouthshire*, p. 6.

[25] Pryce Jones, *Kingfisher of Hope*, pp. 61, 32; see also *Men Without Work*, pp. 112, 126–8, 139–41.

[26] *Annual Report of the King Edward VII Welsh National Memorial Association*, year ending 31 March 1922, p. 55.

ical fitness, such as milk and other dairy products, eggs, and green vegetables'.[27] Girls paid the price for these dietary disadvantages and experienced more 'defects' such as anaemia, blepharitis, defective vision and postural 'deformities' such as curvature of the spine and flat feet.

However, this 'pessimistic' interpretation needs to be qualified by the recognition that those families which were able to earn a regular wage, and maintain a high per capita income, were able to eat relatively well during the Depression. The diet set out in Table 3.2 is that of the family of Eileen Baker who grew up in the Swansea valley; it is probably typical of the diets of more fortunate families. Baker was one of two children of a railwayman who, although not earning wages as high as those of miners or tinplate workers, was in regular employment throughout the interwar period.

A number of features of this diet are immediately noticeable. First, in comparison with the diets of the unemployed, the consumption of meat by Baker's family seems fairly high and, in addition, the weekly diet included some fish, thus ensuring a supply of first-class protein. Laverbread is very high in iron, formed a useful addition to the family's usual fare and would have helped to prevent anaemia. Despite this, Baker stated that the consumption of meat by her family was not high but that in better-off families (that is, those of miners or tinplate workers) the wage earner expected a hot meat dish ready for him on his return from work.[28] One way in which this diet was inadequate, however, was in the consumption of fruit. Baker and her brother were only given one orange each a week.[29]

Other sources also suggest that, provided a family obtained a regular income, the standard of diet enjoyed could be sufficient in quantity and almost adequate in nutritional terms. A number of respondents to Jeffrey Grenfell-Hill's enquiries in the 1990s recalled that their diets in the interwar period seemed satisfactory. These consisted of the children of a colliery examiner, a boilerman and a steelworker. Referring to a standard of life that allowed milk to be

---

[27]   Rhondda UD, RSMO (1935), pp. xlvi–xlvii; (1936), pp. xliv–xlv; (1937), pp. xlix–liii; (1938), p. xlix.

[28]   Eileen Baker, 'Yan Boogie'. *The Autobiography of a Swansea Valley Girl* (Pretoria, 1992), p.5, fn.4; the western part of the coalfield was more economically buoyant than the eastern and central parts of the coalfield during the interwar period.

[29]   Ibid., p. 7.

Table 3.2. Typical diet of Eileen Baker's family, Ystalyfera, during the interwar period

Day	Breakfast	Dinner	Tea
Monday	Cereal (summer), porridge (winter)	Bubble and squeak pudding (usually suet 'roly-poly'); tea or water	Home-made cake with tea; bread and butter or dripping; (bed-time) cocoa with a little milk and boiling water
Tuesday	As above	Minced meat pie with potato top	As above
Wednesday	As above	Liver and bacon, tripe and onions; cawl (winter); pudding	As above
Thursday	As above	Soup with suet dumplings; pudding	As above
Friday	As above	Fish (often in pie) with potatoes	As above
Saturday	As above	Bacon; laver bread; (occasionally) egg and chips	As above
Sunday	As above	Full roast beef and roast potatoes; Yorkshire pudding, gravy and vegetables; rice pudding or, for a treat, tinned fruit and custard; tea or water	As above

Source: Eileen Baker, 'Yan Boogie' (Pretoria, 1992).

delivered daily, the first of these commented, 'Aye, we used to live well. There was no question of it.'[30]

The pessimistic interpretation needs to be qualified by the recognition of further strategies implemented by working-class families to maximize the amount and quality of food available. For example, the possession of an allotment could transform the diet of a family. A school medical officer in Cardiff observed a striking contrast between the children of those families who had a garden or an allotment and those who had neither.[31] Another school inspector

[30] J. Du C. Grenfell-Hill, 'Mother and infants in south Wales, 1900–1930' (unpublished University of Wales Ph.D. thesis, 1993), 265–7 (testimony of 'Lena' from Abertillery).
[31] Cardiff CB, RMOH (1940), p. 77.

was apparently able to tell by sight those children whose parents had allotments, owing 'to their different aspect'.[32] Statistics on the numbers of allotments in south Wales are scarce but it seems likely that allotments were more numerous in the towns and villages of the coastal plain where there was some available land.[33] In the steep, sloping valley communities, where available land was scarce, allotments were fewer and, being squeezed into whatever space could be found between the ubiquitous coal tips, were not very productive. The communities of the eastern and central coalfield were denied the large gardens to which householders in western Glamorgan and in the rural areas had access. Nevertheless, some allotments existed in most areas and it was noted that allotment holders 'multiplied their agricultural efforts' in the wake of the lockout of 1926.[34] Cheap food was increasingly important as unemployment and economic difficulty increased, and certain charitable bodies organized allotment societies for the unemployed.[35]

Another way in which families augmented their diet was by the rearing of pigs. Pig keeping was common in some coalmining communities of south Wales but probably declined during the interwar period. Every part of a pig was used and it was possible to rear a pig on household waste and scraps. Once slaughtered, pieces were distributed to neighbours and to families which had given meat, eggs or vegetables in the past.[36] More common than pig rearing was the practice of keeping poultry. An investigation into food consumption in the Rhondda in the 1930s found that the proportion of imported eggs to home-produced eggs was low. 'But', it was stated, 'nobody thoroughly familiar with the Rhondda Valley would express much surprise at the relative proportions, for backyard poultry flocks are fairly common.'[37] J. Gilmore-Cox, the superintendent of Infant Welfare Administration in Gelligaer, noted that some families possessed goats and were able to give their children 'rich and good' goat's milk. Since the fresh milk supplied in the area was invariably found to be dirty and carried the threat of infection, Gilmore-Cox advocated that 'Every effort should be

[32]   Save the Children Fund, *Unemployment and the Child*, p. 26.
[33]   *Welsh Housing and Development Yearbook* (1925), 74.
[34]   H. W. J. Edwards, *The Good Patch* (London, 1938), p. 116.
[35]   *The Friend*, 69, 37 (1929), 819; however, Jennings, *Brynmawr*, p. 187, noted that the cost of maintaining an allotment was only partly met by charitable funding.
[36]   Museum of Welsh Life Sound Archive, Tape 7224, Lorna Rubbery, Rhyd-y-Car.
[37]   Harry, 'Meat consumption in the Rhondda Valley', 86.

made to promote goat-keeping among the people who have suitable surroundings'.[38] Therefore, for those families with allotments or backyard animals, produce such as eggs, milk, vegetables, potatoes and sometimes meat, if it was not sold, formed an important, if unquantifiable, addition to their diets. Such additions pose a methodological problem in any attempt to assess diets according to patterns of expenditure.

Disparities in food expenditure according to social class, or between the employed and unemployed, are relatively easy to establish but do not reveal a great deal about the nutritional adequacy of the diets of the unemployed. Major methodological problems are inherent in any attempt to assess diets in past societies according to modern nutritional science since precise assessments of the nutritional adequacy of the food consumed by populations or individuals cannot be made. Furthermore, ideas about nutritional adequacy have changed over time and any attempt to assess standards of diet in the past would fail to acknowledge contemporary definitions of an adequate diet. Therefore, diets in interwar south Wales are here assessed according to contemporary criteria drawn up by nutritional scientists in the interwar period.[39]

The well-known feeding experiments of the National Birthday Trust Fund in the 1930s provide a number of insights into this issue and usefully reveal the economic situation of some Rhondda families during the 1930s. Lady Williams, in an article about the scheme, claimed that the majority of those receiving aid from the Fund had less than 4s per head each week to spend on food (Table 3.3). The amounts available for food after other expenses had been covered were inadequate, to say the least. The British Medical Association's estimate of 5s 11d per man and 4s 11d for a woman as the cost of a minimum diet was clearly not being attained by these families.[40] Nor were they attaining the even lower standards esti-

[38] Gelligaer UD, RMOH (1923), p. 18.

[39] On interwar dietary surveys see Mayhew, 'The 1930s nutrition controversy'; Gazeley, *Poverty in Britain*, pp. 72–6.

[40] Mayhew, 'The 1930s nutrition controversy', 451. It has long been argued that the feeding experiments of the Fund constitute evidence of the extreme poverty and poor nutritional status of working-class women in south Wales, but A. Susan Williams has demonstrated that these experiments were methodologically flawed and inconclusive: *Women and Childbirth in the Twentieth Century: A History of the National Birthday Trust Fund, 1928–93* (Stroud, 1997), pp. 81–98; and 'Relief and research: the nutrition work of the National Birthday Trust Fund, 1935–9', in David F. Smith (ed.), *Nutrition in Britain: Science, Scientists and Politics in the Twentieth Century* (London, 1997), pp. 99–122.

Table 3.3. Cases assisted by the National Birthday Trust Fund in the Rhondda
Valley, 1930s

Family	Income			Amount left for food after various outgoings		Amount per head	
Mrs K. (Wattstown). Seven in family	£2	1s	0d	15s	2d	2s	2d
Mrs O. (Treherbert). Seven.	£1	18s	0d	22s	0d	2s	9d
Mrs P (Gelli). Ten	£2	3s	6d	30s	6d	3s	¹/₂d
Mrs M. (Cwmparc). Three		19s	6d	3s	8d	1s	10d
Mrs T. (Penygraig). Four		28s	0d	7s	10d	1s	11¹/₂d

Source: Lady Williams, 'Malnutrition as a cause of maternal mortality', *Public Health*, 1, 50
(October 1936), 14.

mated by the 'Hungry England' inquiry of 1933 in the *Week-End
Review*, which estimated that 5s a week for a man, 4s 2d for a
woman and 2s 9d to 4s 10d for children according to age, were the
minimum costs of a 'practical diet'.[41]

John Boyd Orr rejected the idea of a 'minimum diet' in his well-
known work of 1936, and instead adopted a dietary standard which
provided optimum requirements for health. Boyd Orr classified the
population according to six income groups and estimated the
weekly per capita food expenditure of each group. He asserted that
an average weekly expenditure of 4s per head or less on food meant
a diet deficient in all necessary constituents. The amounts of
protein, fat, carbohydrates, vitamins and minerals necessary to
maintain 'a state of well-being such that no improvement can be
effected by a change in the diet' were not possible at this low level of
expenditure.[42] And yet it is clear that many of the women aided by
the feeding scheme in the Rhondda existed on diets well below this
inadequate standard. By whatever standards the diets of these
expectant mothers in the Rhondda are judged, it seems clear that
they were not receiving adequate nutrition to enable them to face
the rigours of pregnancy safely.

However, the feeding scheme purposely sought to aid those
women most in need and so the cases quoted by Williams can
hardly be said to be representative. These were probably the worst

[41] Mayhew, 'The 1930s nutrition controversy', 449.
[42] Boyd Orr, *Food, Health and Income*, p. 12.

Table 3.4. John Boyd Orr's classification of the population of England and Wales by income groups and food expenditure per person

Group	Income per head per week	Estimated average expenditure on food per person	Estimated population of group	
			No.	%
I	Up to 10s	4s	4,500,000	10
II	10s to 15s	6s	9,000,000	20
III	15s to 20s	8s	9,000,000	20
IV	20s to 30s	10s	9,000,000	20
V	30s to 45s	12s	9,000,000	20
VI	Over 45s	14s	4,500,000	10
Average	30s	9s	–	–

Source: Boyd Orr, *Food, Health and Income*, 21.

cases in the Rhondda with the lowest weekly per capita expenditure on food. If Boyd Orr's standard is applied to various investigations carried out during the 1930s, a better idea of the adequacy of diets in interwar south Wales may be obtained. An investigation carried out by Dr W. Powell Phillips, deputy school medical officer of Cardiff in 1936, focused upon families whose nutritional status was categorized either as 'excellent' (Group A) or as 'bad' (Group D).[43] Families in Group A spent on average just over 5s 8d per person per week on food. This was the group of families chosen by the public health authorities because of the 'excellent' nutritional status of their children, but these families would have been placed in Boyd Orr's group II and, by this standard, would have experienced a diet adequate in proteins and fat but inadequate in terms of calories, calcium, phosphorous, iron and Vitamins A and C. Cardiff families placed in Group D, selected because their children were found to be of 'bad' nutritional status, spent on average 3s 8½d per person per week and would have been placed in Boyd Orr's income group I. According to this standard, the diets of these families were inadequate for perfect health in all the constituents considered (that is, protein, fat, calories, calcium, phosphorous, iron and Vitamins A and C).[44]

[43] Cardiff CB, RMOH (1936), pp. 148–52
[44] On the adequacy of diets according to Boyd Orr's classification, see Boyd Orr, *Food, Health and Income*, pp. 33–6.

The twenty-one Rhondda households studied by Harry and Phillips in July 1936 where the head of the family was unemployed spent on average about 3s 11d per person per week, thus placing them too in Boyd Orr's group I. Their diets would also have been inadequate in all the constituents considered. The eight households where the head was unemployed, but where there were supplementary earners, spent about 5s $3^{1}/_{2}$d per head per week on food, thereby placing them in Boyd Orr's income group II. The last group of seventeen Rhondda families where the head of the household was in employment spent on average about 7s 11d per person per week, which placed them in Boyd Orr's group III. Their diet would have been adequate in calories, protein and fat but inadequate in calcium, phosphorous, iron and Vitamins A and C.[45]

Therefore, if the criteria by which diets are assessed are changed to an ideal standard whereby 'a state of well-being such that no improvement can be effected by a change in the diet', it is clear that these families from Cardiff and the Rhondda fell far short of enjoying adequate diets. Twenty-one of a sample of forty-six Rhondda families (46 per cent) studied, and stated to be representative of the Rhondda valleys as a whole, existed on diets that were nutritionally inadequate in every respect. Even those Rhondda families whose heads of household were in employment experienced diets that were inadequate in certain respects. As John Burnett points out, the absence of the requirements for perfect health experienced by families in the lower groups of Boyd Orr's classification did not necessarily imply starvation or even malnutrition. But it does seem likely that such families which existed on diets that were inadequate in the constituents mentioned by Boyd Orr bore a heavier burden in ill health and premature death than families which could afford more adequate diets.[46]

While it is possible to demonstrate dietary inequalities by examining the differences in food expenditure between different households, and while inequalities within families can be illustrated though an examination of cultural attitudes, it is more difficult to ascertain the effects of unemployment and poverty on the nutritional status of the population over time. Sources which can offer certain insights are the medical inspections of schoolchildren.

---

[45]   Weekly per capita food expenditure of Rhondda families calculated from Harry and Phillips, 'Household budgets in the Rhondda', table III, 88.

[46]   Burnett, *Plenty and Want*, p. 270.

Public health authorities reasoned that since children were one of the most vulnerable sections of the population it was here that insufficient nourishment would manifest itself. However, care must be taken not to draw too many conclusions about the diets of the whole population from this particular section of it since many parents sacrificed their own share of the family's food resources to improve the diets of their children. The nutritional status of school-children might over-state the nutritional status of the population as a whole. Furthermore, the use of evidence relating to the nutritional status of children during the interwar years is problematic. Judgements as to whether or not a child was malnourished could be subjective and therefore misleading. Each medical examiner judged a child against the normal standard in his or her area, and so comparisons between different areas of the country are difficult to make.

There was too a political dimension to the findings of the medical inspections. Charles Webster has pointed out how local medical officers purposely painted a more optimistic picture of the extent of malnutrition than was the case for fear of censure by governments intent on portraying their policies in a favourable light.[47] In poverty-stricken areas such as Aberdare and Ebbw Vale during the depths of the Depression in 1932 and 1933, for example, not a single child was classified as having 'Bad Nutrition'.[48] For these various reasons, the subjective judgements of school medical officers are of limited value in ascertaining the nutritional status of the child population.

Height and weight measurements are a much surer guide to the nutritional status of a population than the subjective judgements of medical examiners. As Phyllis Eveleth and James Tanner have written:

> A child's growth rate reflects better than any other single index, his status of health and nutrition; and often indeed his psychological situation also. Similarly, the average value of children's heights and weights reflects accurately the state of a nation's public health and the average nutritional status of its citizens.[49]

---

[47] Webster, 'Healthy or hungry thirties?', 110–29.
[48] Ibid., 114.
[49] Phyllis B. Eveleth and J. M. Tanner, *Worldwide Variation in Human Growth* (Cambridge, 1976), p. 1.

Furthermore, dietary factors exert a powerful influence on the final height attained by a person; prolonged periods of malnutrition during childhood produce shorter adults. Therefore, the assessment of nutritional status through measurements of height represents a useful method by which to measure the standard of living of a population.[50] Similarly, measurements of weight can be used as an index of nutritional status although this data is more problematic. Its major flaw is that the normal daily variation in weight due to water balance is considerable when compared to variations in height.[51] Inaccurate weighing instruments would compound this problem. Nevertheless, averages of many hundreds of measurements can serve to even out the discrepancies in individual cases and so measurements of weight can prove useful.

The use of height and weight measurements as an indicator of the nutritional status of a population is further complicated by the influence of heredity. Genotype determines the potential of a person or a people to attain a certain height and weight, and environmental factors such as diet and disease determine how much of that potential is realized.[52] Therefore, while the differences in height between two populations might be determined to some extent by dietary factors, the influence of heredity and genetic factors cannot be ruled out. On the other hand, Floud, Wachter and Gregory argue that variations in height within very broad racial groups are primarily the product of environmental factors. Measurements of height and weight over time are useful, as are comparisons between different sections of the population at any point in time.

In surveys of adult physique in Britain, Welsh people have continually been found to be the shortest. A survey conducted by Dr John Beddoe for the Anthropological Society of London in 1869 found that the average Scotsman was the tallest and heaviest followed by the Irishman, the Englishman and lastly the Welshman.[53] Welsh recruits during the First World War were seemingly shorter than soldiers from other parts of Britain and also their German counterparts, and by the 1980s Welsh adult males were

[50]   Roderick Floud, Kenneth W. Wachter and Annabel Gregory, *Height, Health and History: Nutritional Status in the United Kingdom, 1750–1980* (Cambridge, 1990), p. 19.

[51]   B. J. Harris, 'Medical inspection and the nutrition of schoolchildren in Britain, 1900–1950' (unpublished University of London Ph.D. thesis, 1989), 289.

[52]   Floud, Wachter and Gregory, *Height, Health and History*, p. 5.

[53]   Quoted ibid., p. 199.

Figure 3.1. Cartoon which publicized the importance of nutrition during childhood, 1927

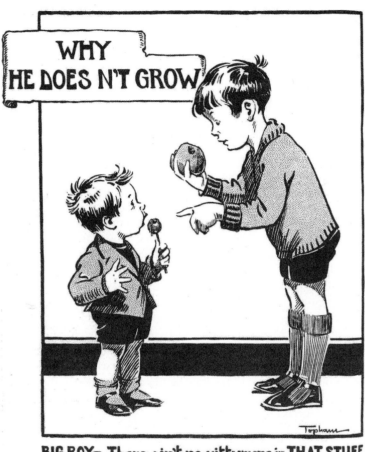

Source: Maternity and Child Welfare, 11, 11 (1927), 356.

still the shortest in Britain.[54] Anecdotal evidence from the interwar
period tended to confirm this pattern. People in the prosperous
communities of south-east England who were spectators of the

[54]   Gervase Phillips, 'An army of giants: height and medical characteristics of Welsh
soldiers, 1914–1918', *Archives*, 12, 97 (1997), 142–3, 144; Floud, Wachter and Gregory, *Height,
Health and History*, p. 203.

Hunger Marches of the 1930s often commented at the shock they received when they saw how short were the miners of south Wales.[55] The relatively smaller stature of Welsh people took on an added significance during the interwar depression:

> because the physique of Welsh people has been undermined by the prolonged privations of unemployment, and undersized anaemic youths and girls are the chief representatives of our country in England today, there has grown up among a certain class an idea that the Welsh race itself is degenerate and unfit, and should not be allowed to multiply further.[56]

Schoolchildren were, of course, the only section of the population to be systematically measured each year and the statistics obtained from the annual reports of school medical officers can be used to plot trends in the nutritional status of the population. Although all school medical officers were required to measure the heights and weights of children in the local education authority areas there was no requirement to publish them. Of the fifteen local education authorities in south Wales, only Rhondda and Barry school medical officers published height and weight measurements throughout the interwar period; the officers of Cardiff, Monmouthshire, Ebbw Vale and Abertillery published measurements for most years in the period, while the remaining officers published none at all.

Data relating to the height and weight measurements of children in south Wales reveals a number of trends.[57] Considerable variation from one year to the next in the Abertillery figures suggests that the way in which the measurements were taken varied and are, therefore, not reliable. The Ebbw Vale figures are recorded to the nearest inch and pound and so mask small changes in the average figure. The measurements for Barry suggest a very gradual increase in both height and weight throughout the interwar period. In the case of the Rhondda, a gradual increase in the heights of children of different ages can be detected beginning in the late 1920s to early 1930s.[58] This is borne out by the findings of Bernard Harris, who

---

[55] Ibid., p. 2; F. Zweig, *Men in the Pits* (London, 1948), p. 4, argued that miners were of short stature generally and that this was a 'sort of adaptation to the mines'.

[56] Lady Williams, 'Modern theories of nutrition in relation to Welsh migration', *Public Health in Wales*, Addresses delivered to the Welsh School of Social Services, Llandrindod Wells, 10–13 August 1936, p. 56.

[57] For more on the height and weight data of children in south Wales, see Thompson, 'Social history of health', 389–400.

[58] The Monmouthshire school medical officer noted that school children in the county were taller and heavier in 1931 than comparably aged children in the county in 1913 and

examined the influence of unemployment on the physiques of schoolchildren throughout Britain.

Harris found that the children living in areas such as the Rhondda, Bradford and Leeds which experienced high levels of unemployment were generally shorter and weighed less than children in areas such as Cambridge or Croydon, where unemployment was less severe.[59] Furthermore, although areas such as the Rhondda shared in the secular increases in height and weight that all areas experienced in the period *c.*1910 to 1950, the rate of increase was more gradual, and therefore regional inequalities intensified over the period.[60] However, while Harris was able to show that high levels of unemployment were inversely associated with child physique, he also made the point that unemployment did not necessarily determine stature. By the use of regression analysis Harris argued that in places like the Rhondda unemployment was not the only determinant of the heights of children and that these areas would have experienced a low standard of health even without economic depression.[61]

In contrast, the Monmouthshire school medical service was firmly of the opinion that the economic fortunes of an area were generally reflected in the heights and weights of the children. In an investigation published in 1931 it was found that the children of the New Inn to St Dials area, in the lower part of the Eastern valley, were the heaviest and tallest in the county. This was an area in which the steel and tinplate works were described as 'fairly thriving'. In contrast, areas like Rhymney, Blaina, Nantyglo and Blaenavon, at the heads of the valleys, which had suffered economic dislocation to a greater degree, contained the shortest and lightest children in the county.[62]

The survey also found that children from the rural areas of eastern Monmouthshire were generally taller and heavier than chil-

---

1921; Monmouthshire Education Committee, *Annual Report of the Medical Inspection Department* (1931), p. 86.

[59] Harris, 'Medical inspection and the nutrition of schoolchildren in Britain', 184; Bernard Harris, 'The height of schoolchildren in Britain, 1900–1950', in John Komlos (ed.), *Stature, Living Standards, and Economic Development: Essays in Anthropometric History* (London, 1994), pp. 25–38.

[60] Harris, 'Medical inspection and the nutrition of schoolchildren in Britain', 183.

[61] Ibid., 271–2.

[62] Monmouthshire Education Committee, *Annual Report of the Medical Inspection Department* (1931), appendix II, 'Special report upon the state of nutrition of the school children in Monmouthshire'.

dren from the urban districts of the western part of the county.[63] This perplexed the author of the survey who asked: 'Why is the country child so much better physically than the town child? Country folk are as poor as town dwellers, and have not plentiful supplies of butter, milk and eggs.'[64] A further survey carried out in September 1934 found that:

> There is evidence in the rural areas that some of the children are getting sufficient quantities of food necessary to appease their hunger, but are not getting the quality essential for the healthy development of growing youth. Even in cases where the parents of the children concerned are comparatively well off, e.g., having many head of cattle, poultry, etc., the children were found to have little or no milk or even eggs in their daily diet.[65]

Similarly, the survey found that there was a marked lack of meat and protein in their diet, with some children receiving no meat at all and others only occasionally. The survey concluded that malnutrition in the rural areas was due to the low wages of the rural workers, the large size of some families, the difficulty of obtaining sufficient milk and the long distances which schoolchildren in rural areas had to travel to school.[66] Nevertheless, various other studies conducted during the 1930s commented on the better nutritional status of rural children in relation to urban children.[67] Thus, despite the inadequate diets of rural children, the survey of 1931 found that, in Monmouthshire at least, they were heavier and taller than their urban counterparts. If the diets of rural children were inferior to those of urban children, other environmental factors were acting to make their stature greater than that of urban children. Environmental pollution, physical topography and disease ecology were only some of the factors that influenced this phenomenon.

The causes of the increases in stature of children in the interwar period are difficult to determine. They are unlikely to be as the result of school-feeding schemes which were instituted during the interwar period since, as Charles Webster has shown, the provision

[63] Earlier surveys had concluded that the nutritional status of rural children was inferior to that of urban children and so the findings of the investigation of heights and weights in 1931 came as a surprise to the public health authorities; see Monmouthshire Education Committee, *Annual Report of the Medical Inspection Department* (1922), appendix III; (1925), p. 10.

[64] Monmouthshire Education Committee, *Annual Report of the Medical Inspection Department* (1931), pp. 87, 89.

[65] Monmouthshire Education Committee, *Annual Report of the Medical Inspection Department* (1934), p. 51.

[66] Ibid.

[67] Monmouthshire Education Committee, *Annual Report of the Medical Inspection Department* (1937), pp. 49, 62.

of school meals varied from one district to another and only catered for a small proportion of the total school population in any area.[68] Even in south Wales, an area which provided school meals more generously than other parts of England and Wales, only a third of the school population in the most depressed areas were receiving meals or milk by the mid 1930s, which seems impressive until it is recognized that between a third and a half of children found to be malnourished at that time were not receiving meals or milk.[69]

A significant factor in the increases in heights and weights was the decrease in the threats posed by infectious diseases. Infection affects nutritional status in a number of ways but generally it serves to limit the rate at which infants and children increase in height and weight and can even cause a decrease in weight.[70] Therefore, the increases in height and weight were, at least in part, caused by the decline in the number and severity of cases of infectious diseases which had been occurring in the decades before the 1920s and which continued in the interwar period. The efforts of public health officials to notify, isolate and treat cases of infectious disease were influential in the decrease of infections. This helps to explain the differences in height and weight between urban and rural children since children in the more sparsely populated agricultural areas encountered fewer potential contacts and were much less subject to the threat of infectious disease.

It is more difficult to determine whether improvements in the nutritional intakes of children in interwar south Wales were the cause of the increases in stature. A clue might be offered by the milk consumption figures published by the Rhondda medical officer in his annual reports (Figure 3.2). Despite the poverty of the interwar period, the per capita consumption of milk in the Rhondda doubled, albeit gradually and from a low base. The average per capita consumption was still only a third of a pint by the late 1930s. Nevertheless, in the case of this one nutritious foodstuff for which data is available to assess the pattern of consumption over time, it would seem that levels of consumption improved during the interwar period. The extent to which this was also true of other foodstuffs is unclear.

---

[68] Webster, 'Health, welfare and unemployment', 213–18.

[69] Ibid., 217.

[70] Floud, Wachter and Gregory, *Height, Health and History*, pp. 245–6.

Figure 3.2. Estimated daily per capita milk consumption in the Rhondda Urban
District, 1915–39

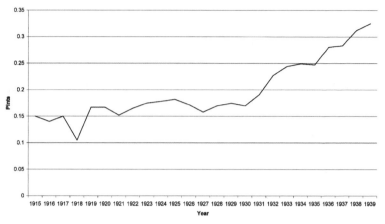

Source: Rhondda UD, RMOH (1920–39).

Numerous factors influenced a family's standard of diet. These
factors varied considerably in nature and extent, as well as over time
and geographically. Nevertheless, considerable differences evidently
existed in the standards of diets of different families and this was
mainly as a result of their differing levels of income. Income was by
far the most important determinant of standards of diet. The
unemployed and low-income families existed on diets that were
wholly inadequate according to optimal nutritional standards and
even fell below the minimum diets set by the government and other
bodies and authorities in the 1930s. Even families noted for the
excellent nutritional status of their children were found, on closer
inspection, to exist on diets that were inadequate when judged by
the British Medical Association's minimum standard. Within families, women and older girls bore the brunt of any shortages in food.

On the other hand, certain pieces of evidence tend to suggest
that nutritional standards were improving gradually throughout the
1920s and, more especially, the 1930s. Food prices fell during the
interwar period and, while this was of some benefit to the unemployed and the poor, it allowed those with an adequate income
to enjoy a reasonably wholesome diet. For those in work, the

interwar period, even in south Wales, was a time of improving nutritional standards. Moreover, the amount of fresh milk consumed in the Rhondda per head of population increased between 1915 and 1939 and, more tellingly, the physique of school-children seems to have improved to some extent. This view needs to be balanced against the fact that both indices began from a low base and increased more slowly than elsewhere. Economic depression served to slow down the improvement in standards and to intensify inequalities compared to more prosperous areas of Britain. The people of south Wales might, in some ways, have been 'better off' than their counterparts in the Victorian and Edwardian periods but continued to lose ground in comparison with working-class families in other parts of Britain.

IV

'HEART-BREAK HOUSES?':[1] HOUSING CONDITIONS AND HOUSE BUILDING

A fit house should be:

(1) free from serious dampness;
(2) satisfactorily lighted and ventilated;
(3) properly drained and provided with adequate sanitary conveniences and with a sink and suitable arrangements for disposing of slop water; and
(4) in good general repair;

and should have

(5) a satisfactory water supply;
(6) adequate washing accommodation;
(7) adequate facilities for preparing and cooking food; and
(8) a well-ventilated store for food.

(Ministry of Health, *Manual on Unfit Houses and Unhealthy Areas* (London, 1919), p. 10)

The influence of housing on standards of health in interwar south Wales is even more difficult to discern than the influence of diet. There is no way of measuring objectively the quality or comfort of housing. A number of crude indicators of housing standards are available, such as levels of overcrowding or multi-occupation, but for the most part judgements on the quality of housing are inescapably subjective. The slum clearance programmes drawn up by local authorities, for example, tell us very little about the nature and extent of slum property in particular areas, even if an objective definition could be devised, and more about the opinions of sanitary inspectors and medical officers, the political will and financial capabilities of the local authority, and the level of housing demand in a particular district. Nevertheless, the vast majority of people spent a considerable proportion of their time in the home and the nature of that home had important implications for the health and

---

[1] *South Wales Evening Express* (16 July 1927), 1.

life-chances of the population. Housing standards had an important influence on certain diseases, especially tuberculosis, and it is therefore necessary to ascertain the nature of housing in south Wales and the ways in which housing conditions changed during the interwar period.

The first thing to note is that south Wales, in common with most other parts of Britain, faced a housing shortage in the early 1920s. House building was suspended during the war as efforts were directed towards the war effort, but even prior to this house building experienced a cyclical downturn in the years before the First World War, both in British terms and in south Wales.[2] The scale of the shortage can partly be gauged by the fact that in the intercensal period 1911–21 the number of 'private families' in Glamorgan increased by 41,085 (18.4 per cent), and by 17,647 (22.4 per cent) in Monmouthshire while the number of dwellings increased by only 21,176 (10.4 per cent) and 9,525 (13.1 per cent) respectively.[3] A fall in family size and an increase in the number of families led to a predictable increase in overcrowding. The percentage of 'private families' with more than two persons living per room increased from 6.1 per cent to 7.9 per cent in Glamorgan and from 7.5 per cent to 8.8 per cent in Monmouthshire in the same period.[4]

Medical officers noted the growing problem in their annual reports. The Mountain Ash medical officer recorded that overcrowding was rife in his district and had become pronounced in the period 1914–20 because of the cessation of house building, while his colleague at Maesteg commented in 1923 that the housing stock in the district in 1914 had been well below actual requirements. Since that date, he continued, private enterprise had been stagnant and instead of an average of 100 houses per year being built, which would have resulted in about 1,000 houses in the ten-year period, only 126 had been built, including 66 houses built by the council.[5] Moreover, the suspension of repairs to the housing stock during the war meant that the condition of houses had deteriorated and they were less sanitary in 1918 than in 1914.[6]

[2]   Martin J. Daunton, 'Introduction', *Councillors and Tenants: Local Authority Housing in English Cities, 1919–1939* (Leicester, 1984), p. 7; Malcolm J. Fisk, *Housing in the Rhondda, 1800–1940* (Cardiff, 1996), pp. 85–6.

[3]   Census 1921, County of Glamorgan, p. xx; County of Monmouth, p. xix.

[4]   Ibid.

[5]   Mountain Ash UD, RMOH (1920); Maesteg UD, RMOH (1923), p. 5.

[6]   NLW, E. L. Chappell papers, Ministry of Health, Repairs to Property Investigation, General Report (undated).

Despite the general increase in overcrowding and the overall deterioration in the housing stock in the period up to 1920, standards of housing varied across the region. An article by the housing reformer Edgar Chappell published in 1920 surveyed the extent of insanitary property in south Wales and his analysis remained relevant for the rest of the interwar period.[7] He began by pointing out that the amount of unfit property in the industrial areas of Wales was small in comparison with other coalfields in Britain. Housing conditions in south Wales were not as bad as those in the Durham and Northumberland coalfield nor were standards in the large towns of south Wales as insanitary as those in cities such as London, Liverpool, Leeds and Glasgow. Chappell, as many others after him have done, attributed this comparative lack of insanitary conditions to the relatively late development of the coal industry in Wales.[8] Nevertheless, though relatively sanitary in comparison with other coalfields and large cities, there were in south Wales certain areas which contained a considerable number of dilapidated and unfit houses.

Most insanitary property was situated at the extremes of the coalfield near the outcrops. Along the eastern and northern outcrops, the impetus of the early coal industry and the iron industry of the late eighteenth and early nineteenth centuries had produced a string of townships stretching from Pontypool in the east to Ystalyfera in the west and including Garndiffaith, Blaenavon, Nantyglo, Ebbw Vale, Tredegar, Rhymney, Merthyr and Aberdare. These towns, developed over a century earlier, before the introduction of by-laws or standards governing house building, were characterized by a large amount of unfit property by the early twentieth century. They included a large proportion of small, badly built cottage property, concentrated into small areas and accompanied by large numbers of cellar-dwellings and back-to-back houses.

Similarly, along the southern outcrop of the coal measures, towns and villages stretching from Burry Port to Maesteg, and including Llanelli, Swansea, Neath and Cwmavon, formed a second area of housing of a 'slummy' character. The iron, copper and, later, tinplate industries were responsible for the development of urban

[7] Edgar Chappell, 'The housing problem in Wales', *Welsh Housing and Development Association Yearbook* (1920), 33–66.

[8] See also Ministry of Health, *Report on Maternal Mortality in Wales* [Cmd. 5423], 1936–7, xi, p. 12; Davies, *History of Wales*, p. 403.

communities in these localities. The quality of housing, in both these areas at least, was partly determined by its age. It was stated in 1931, for example, that of the 10,990 houses in the Aberdare Urban District on the northern outcrop, 2,750 were erected a century earlier and 3,500 eighty years previously, while in Swansea on the southern outcrop 35 per cent of pre-war housing was 50 to 100 years old and 15 per cent was 75 to 100 years old.[9] The medical officer of Tredegar referred to the inhabitants of houses over a century old in his district as 'inmates'.[10]

Apart from these outcrop districts, Chappell observed that insanitary property was also present in the relatively modern mining villages nearer the centre of the coalfield, but in most cases this was not due to the age of the dwellings but rather to poor building techniques or the neglect and misconduct of the tenants.[11] Furthermore, many houses suffered the effects of mining subsidence, which predisposed them to damp penetration and premature dilapidation, through cracked walls, ceilings, windows, floors and roofs. In some cases subsidence caused major structural damage and was sufficient to require the complete renovation of a house. Harold Callender, the London correspondent of the *New York Times*, saw the subsidence that affected so many villages in south Wales as symbolic of the economic depression. In an article on the Nantyglo and Blaina area in 1938, he wrote that:

> As a mine first builds a house for its workers, then cuts away the coal upon which it stands, so the coal industry first developed and largely populated South Wales (whose inhabitants increased tenfold in a century), then retreated, depriving much of that population of its economic foundation. South Wales, like its undermined valleys, is a region in the process of subsidence; for the industry that sustained it has shrunk and many communities dependant upon coal have sunk into dilapidation.[12]

The South Wales Regional Survey Committee found that in some areas the surface had been depressed by as much as 15 feet or more during a period of about forty years. Subsidence, it noted, was marked along the northern rim of the coalfield, where workings were relatively shallow, and over the steeper measures along the

---

9   *Western Mail* (17 June 1931), 9; Swansea CB, RMOH (1930), p. 91.
10   Tredegar UD, RMOH (1932), p. 25.
11   Chappell, 'Housing problem in Wales', 37–8.
12   *New York Times Magazine* (10 April 1938), 7.

southern outcrop. Roadways, gas and water mains, sewers, bridges, tramways and, of course, housing, all suffered the adverse effects of the unstable foundation upon which much of south Wales had been built.[13]

In any assessment of the implications of housing for health, consideration of the internal environment is important. South Wales showed marked variations from other areas of Britain in its architectural styles and internal configurations, but there was also diversity within the region. Most typical of south Wales was the terraced housing of the mining valleys, which was the product of the 'by-law period' of house building that occurred in the half-century or so before the First World War. Situated in two-storied terraces that followed the contours of the valleys, the high densities of such houses reflected the lack of available flat building land and the high cost of building on such undulating land. The houses had a narrow frontage of a room's width and a deep extension of two rooms. Typically provided by building clubs or speculative builders, these houses consisted of a front room (or parlour), a living room and, maybe, a scullery extension on the ground floor and two or, more probably, three bedrooms on the first floor.[14] The vast majority were without bathrooms, and WC facilities were often shared and situated outdoors. Only 6 per cent of houses in the Rhondda valleys, for example, possessed bathrooms by 1930.[15] These houses were in most cases without any forecourts and had only a limited amount of garden space at the back, if any at all. Very frequently, the space at the back of the houses was hemmed in by embankments which prevented the circulation of air.

Along the heads of the valleys area there was a high concentration of much older property, built in the period before building by-laws were introduced and characterized by a number of insanitary house types, such as cellar-dwellings, back-to-earth and back-to-backs.[16] The houses were smaller than the more recently built houses in the coalfield, had a lower headroom, smaller

[13]   Ministry of Health, *South Wales Regional Survey Committee* (London, 1921), pp. 28–9.
[14]   Fisk, *Housing in the Rhondda.*
[15]   Rhondda UD, RMOH (1930), p. 98.
[16]   On these insanitary house-types in south Wales, see Angus Calder and Dorothy Sheridan (eds), *Speak for Yourself: A Mass-Observation Anthology, 1937–49* (London, 1984), p. 109; Nantyglo and Blaina UDC, Sanitary Inspector's Report Book, 17 January 1924; Tredegar UD, RMOH (1925), p. 12; Pontardawe RD, RMOH (1930), p. 13; Rhondda UD, RMOH (1930), p. 99; *Western Mail* (11 May 1933), 11.

windows and were often inadequately lit and ventilated. It was reported that in the north and central wards of Nantyglo and Blaina there were streets of houses with only one living room and one bedroom and even three inhabitants made them over-crowded.[17] In the anthracite district of west Glamorgan, houses were more likely to be detached or semi-detached, reflecting the more gradual development of the coal industry and the greater amount of flat building land.[18] The rooms of these houses were more spacious and the houses were more likely to possess relatively large gardens in comparison with the houses of the central and eastern part of the coalfield. Rural areas such as Gower, the Vale of Glamorgan and the eastern parts of Monmouthshire were characterized by sparsely scattered farms and hamlets with houses that could be as much as 200 years old. They often possessed primitive sanitary conveniences (although these were gradually replaced during the interwar period) and small, often damp, rooms that were inadequately lit or ventilated. Typically, they consisted of only one living room and two bedrooms,[19] with the result that overcrowding was qualitatively different in rural areas and was more often due to the smallness of the houses rather than to the size of the family or the practice of sub-letting.[20]

Of the larger towns in south Wales, Cardiff was characterized by large houses with many large rooms, which caused rents to be high and contributed to the high level of multi-occupation found in the town.[21] Built in the late nineteenth century, most houses in Cardiff and Barry were relatively modern, well-designed and well-built and this partly accounted for the small amount of slum clearance that was necessary in the 1930s. In Swansea, on the other hand, there existed a great deal of insanitary property and the bulk of the houses were of the four- or six-room type. The six-room type usually consisted of the four-room type with a back extension consisting of a downstairs kitchen and a tiny bedroom upstairs. Some of the four-room type consisted of the old one-up, one-down

---

[17]   Nantyglo and Blaina UD, RMOH (1932), p. 13.

[18]   Philip N. Jones, *Colliery Settlement in the South Wales Coalfield 1850 to 1926* (Hull, 1969).

[19]   Monmouth RD, RMOH (1930), p. 7, stated that a 'large majority' of working-class housing was of this size; Monmouth MB, RMOH (1930), p. 5, stated that about 50 per cent of the houses in this district were of this type.

[20]   Monmouth RD, RMOH (1936), p. 7.

[21]   Cardiff CB, RMOH (1922), p. 46.

house type with a lean-to extension at the back.[22] None of these had much space at the rear and suffered a lack of through ventilation as a result, while many of them had front doors which opened straight into the living room, which made them unpopular. By 1930 Swansea still had 150 houses situated in 27 narrow courts. The medical officer considered all these types to be unsatisfactory.[23]

There was great variety in the house styles and internal layouts of the houses in south Wales to determine the use to which domestic space could be put. In addition, cultural and social factors helped to dictate how internal space could be utilized by its inhabitants. There were no typical households in south Wales, but certain common characteristics can be discerned. The interior was divided into a number of strongly demarcated spaces, each classified according to a particular use and the contents it contained.[24] Kitchens, or living rooms as they were more often known, were the focus of working-class households and the room in which daily life was lived. The living room was the room in which the family meals were prepared and consumed and, because of the almost total lack of bathrooms and even sculleries in houses in south Wales, it was also the place in which the cleaning of clothes and the bathing of bodies took place. Numerous medical officers commented on the high number of infant deaths which occurred from scalding in baths of boiling hot water.[25] The preparation of these baths also took its toll on the women of the households as the daily toil of lifting and carrying large pans of water could cause women to strain themselves.[26] Medical officers argued that pithead baths would give mothers more time to devote to the care of their infants and would cause a decrease in infant mortality. Fires were coal fuelled and continually coated everything in the living room with a fine film of dust. On cold, wet days clothes had to be dried in the house, and in

---

[22]   Swansea CB, RMOH (1930), p. 91.

[23]   Ibid.

[24]   R. J. Lawrence, 'Domestic space and society: a cross cultural study', *Comparative Studies in Society and History*, 24 (1982), 104–30.

[25]   Deirdre Beddoe, 'Munitionettes, maids and mams: women in Wales, 1914–1939', in John, *Our Mothers' Land*, pp. 203–4; see for example Maesteg UD, RMOH (1921), p. 6; (1922), p. 4.

[26]   Neil Evans and Dot Jones, '"A blessing for the miner's wife": the campaign for pithead baths in the South Wales Coalfield, 1908–50', *Llafur*, 6, 3 (1994), 6; Beddoe, 'Munitionettes, maids and mams', pp. 203–4.

front of the fire especially, creating a damp, steamy atmosphere that predisposed inhabitants to respiratory disease.[27]

The kitchen was situated at the back of the house where the everyday processes of eating and cleaning could take place in a private environment, hidden from prying eyes, and allowing the image of respectability to be preserved. Edith Davies of Ynysybwl, for example, has commented:

> I suppose we were a typical miner's family in that we used the back kitchen as a living room cum dining room, bathroom, laundry room and play-room rolled into one. Simply furnished it contained a scrubbed kitchen table, a sofa along one wall placed behind the table where we children sat for meals, a wooden armchair and one kitchen chair. The focal point was the fireplace where burnt a cosy coal fire and around which we sat as a family in the evenings.[28]

Many families possessed a 'best room' or parlour at the front of the house which served as the respectable image that the family presented to the outside world. This room was used on special occasions such as weddings, birthdays and funerals, or to receive important visitors such as the local minister or doctor. That the parlour was so little used at a time of housing shortage and overcrowding caused concern among public health authorities.[29]

The need to preserve the parlour as the 'best room' could sometimes exacerbate overcrowding of bedroom accommodation. The medical officer of Pontardawe found that the Overcrowding Act of 1936 could not abate many cases of overcrowding in his district because of the way in which the Act considered parlours appropriate as sleeping quarters. Families in his district, he commented, would not tolerate the conversion of parlours into bedroom accommodation and, in consequence, overcrowding was exacerbated.[30] The sanctity of the parlour was important enough for some families to acquiesce in the overcrowding of bedroom accommodation.

Numerous examples of bedrooms containing anything up to a dozen people, or beds sleeping half a dozen individuals, could be quoted. Dr Bruce Low gave an example of a house found in Nantyglo during an investigation into an outbreak of typhoid fever

---

27   Port Talbot MB, RMOH (1922), p. 47.
28   Davies, *The Innocent Years*, p. 31.
29   Monmouth CC, RMOH (1921), p. 22.
30   Pontardawe RD, RMOH (1936), p. 20.

in 1924 that had a bedroom sleeping brothers aged 19, 11, 10, 10, 6 and 4 in one bed and sisters aged 17, 16, 7 and 1 in another bed.[31] Parents in Newport complained that the education of their children was seriously handicapped by the unsatisfactory sleeping arrangements they had to endure.[32] In a few instances, parlours and even kitchens were used as sleeping quarters, suggesting that the desire to order the internal environment according to certain ideals was often frustrated by the effects of poverty or large family size. Although these are the most extreme examples, it was certainly not uncommon for bedroom accommodation to be shared. In Cardiff in 1924, for example, an examination of the sleeping arrangements of new cases of pulmonary tuberculosis found that 161 out of 301 cases shared a bed with another person, while 193 out of the 301 shared a bed or bedroom. There were 194 contacts sleeping in the same beds as these 161 cases and 173 who slept in the same bedroom but not in the same bed.[33] This pattern improved only very slightly during the 1920s and 1930s, and by 1939 still only 50 per cent of new cases had a bedroom to themselves.[34]

Multi-occupation exacerbated the problems of overcrowding. It severely disrupted the demarcation of domestic space because of the need to share certain facilities and the resulting decrease in the amount of space available to each family. The phenomenon of multi-occupation varied in intensity throughout Britain but was marked in south Wales and even intensified during the interwar period. The Merthyr medical officer was of the opinion that 'Overcrowding as understood years ago has changed from individual lodgers to the houses containing two or more families', while other medical officers noted an increase in multi-occupation in the early 1920s.[35] According to the census of 1921, 29 per cent of families in Glamorgan and 28 per cent of those in Monmouthshire were living at a density of two or more families per dwelling.[36] Furthermore, multi-occupation was not confined to larger houses. A survey of housing in Rhymney in the mid 1920s established that there were 129 families each living in one room, forty-seven

[31]   Bruce Low, Untitled report to the Senior Medical Officer on the Sanitary Administration of the Nantyglo and Blaina UD, p. 2.

[32]   Newport CB, RMOH (1921), p. 45.

[33]   Cardiff CB, RMOH (1924), p. 20.

[34]   Cardiff CB, RMOH (1924–39).

[35]   Merthyr CB, RMOH (1922), p. 38; Rhondda UD, RMOH (1920), pp. 86–7.

[36]   Census of England and Wales, 1921, Glamorgan p. xiii; Monmouthshire p. xii.

instances of two families occupying one room and even one case of three families living in one room.[37]

With the fall in population that began in the late 1920s and the increase in the number of houses which were being built annually, the situation eased somewhat, but the census of 1931 nevertheless revealed that 28 per cent of families in Glamorgan and 23.3 per cent in Monmouthshire still shared a house.[38] The highest levels of multi-occupation in south Wales were found in Cardiff where 40.9 per cent of families lived in apartments in 1931.[39] By using this definition of overcrowding it is possible to see the inadequacy of the traditional census standard that ranked south Wales as a region characterized by low levels of overcrowding.[40] The difference between these two standards was clearly illustrated by the applications for council houses received by the Swansea Borough Council in 1930. Of 3,347 applications received, 888, or 26.5 per cent, were overcrowded according to the census standard of houses with more than two persons per room. In contrast, 2,554 families (76.3 per cent) were overcrowded according to the standard of two or more families per house.[41]

Houses inhabited by more than one family were usually 'without separate family amenities, without separate and proper accommodation for cooking, for storage of food, for washing or separate closet accommodation'.[42] Families were forced, for example, to cook on open parlour grates not intended for such use. Families were also forced to share one privy or closet and it was in such conditions that the cleansing of the convenience was sometimes neglected. In Tredegar, it was found that families which occupied the front half of the back-to-back houses in the town were deprived of the use of the closet situated at the back of the house and were forced to deposit 'much offensive matter' in the street.[43]

Multi-occupation could also be a source of tension and worry for the families involved. The medical officer of Newport noted how the sharing of cottages by families not kindly disposed to each other

[37]   Monmouth CC, RMOH (1925), p. 19.
[38]   Census of England and Wales, 1931, Glamorgan p. xi; Monmouthshire p. xii.
[39]   Ibid., Glamorgan, p. 12.
[40]   A mistake made by Stephen V. Ward, *The Geography of Interwar Britain: The State and Uneven Development* (London, 1988), p. 29.
[41]   Swansea CB, RMOH (1930), pp. 92–3.
[42]   Ibid.
[43]   Tredegar UD, RMOH (1925), p. 12.

caused 'a large amount of unhappiness and even ill-health owing to constant worry'.[44] Local newspapers are full of court reports of disagreements and even violence between tenants and their sub-tenants caused by the inability to cooperate in the shared use of facilities.[45] Even among those households that sub-let a part of their accommodation to relatives, the difficulties could cause friction and distress. An investigation carried out by the Save the Children Fund in 1933 found that poverty caused many young families to live with their in-laws with the result that 'the old and the young couples get on each others' nerves, quarrels result, and an atmosphere is created which is generally bad for the children'.[46] More importantly, such conditions of multi-occupation or insufficient domestic space often had important consequences for childbirth and deaths. The medical officer of Blaenavon observed that:

> It is not uncommon to find in the case of a mother giving birth that the child has to be delivered by the nurse or doctor in an only bedroom which is of necessity the only sleeping place of sometimes three, four, and often more children of varying ages. Should the birth take place during the hours of the night or early morning, which is often the case, the children must be roused from their slumber and removed to the houses of relatives or friends, which is not always possible, or remain in the bedroom during this trying and difficult period.[47]

Similarly, a death in a family living in overcrowded conditions was made even more traumatic because of the inability of many families to lay out the body of the deceased in a spare room. In such cases a relative's or neighbour's house was sometimes used.[48] Where a family did have a parlour in which to lay the body, the corpse might remain in the house for a number of days, which also alarmed public health authorities, especially in the case of deaths from infectious disease.[49]

For various reasons the sanitary condition of large numbers of houses deteriorated as a result of the interwar depression. First, local authorities inhibited by financial considerations did not

---

[44]   Newport CB, RMOH (1921), p. 44.
[45]   See for example *Free Press of Monmouthshire* (3 February 1928), 9; (23 September 1932), 3; also, B. L. Coombes, *Miners Day* (London, 1945), p. 74.
[46]   Save the Children Fund, *Unemployment and the Child*, p. 29.
[47]   *The Times* (5 August 1929), 15.
[48]   See for example *Western Mail* (11 March 1924), 9.
[49]   *The Times* (5 August 1929), 15.

employ the number of sanitary inspectors that the size of districts warranted. For example, Dr Bruce Low, in a review of the sanitary administration of the Abersychan Urban District, recommended that a letter be sent to the district council advising that a second sanitary inspector be appointed. 'If the finances of the Council at the present time do not justify the expense immediately', he wrote, 'they should keep in mind the necessity and, as soon as their circumstances permit them, make the new appointment.'[50] The financial difficulties of Nantyglo and Blaina Urban District Council meant that the usually full-time sanitary inspector had to spend three-quarters of 1924 with another department, with the result that very little work was done in that year.[51] In addition, sanitary inspectors and medical officers were often advanced in age or varied in the energy which they devoted to their duties.[52] Other housing inspectors were forced to adopt a much lower standard when assessing houses because the closing of a house decreased the housing stock and increased the overcrowding in a district. Therefore, house-to-house inspections often suffered as a result of the inadequacies of sanitary departments with the result that owners were not required to maintain their property.

Even when sanitary authorities were active in inspecting houses and taking measures to compel work to be done, various factors could frustrate the process of repair. First, private landlords were often very reluctant to spend money at a time of economic uncertainty.[53] As tenants built up arrears, landlords were unwilling to invest in housing on which they saw no prospect of increased income in the form of higher rents. The Rent Restriction Act of 1915 meant that no matter how much a landlord spent on repairs, the rents of houses subject to the Act could not be raised. In fact, local authorities similarly cut expenditure on repairs to the houses they owned, particularly those whose tenants were in arrears with their rent payments.[54]

[50]   NLW, Welsh Board of Health collection, Box 3, R. Bruce Low, Report on the sanitary circumstances of the Abersychan Urban District, 11 February 1929.

[51]   Nantyglo and Blaina UD, RMOH (1924), p. 2.

[52]   See for example NLW, Welsh Board of Health collection, Box 55Q, R. Bruce Low, 'Inspection of a sanitary district (Monmouth RD)', 6 May 1925. Low commented that 'Both the inspectors are old men and we cannot expect much of them in the way of initiative'.

[53]   See for example Gelligaer UD, RMOH (1927), p. 41.

[54]   See for example West Glamorgan Record Office, Neath RDC, Housing and Town Planning Committee minutes, 2 December 1929; Swansea CBC, Housing of the Working Classes Committee minutes, 20 March 1923.

Houses whose leases were soon to expire created a further problem. These invariably presented the most pressing housing problem in many communities, especially in those districts situated along the northern rim of the coalfield and in the area from Port Talbot to Swansea, where many leases of ninety-nine years' duration were due to expire during the interwar period. For example, at the end of the First World War, 400 leases were due to expire in Aberdare, while hundreds more were due to lapse in Nantyglo.[55] In these cases, local authorities did not feel justified in forcing owners to spend large amounts of money on repairs, and so property tended to deteriorate rapidly 'towards the fag end of leases'.[56] For the same reasons, authorities did not feel justified in compelling owners of houses scheduled for slum clearance in the 1930s to make repairs, despite the fact that houses were often designated for clearance in 1933 but not scheduled for demolition until the end of the decade.

In addition to those landlords who were unwilling to make repairs, there were a great many who were unable to do so.[57] Many small-scale landlords owned only one or two houses and were themselves in a very difficult financial situation.[58] Some were unemployed miners and the landlord of one house in Blaina, described by the medical officer as a 'saturated, rotting mess', was himself an inmate of the workhouse.[59] Owed huge amounts in arrears and themselves very poor, there was no chance of landlords carrying out repairs to many houses. It is noticeable that in some of the worst rows of houses no rent had been paid for many years.[60] Thus, in those areas which suffered most from unemployment, housing conditions deteriorated as local authorities were unable to enforce a high standard of fitness and house owners were too impoverished to carry out repairs.

Financial capability determined not only the quality of the house which a family could afford but also its location. Houses situated in a healthy environment possessed higher rents than those which

---

[55]   Chappell, Repair of Houses Investigation, Aberdare and Nantyglo and Blaina.

[56]   Ibid., Nantyglo and Blaina.

[57]   See for example Merthyr CB, RMOH (1936), pp. 10–11.

[58]   See for example Port Talbot MB, RMOH (1926), p. 48; Penybont RD, RMOH (1930), p. 54.

[59]   *South Wales Weekly Argus* (4 Oct. 1924), 3.

[60]   See for example Bruce Low, Untitled report on the sanitary administration of the Nantyglo and Blaina UD, p. 1.

suffered the effects of air pollution, inadequate sanitary systems and a generally unwholesome environment of unmade roads and pavements, rubbish tips and inadequate leisure amenities. Following his survey of the housing situation in Maesteg in 1926, Dr Bruce Low observed that 'A disconcerting feature of the housing position is that tenants are leaving good houses and are clamouring for hovels owing to the cheaper rent.'[61] This example demonstrates that, for many families, migration to cheaper rented property was a means of self-relief from poverty.[62]

Poverty-stricken families faced obstacles in their attempts to improve their housing conditions by moving to a better type of house. As the medical officer of Barry commented, 'It is obvious that private owners cannot and will not provide for the class of tenant that can be termed as forming the "submerged tenth".'[63] Not wanting to take in tenants with a history of defaulting on rent, landlords insisted on inspecting an applicant's rent book or else sought a reference from his or, less commonly, her previous landlord.[64] Landlords often refused to rent their houses to large families[65] and even to those families afflicted with tuberculosis.[66] The Rhondda medical officer observed in 1929 that: 'though there is a considerable number of vacant premises in the district the rents demanded or conditions imposed by the owners preclude their occupation by tenants with large families and proportionately inadequate incomes.'[67] Therefore, the poverty of certain families prevented them from improving their housing conditions even if their financial situation had improved. Their 'history . . . [was] such that little encouragement [was] given to private owners or the Local Authority to provide them with suitable dwellings'.[68]

A further way in which poverty influenced housing conditions was that the poorest were the most likely to resort to sub-letting. In

[61]   NLW, Welsh Board of Health collection, Box 49Q, R. Bruce Low, Report on the sanitary circumstances of the Maesteg Urban District, 9 February 1926, p. 24; see also Penybont RD, RMOH (1927), p. 53.

[62]   A point made by S. J. Page, 'The mobility of the poor: a case study of Edwardian Leicester', *The Local Historian*, 21, 3 (1991), 118.

[63]   Barry UD, RMOH (1925), p. 32; the phrase 'submerged tenth' has strong eugenicist connotations.

[64]   Colin G. Pooley and Jean Turnbull, *Migration and Mobility in Britain since the Eighteenth Century* (London, 1998), pp. 233–4.

[65]   *Western Mail* (11 May 1933), 11.

[66]   Newport CB, RMOH (1925), p. 42.

[67]   Rhondda UD, RMOH (1929), p. 87.

[68]   Barry UD, RMOH (1927), p. 21.

the Penybont Rural District, houses occupied by single families were being vacated due to the inability to pay rent and the families moved into apartments in other houses.[69] Tenants could decide to sub-let rooms or utilize the space themselves as their family composition or economic conditions changed.[70]

In short, there existed a massive need for better housing accommodation in south Wales during the early 1920s. Large amounts of insanitary property and a significant degree of overcrowding demonstrated this need. The great need for new houses was reflected in the large estimates that were made by local authorities in accordance with the terms of the Housing Act of 1919. Various sources give different estimates. The National Housing and Town Planning Council estimated that 45,161 houses were required in Glamorgan and 21,436 in Monmouthshire, of which it was expected that the local authorities would build 40,272 and 20,306 houses respectively.[71] Therefore, it was estimated in 1919 that between 60,000 and 70,000 houses needed to be built in south Wales.

The large amount of insanitary property and the dearth of houses which affected all areas of south Wales to a greater or lesser degree meant that the ability of local authorities to make houses available and replace insanitary property was of great importance to the health and welfare of a large number of families. The number of people whose standard of life could be improved by access to a new council house was determined by the success with which councils could overcome the problems besetting them and successfully provide houses. While private enterprise provided some houses to let in interwar south Wales, the number built was probably fewer than the total built by local authorities.[72] Nevertheless, in

---

[69]   Penybont RD, RMOH (1927), p. 53.

[70]   Anna Davin, *Growing up Poor: Home, School and Street in London, 1870–1914* (London, 1996), pp. 29–38.

[71]   National Housing and Town Planning Council, *Programme of Housing and Town Planning Conference for Wales and Monmouthshire*, 8–9 July 1921, at Llandrindod Wells; these included the associated county boroughs in each of the two counties; slightly higher estimates were given in A. L. Thomas, 'Housing and Town Planning Act (1919). Progress of Housing in Wales and Monmouth to December 31st, 1921', *Welsh Housing and Development Association Yearbook* (1922), 22.

[72]   Detailed records of the activities of private enterprise in the provision of houses are scarce but J. L. Marshall, 'The pattern of housebuilding in the inter-war period in England and Wales', *Scottish Journal of Political Economy*, 15, 2 (1968), 189, has found that of the 33,076 houses of a rateable value of up to £26 built in Wales in the period 1 October 1933 to 31 March 1939, 7,770 or 23.5% were to let.

Figure 4.1. Houses built by local authorities in England and Wales, 1919 to 31 March 1940, expressed as a rate per 1,000 persons (1939 population)

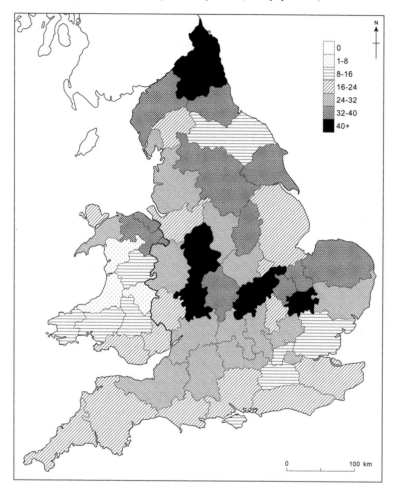

Source: Calculated from statistics in Marshall, 'Pattern of housebuilding', 199–200; *Registrar-General's Statistical Review of England and Wales* (1939).

a British context, it is apparent that local authorities in Wales built relatively few houses in the interwar period.

Of the 13 Welsh counties, only Denbigh and Flint achieved a rate of house building greater than the average for England and Wales as a whole. Glamorgan and Monmouthshire compared favourably with the rural areas of Wales and yet they fell far short of the average rate for England and Wales as a whole, reflecting both the impoverished nature of the local authorities in south Wales and the reluctance of the Ministry of Health to sanction housing schemes in areas suffering depopulation and local authority indebtedness. Owing to the large volume of unemployment in Nantyglo and Blaina, for example, the Ministry announced in 1923 that it had refused to sanction more houses.[73] In the period following the lockout of 1926, the Ministry attempted to keep a tight grip on the expenditure of councils in mining areas throughout Britain. Gelligaer Urban District Council, for example, submitted a five-year building programme for the erection of 2,000 houses to the Ministry in 1927, but only obtained sanction for fifty houses. As a result the council contemplated no further schemes and its Housing Department was closed.[74]

In total, local authorities in south Wales built almost 32,000 houses during the twenty-year period between the wars. Measured against the population and the existing housing stock, considerably fewer houses were built than the average for England and Wales as a whole (see Table 4.1). These broad generalizations hide wide variations in south Wales and closer examination serves to show how the activities of a small number of authorities in the region made up a large proportion of the total number of houses built. They also serve to show how housing need, however defined, was not matched by the ability of authorities to build sufficient houses. The county boroughs of Cardiff (29.8 houses per 1,000 persons) and Swansea (31.39 per 1,000) maintained a high level of house building during the interwar period.[75] These two districts, while only containing 20–25 per cent of the population, built about 35 per cent of the total number of houses built in interwar south Wales. Their diverse and relatively more buoyant economies, their high rateable values and low rate poundage meant that the councils were in a position to take advantage of the central government subsidies offered for the purpose of house building.

Newport (13.13 per 1,000) built relatively few houses under the various Housing Acts but did make loans available to private builders under the Housing Act of 1923. In this way it provided an

---

[73]   *Western Mail* (24 March 1923), 9.
[74]   Gelligaer UD, RMOH (1927), p. 41.
[75]   See Appendix 4.1.

Table 4.1. Houses built in south Wales and England and Wales, 1919–39

	Total houses built 1919–39	Rate per 1,000 persons (1939 pop.)
Glamorgan (with CBs)	24,393	21.07
Monmouthshire (with CBs)	7,417	18.56
England and Wales	1,159,305	27.96

Source: Marshall, 'Patterns of housebuilding', 199–200.

additional 2,433 houses in the late 1920s both within and outside the borough boundary. The medical officer of nearby Magor Rural District recorded how his council was offering a subsidy of £75 to private builders for every house built but that the Newport council was offering £110 for every house built in his district, providing they were within half a mile of the borough boundary.[76] Many houses were provided by private enterprise in the rural areas bordering Newport in the interwar period and the same was true of both Cardiff and Swansea.

Councils in the western part of Glamorgan also maintained high rates of building activity. Llwchwr (27.04), Pontardawe (27.12), Neath MB (24.80), Port Talbot (31.62) and Glyncorrwg (31.67) all achieved high rates of building, reflecting the relatively more favourable economic circumstances which they experienced during the interwar period.[77] Significantly, with the exception of Glyncorrwg, these were also areas that witnessed a great deal of private house building activity. Figure 4.2 shows the geographical distribution of building activity throughout south Wales. It is evident that the rural districts of Penybont (38.57), Cowbridge (25.92) and Llantrisant and Llantwit Fardre (35.77) also achieved high rates of council house building.

In Glamorgan, the urban districts of Maesteg (8.21), Ogmore and Garw (8.84), Aberdare (12.83), Mountain Ash (8.10), Pontypridd (14.93) and the county borough of Merthyr (12.92) built relatively few houses, despite the great need identified by surveys made in 1919 and the annual reports of their medical officers

[76]   Magor RD, RMOH (1923), p. 8.
[77]   That local authorities could take a great deal of pride in their building activities was shown in 1939 when the Pontardawe RDC built its 1000th house. A tablet recorded this 'outstanding achievement' at Alltygrug Road, Ystalyfera, and the house was appropriately named 'Y Filfan'; Pontardawe RD, RMOH (1939), p. 40.

Figure 4.2. Houses built by local authorities in south Wales, 1920–38, per 1,000 persons (1939 population)

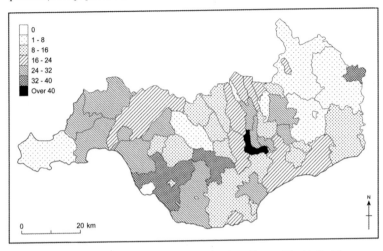

Source: Based on figures in annual reports of the medical officers of health for Glamorgan CC, Monmouthshire CC and individual districts (1920–39); for key, see Maps 1 and 2.

throughout the period. Local authority indebtedness and the attitude of the Ministry of Health meant that councils were frustrated in their attempts to provide houses. Political will was rendered meaningless by the economic dislocation suffered in these areas. This is most clearly demonstrated by the record of 'red' Rhondda. Despite the massive need for houses constantly expressed by its medical officer and the commitment of the council to the welfare of its population, Rhondda Urban District Council was able to build only around 300 houses in the interwar period, a rate of 2.48 houses per 1,000 persons, well below nearly every other area of south Wales. Other authorities that built very few houses were Porthcawl and Usk, which built no houses at all,[78] and the rural areas of Gower and the eastern parts of Monmouthshire.

The mining districts of the western valleys of Monmouthshire were able to build more houses than their Glamorgan counterparts. The urban districts of Bedwellty (27.09), Mynyddislwyn (30.15),

[78] Private enterprise was sufficiently active in Porthcawl, it was stated, that no houses needed to be built by the council.

Pontypool (27.79) and Cwmbran (24.89) maintained relatively high levels of activity, although the districts at the heads of the valleys built at lower than average rates. Most impressively, the district of Bedwas and Machen achieved the highest rate of any authority in south Wales. It built at a rate of 47.47 houses per 1,000 persons, a rate more than twice the county average and, while in absolute terms this only represented 386 houses, its record was still notable. Part of the reason for this high level of building activity was the relatively better economic conditions of the Rhymney valley. This had been a rapidly expanding area in the two decades before 1920 as large-scale colliery development caused a massive increase in population and a concurrent involvement in house building on the part of colliery companies such as Powell Duffryn and the Tredegar Iron and Coal Company. The 'model villages' of Oakdale and Markham, located near the Rhymney valley, were a result of this involvement. This colliery development came much later than the opening up of the coal reserves elsewhere in south Wales and even continued into the 1920s. In fact, the Rhymney valley was one of the few places in south Wales to witness the sinking of new pits in the 1920s. This late development and relative prosperity meant that houses were still being built during the interwar period, and with unemployment at more manageable levels than the steam-coal producing areas of Glamorgan,[79] the local authorities were able to achieve a higher rate of house building.

As a result of these factors and as further evidence of economic conditions, the western valleys of Monmouthshire suffered less depopulation during the interwar years than those districts of Glamorgan which had built so few houses. Bedwas and Machen, for example, had a population of 8,487 in 1921; it had fallen only to 8,307 by 1939.[80] Bedwellty lost about 10 per cent of its population of 30,000 enumerated in 1921 while Mynyddislwyn's population had only declined from 14,900 to 13,100 in the same period. On the other hand, in those areas of Glamorgan that had built very few houses, emigration was considerable with many of the most depressed districts haemorrhaging as much as a quarter of their people. Significantly, the population of the Rhondda fell from 162,000 in 1921 to an estimated 119,600 in 1939, a fall of over 25

[79]   See Board of Trade, *An Industrial Survey of South Wales* (London, 1932), pp. 31–8, 51.
[80]   Census 1921; *Registrar General's Statistical Review* (1939).

Figure 4.3. House-building rates of Glamorgan and Monmouthshire administrative counties per 1,000 population (1921 Census), 1920–39

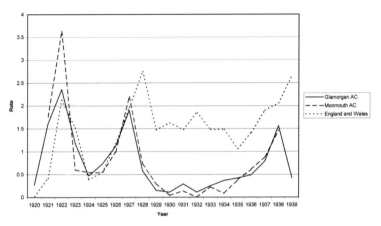

per cent. It is also significant that of those mining districts of western Monmouthshire, Abertillery had an extremely low rate of building activity (5.73) and was a district that suffered high levels of depopulation (from 39,000 people in 1921 to 28,000 in 1939, a fall of about 28 per cent). Therefore, it would seem that depopulation either convinced local authorities that the building of houses was unnecessary or, more likely, it led the Ministry of Health to deny approval for local authority schemes in such depressed areas.[81]

Population pressure undoubtedly influenced the pattern of house building in south Wales but further evidence that the poverty of the local authorities was also a strong factor is provided by Figure 4.3. It is evident that local authorities in the two administrative counties were able to build at a slightly higher rate than the average for England and Wales as a whole in the early 1920s. This was because the Housing Act of 1919 limited the financial contribution of local authorities to the product of a penny rate and any expenditure incurred in excess of this was to be provided by Exchequer funds. This negligible, token amount which local authorities incurred meant that the Act was redistributive among regions as taxes paid in more prosperous regions of England and Wales were paid out to less affluent areas in the form of house-building subsidies. In theory

[81]   Ward, *Geography of Interwar Britain*.

at least, local authorities were not constrained by their financial circumstances and could build as many houses as were needed. It is evident from Figure 4.3 that local authorities in south Wales took advantage of this central government funding to a significant degree, as the peak in building activity in 1922 clearly shows. The cut-backs in government expenditure in the two or three years that followed affected south Wales in the same way as they affected England and Wales. Subsequent housing legislation departed markedly from the redistributive element of the 1919 Act, generally limiting the Exchequer's contribution to a flat-rate subsidy or lump sum for every house built and, in the 1930s, for the number of persons rehoused from certain classes of houses. As economic conditions deteriorated in south Wales from the late 1920s so the level of building fell drastically in comparison to other areas of Britain. Local authorities were forced by government legislation to tax their own depressed communities to provide badly needed houses. In this way, regional disadvantage was exacerbated and derelict areas such as south Wales, with their low rateable value and high rate poundage, languished as central government failed to deal effectively with the problems besetting them.

Any evaluation of the extent to which the house-building activities of local authorities improved the living conditions of the population needs to take the Housing Act of 1930 into account. The Act made central funds available for the specific purpose of slum clearance and, most importantly, linked the subsidy provided to the number of people displaced from the slums and rehoused in new council houses. Since the subsidy was dependent on the number of people rehoused rather than on the number of houses built, councils had a greater incentive to deal with the large families who so often endured the worst living conditions. Economic difficulties led to the Act's implementation being postponed until it was reactivated in 1933. Authorities in south Wales, as in the rest of England and Wales, were required by the terms of the Act to prepare schedules for the clearance of all slums in their areas in the five-year period 1934–8. The Act, however, did not adequately define a 'slum' and so local authorities were free to apply the Act to as many or as few houses as they saw fit. As a result, the slum clearance schemes of the local authorities give only a very general indication of the distribution of slum housing throughout the country. Nevertheless, local authorities in south Wales submitted schemes for the demolition of 5,647 houses in five years. Of the county boroughs, Swansea planned to clear 1,317 houses, Newport 140 and Merthyr 482.[82] Cardiff planned to demolish 203 houses and, although it surpassed this figure by over 50 per cent, this left the city with the lowest slum clearance totals of any city of comparable size in England and Wales.[83] This, in part, reflected the late development of Cardiff relative to other towns of a similar size and the resultant lack of slum housing.

Other large schemes in south Wales included 500 houses to be demolished in Aberdare, 263 in Port Talbot, 258 in the borough of Neath, 220 in Risca, 201 in Ebbw Vale and 200 in Pontypridd. These figures, it must be remembered, were derived from the considerations of the medical officers, sanitary inspectors and councils of the various districts and therefore do not represent the amount of insanitary property in each area. The fact that many local authorities subsequently increased their programmes is evidence that the initial schemes underestimated the amount of slum housing in south Wales.

Despite these increases, many local authorities could not build the numbers they first enumerated in 1933. Of the county boroughs, Cardiff and Swansea had achieved their targets by the end of 1938, while Merthyr had built only 232 of the 482 it had originally planned and was well short of the 566 to which it subsequently increased its scheme.[84] By the end of March 1940, however, Merthyr had built 426. Newport was even further short of its projections by the end of 1938, having built only 68 of the 140 it had originally scheduled. The Rhondda Urban District is the only other district for which comparable statistics are available. By the end of 1938 it had built 47 of the 164 it had planned and had not improved on this figure by March 1940.[85] Economic conditions had an adverse effect on the building programmes of the various local

<hr/>

[82]   *Particulars of the Slum Clearance Programmes furnished by Local Authorities* [Cmd. 4535], 1933–4, xxi; Swansea's scheme is not listed in these returns but the annual report of the medical officer for 1933 states the number of houses to be demolished as 1,317.

[83]   J. H. Jennings, 'Geographical implications of the municipal housing programme in England and Wales 1919–39', *Urban Studies*, 8, 2 (1971), 133.

[84]   Marshall, 'Pattern of housebuilding', 202.

[85]   A report published in 1946 recorded that, of the 32 local authorities on the coalfield for which it had details, 26 still had slum clearance schemes outstanding from the 1930s, amounting to 2,367 houses; see Ministry of Fuel and Power, *South Wales Coalfield Regional Survey Report* (London, 1946), p. 207.

Table 4.2. Increases in local authorities' slum clearance schemes in south Wales, 1933–8

	Houses to be demolished under 1933 plan	Revised programmes by 30 June 1938
Glamorgan AC	1,857	2,781
Monmouth AC	1,648	2,496
Cardiff CB	203	217
Merthyr CB	482	566
Swansea CB	1,317	1,317
Newport CB	140	162
Total	5,647	7,539

Source: Particulars of Slum Clearance Programmes furnished by Local Authorities; Ministry of Health, *Inquiry into the Anti-Tuberculosis Service in Wales and Monmouthshire*, 135.

authorities throughout the interwar period and the slum clearance schemes of the late 1930s were no exception. Blaenavon's badly needed slum clearance scheme, for example, was suspended in 1934 owing to the council's financial difficulties.[86] Therefore, it is clear that many authorities were not able to build as many houses as were necessary nor at comparable rates to other parts of Britain.

The extent to which the houses that were built effectively 'solved' the housing problem is difficult to ascertain. It does seem that the worst cases of overcrowding were abated to some extent during the 1930s as the 'Overcrowding Act' of 1935 served to focus attention on the matter and linked central funding to the number of families that were rehoused from overcrowded conditions. Furthermore, increasing emigration eased the population pressure that had been so evident during the 1920s, although the problem was not abated to the extent that the scale of emigration might suggest. As the population left south Wales during the late 1920s and 1930s so the number of uninhabited houses increased. While houses were becoming available to some degree, families were still too impoverished to afford the normal rents of many houses and sub-letting continued on a large scale.[87] This problem was exacerbated by the workings of the Rent Restriction Act which meant that in many

[86]   Blaenavon UD, RMOH (1934), p. 11. Blaenavon restarted its scheme in 1939 but was only able to build 38 of its original plan for 60 houses.
[87]   See for example Rhondda UD, RMOH (1937), pp. 114–15; (1938), p. 110.

cases where a house was vacated, the rent to be charged increased dramatically.[88]

Furthermore, the nature of the emigration that took place meant that it was often the younger adult members of large families and small families living in 'apartments' that left the stricken areas, thereby not freeing up houses by their departure.[89] The house-building programmes of local authorities were evidently not enough to eliminate all overcrowding. Even in Bedwellty, whose council maintained a higher than average rate of building, over-crowding was rife as late as 1936. The overcrowding survey of 1935 had shown that only twenty houses were overcrowded by the stand-ard it used, and, of these, only one was a house owned by the council.[90] That the standard employed by this survey was nonsens-ical was shown by the medical officer's annual report of the following year; it stated that in Aberbargoed, 21 per cent of the houses were occupied by two or more families, while in Cefn Fforest and Blackwood 16 per cent and 10 per cent of the houses were similarly overcrowded. Of the council's houses, 23 per cent were inhabited by two or more families.[91] Local authorities in south Wales, therefore, did not build houses in sufficient number nor were the houses that were built erected in those districts of greatest need.

Despite the low number of houses built in south Wales, those built by local authorities made significant improvements to the living conditions of the families fortunate enough to gain a house. The external environment was transformed as houses were built on low-density estates, designed according to garden-village principles; they possessed large gardens, grass verges and wide, open streets. Despite the fact that local authorities in south Wales built relatively few houses during this period, the large estates erected made a significant impact on the urban environment. At Townhill in Swansea, 2,336 houses had been completed by the end of November 1939 with a further 1,364 completed on the adjoining Mayhill estate.[92] The borough council was apparently concerned to

[88] See Aneurin Bevan's speech in the House of Commons, reported in *Western Mail* (4 July 1930), 9.

[89] Rhondda UD, RMOH (1936), p. 99.

[90] Ministry of Health, *Overcrowding Survey* (London, 1936), p. 153.

[91] Bedwellty UD, RMOH (1936), pp. 42–3.

[92] West Glamorgan Record Office, Swansea CBC, Housing of the Working Classes Committee minutes, 29 November 1939.

give 'each house a view of the wonderful panorama, either of the sea and the Devonshire coast, the Gower peninsula, or the Black Mountains and the Brecon Beacons'.[93] In Cardiff the estates of Ely, Mynachdy, and Pengam and Tremorfa consisted of 4,187, 788 and 1,030 houses respectively by 1939 and were situated on the outskirts of the city.[94] Smaller, though still considerable, estates were situated elsewhere in south Wales and remain distinctive features of the urban landscape to this day.

Within the new houses, the relatively spacious bedrooms, the kitchen equipped with modern amenities, and the indoor bathroom, created a domestic environment in marked contrast to the one previously known by the new tenants. For those families rehoused as part of the slum clearance campaign of the 1930s the improvement was even more marked.[95] The massive numbers of applications that councils received is evidence of the attraction that the new houses held for most families. Local authority houses were not without their structural and sanitary problems,[96] and could not wholly make up for the effects of poverty,[97] but both councils and tenants conceived of local authority housing as a massive improvement on the property available from private landlords.[98]

Thus, while housing conditions in south Wales were relatively better than in the other coalfields or towns of Britain, they were nevertheless unsatisfactory. Severe problems had developed by the early 1920s – overcrowding, housing shortage, insanitary property – that were not effectively dealt with in the following years. The economic depression of the 1920s and 1930s served in many cases to exacerbate existing problems and, in other cases, to retard any improvements that might have occurred in a more favourable economic

[93]   Swansea County Borough, *Souvenir of the Opening of the Guildhall* (Swansea, 1934).
[94]   M. C. Bourne, 'A study of council house building activity in post-war Cardiff' (unpubl. M.Sc. thesis, UWIST, 1981), 26–7.
[95]   For a comparable example, see Madeline McKenna, 'The suburbanization of the working-class population of Liverpool between the wars', *Social History*, 16, 2 (1991), 180–1.
[96]   See for example West Glamorgan Record Office, Port Talbot MBC, Sanitary Committee minutes, 19 February 1929; Port Talbot MBC, RMOH (1924), p. 45; *Free Press of Monmouthshire* (14 November 1924), 12.
[97]   Many tenants were forced to sub-let rooms to pay the rent and make ends meet; see Nantyglo and Blaina UD, RMOH (1926), p. 7.
[98]   As a good example, see the approving comments of G. A. Morgan, the sanitary inspector of the Port Talbot Municipal Borough; Port Talbot MB, RMOH (1936), p. 60.

climate. More importantly, these economic difficulties also served to limit the number of houses that were built in interwar south Wales. In this respect, the region was considerably disadvantaged in comparison with the north-east of England, where local authorities were able to take much greater advantage of the housing legislation to build large numbers of houses, although there also existed a greater need for new houses there.[99] Of the houses that were built by local authorities in south Wales, far too few were granted to families in greatest need. It was only with the Housing Acts of 1930 and 1935 that the housing needs of such families were addressed but, again, far too few houses were built to make a significant difference to the living condition of the population as a whole. For these various reasons, it must be concluded that very few improvements were made in standards of housing accommodation in interwar south Wales. In fact, for many families housing conditions actually deteriorated during the two decades as investment in the existing housing stock plummeted.

99   Jennings, 'Geographical implications', 128.

V
'LEPROUS TOWNS': ENVIRONMENT, SANITATION AND LEISURE

It was time, said Orwig, for a great accession of beauty in Elmhill. It was to be expected, he said, that the Industrial Revolution should have left a darkening wake of leprous towns but it seemed to have used Elmhill as a laboratory of new styles.[1]

'Public health' has been defined as 'community action undertaken to avoid disease and other threats to the health and welfare of individuals and the community at large'.[2] The nature and extent of this action constantly change as community perceptions of the dangers to health change. During the late eighteenth and nineteenth centuries public health measures were conceived of in terms of sanitary reform as industrialization and growing urbanization multiplied the environmental threats to the health of the population. Efforts were directed at improving standards of air quality, the successful supply of clean drinking water and the construction of effective means of sewage disposal.[3] By the last quarter of the nineteenth century, the ideological underpinnings of preventive or environmental medicine of this type came to be challenged by the 'germ theory' of medicine, by developments in the biological sciences and by a greater awareness of the implications of poverty, so that by the time of the First World War the role of medicine was perceived by practitioners and public alike to be largely curative in intention and practice, and more concerned with the behaviour and actions of private individuals. Preventive measures came to consist of the notification, isolation and treatment of infectious diseases, and large-scale educational campaigns to educate the public about hygiene and disease. The simultaneous development of health insurance at this time meant that public health officials increasingly

[1]   Gwyn Thomas, *A Point of Order* (London, 1956), p. 55.
[2]   John Duffy, 'History of public health and sanitation in the West since 1700', in Kenneth Kiple (ed.), *The Cambridge World History of Human Disease* (Cambridge, 1993), p. 200.
[3]   Hardy, *Epidemic Streets*, pp. 2–3.

took on a managerial role, coordinating a collection of medical services.[4] Environmental medicine came to be overlooked as Chadwickian ideas of sanitary reform, though admitted and acknowledged, no longer dominated community responses.

Partly as a result of this chronology, the historiography of public health is largely concerned with the period before 1914. There are, of course, very good reasons for this but, nevertheless, it was also the case that environmental improvements were achieved at different times in different parts of Britain and a great deal of work still faced public health authorities in south Wales in the interwar period. Furthermore, sanitary reform did not entail a change from insanitary to ideal conditions. Rather, such reform was a long, drawn-out process whereby improvements were made only gradually, and at varying rates in different places, and in which setbacks and break-downs in systems continued to be characteristic. Conditions in interwar south Wales were often far from ideal despite improvements made during the preceding decades. Sanitation was not a problem that had been solved by the First World War but was a continuing issue that required constant attention. Developments and improvements in sanitary infrastructures and public hygiene continued up until the Second World War and, indeed, beyond. Furthermore, the efficacy of the 'sanitarians' in south Wales varied according to the different environmental problems they encountered. As will become apparent, sewerage systems and water supplies received a great deal of attention, both before and during the interwar years, while other aspects of the environment, namely the state of public places, the condition of rivers and standards of air quality, did not receive this level of attention. Therefore, it is necessary to consider those aspects of public health and the environment usually associated with studies of nineteenth-century conditions.

In addition, the environment of south Wales was inextricably bound up with its fortunes as an economic region. As B. W. Clapp has written, 'Every economic process leaves behind a waste product' and this seems especially apposite in the case of the old, heavy industries that characterized the economies of regions such as south Wales.[5] It was commented that south Wales was the

    [4] Dorothy Porter, 'Public health', in W. F. Bynum and Roy Porter (eds), *Companion Encyclopedia of the History of Medicine* (London, 1993), vol. 2, p. 1257.
    [5] B. W. Clapp, *An Environmental History of Britain since the Industrial Revolution* (London, 1994), p. 13.

'product of coal civilisation', with every aspect of life blighted by this most destructive of extractive industries.[6] In the economic depression of the interwar years the environment took on an added significance as the drab, depressing quality of mining villages was read as a metaphor for the dire economic situation. More importantly, certain aspects of the environment were adversely affected by the inability of local authorities to make expenditure on basic sanitary requirements and it is clear that certain councils were emasculated by the loss of income occasioned by economic decline.

In any consideration of nineteenth-century standards of public health, the supply of water has always been of paramount importance, and yet this variable is rarely considered as a factor in twentieth-century standards of health, or at least not in the developed world. It is more often assumed that the 'problem' of water supply in Britain had been solved by the time of the First World War and is therefore not deserving of study. An examination of water provision in interwar south Wales shows this assumption to be incorrect.

The South Wales Regional Survey Committee appointed by the Ministry of Health in February 1921 found that the sources of water supply in south Wales varied from the very best class of large impounding reservoirs to direct supplies provided by springs and open ditches.[7] Similarly, undertakings ranged from those owned by a single local authority or private owner to joint boards of many authorities and to Statutory Water Companies. It seemed 'as though almost every method of supply and control of water exist[ed] in the area'.[8] Water provision was demand-led as consumers received the water supply they were prepared, or able, to pay for.[9] The four county boroughs of south Wales, empowered by the potentially large amounts of capital at their disposal, were able to erect large reservoirs in the Brecon Beacons to supply their citizens with adequate amounts of relatively clean water, and while they did to some extent augment the supplies of other local author-

---

[6]   NLW, E. L. Chappell papers, South Wales Regional Survey Committee, Statements of Witnesses and Minutes of Evidence, evidence of Cllr John Thomas, Treasurer (Afan Valley) SWMF, p. 3.

[7]   Ministry of Health, *Report of the South Wales Regional Survey Committee*, p. 45.

[8]   Chappell, South Wales Regional Survey Committee, Statements of Witnesses and Minutes of Evidence, Notes for Report, section VIII, Engineering Services, Water Supply.

[9]   W. F. Bynum and Roy Porter (eds), *Living and Dying in London, Medical History Supplement* (London, 1991), p. xv.

ities, these smaller authorities were largely forced to obtain a supply as best they could.[10] Sharp disparities in the quantity and quality of water supplied were experienced and many areas were said to be on the 'famine line'.[11] The Pontypridd and Rhondda Joint Water Board served these two very populous areas while the Pontypool Gas and Water Company supplied the urban districts of Pontypool, Panteg and Abersychan. Other joint boards and statutory companies included the Abertillery and District Water Board, the Rhymney and Aber Valley Gas and Water Company, the Bridgend Gas and Water Company and the Garw Water Company, supplying their respective areas.

Elsewhere, the urban districts of Llanfrechfa Upper, Blaenavon, Ebbw Vale, Tredegar, Mountain Ash, Aberdare, Porthcawl, Maesteg, Glyncorrwg, Margam and Neath all had their own undertakings, consisting mainly of small reservoirs and often supplemented by springs and streams. These smaller undertakings were predictably much less reliable than the large concerns of the county boroughs. Situated largely on the coalfield, these supplies were decreasing in yield due to the effect of subsidence caused by mine workings.[12] This, it was reported, was most marked in the case of the Abertillery and District Water Board. Periods of dry weather provoked severe difficulties, caused water to run short and even led to authorities cutting off the supply at certain times of the day. As the Port Talbot medical officer pointed out, 'This must cause great inconvenience in an industrial district, where the men are working the three shifts around the clock.'[13] In the Ffosmaen and Coedcae areas of the Nantyglo and Blaina Urban District there was no water 'on many hours each day . . . and on four occasions the supply to the District Hospital was cut off during operations'.[14] Since these were relatively high areas the water pressure was not sufficient to supply them and it was not until 1936 that a main was laid to supply Ffosmaen and Coedcae and ensure a constant supply to the hospital. An outbreak of typhoid fever in the district in 1927 was attributed to the use of wells and streams by local people because of the unreliable supply.[15]

[10]   Ministry of Health, *South Wales Regional Survey Committee*, p. 46.
[11]   Ibid.
[12]   Some undertakings disconnected their supply during the night so as to lessen the loss due to subsidence.
[13]   Port Talbot MB, RMOH (1923), p. 53.
[14]   Nantyglo and Blaina UD, RMOH (1926), p. 8.
[15]   Nantyglo and Blaina UD, RMOH (1927), p. 2.

This insufficiency of supply affected all areas of south Wales, apart from the county boroughs, to a greater or lesser degree, most especially in the summer months or in times of drought. This was most apparent in those areas such as the Barry and Ogmore and Garw urban districts and the rural districts of Pontardawe and Penybont that depended to a greater extent on springs for their supply. This insufficiency and the subsequent cut-offs that inevitably occurred each summer had obvious consequences for the daily routines of households, as processes such as food preparation, bathing and washing clothes were made more difficult. It also meant that toilets could not be flushed, thus obviating the benefits that cistern-flushing toilets were supposed to bring and making hand-flushed toilets even more insanitary. Furthermore, insufficiency of supply could prove an obstacle in the way of connecting houses to sewers, as at Cwmavon, Port Talbot, where the water mains did not provide a sufficient supply for flushing purposes and convinced householders that there was no point in connecting to the council's newly laid main.[16] Similarly, rural areas such as the Gower peninsula and eastern Monmouthshire depended to a large extent on unreliable sources. The scattered and isolated nature of the houses and communities of these areas meant that a piped water supply was too costly. The Magor Rural District derived some of its water supply from Newport County Borough Council and public companies such as the Great Western Railway but, in common with other rural areas, had to rely on springs, deep wells, and, more dangerously from a public health point of view, on shallow wells, 'reens' and open ditches for the remainder of its supply.[17]

This was largely the situation in the immediate post-war years but efforts to improve the quality and sufficiency of supply were coming to fruition in the interwar period. The Grwyne Fawr reservoir in the Brecon Beacons, established by an Act of Parliament in 1910, was finally completed in 1928. While only half full when a drought began in that year, the reservoir had sufficient quantity to supply the urban districts of Abertillery, Abercarn, Mynyddislwyn and Risca with an adequate amount of water throughout the year. The 100,000 inhabitants of these districts continued to be well supplied through another drought experienced in 1929 and,

---

[16] Port Talbot MB, RMOH (1925), p. 87.
[17] Magor RD, RMOH (1927), p. 4; 'Reen' was the local name for a ditch containing sluggishly flowing surface water.

indeed, throughout the 1930s.[18] Similarly, the Taf Fechan reservoir was completed and filled by April 1928 and supplied water in bulk to Merthyr, Pontypridd, the Rhondda Water Board, the Rhymney Valley Water Board, Barry and other places.[19] For these areas at least, a constant water supply was assured with the completion of these large schemes.

Residual problems remained, however. The supply of Blaenavon, for example, posed a serious danger for the health of its citizens throughout the interwar period. Its medical officer had informed the council of the advisability of adding to the number of sources of supply and to increasing further the storage capacity of their reservoirs because of the intermittent supply experienced each summer.[20] Some parts of the town, particularly those situated in higher localities, were only able to obtain one hour's supply of water each day and since there was no adequate means of storing water in their houses this proved very inconvenient for the townspeople and was considered unsatisfactory by the public health authorities.[21]

An insufficient supply often had more direct consequences for the health of the population. A drought in the summer of 1921 caused shortages to be experienced in many districts and in the Ogmore valley it was the cause of an epidemic of water-borne bacillary dysentery, mainly affecting children. It was estimated that 700 cases had occurred in the early stages of the outbreak.[22] Such outbreaks did not occur solely within those districts dependent on an unreliable supply. In the summer of 1937 the level in the storage reservoirs of the Swansea County Borough fell and by November there was an increased prevalence of diarrhoea in the districts dependent on the supply.[23]

Another residual problem that endangered public health and caused the authorities great anxiety was that of private water supplies. These supplies, not owned by a local authority, joint water board or statutory water company, existed to a greater or lesser

[18]   Monmouthshire CC, RMOH (1928), pp. 14–15; (1937), pp. 124–5.

[19]   Monmouthshire CC, RMOH (1928), p. 15; R. C. S. Walters, *The Nation's Water Supply* (London, 1936), p. 117.

[20]   Monmouthshire CC, RMOH (1928), p. 16.

[21]   Ibid.

[22]   Glamorgan CC, RMOH (1921), p. 26.

[23]   Swansea CB, RMOH (1937), pp. 79–80; this was probably due to the fact that throughout the interwar period the supplies of the Swansea CB were not filtered in any way.

extent in most areas of south Wales and the dangers they posed are illustrated by a study of the Rhondda valleys. Throughout the early 1920s the medical officer's annual reports commented on the nature of these supplies in various parts of the district. The upper part of Clydach Vale was dependent for its supply on the Cambrian Combine Colliery Company, which also supplied around 300 houses in Llwynypia,[24] while a further sixty-four houses in Pontygwaith derived their water from the Ferndale Brewery Company.[25] Other private supplies existed at Blaenrhondda, Cwmparc,[26] and Ystrad,[27] while at Dinas there were nine separate private supplies still in existence by 1925, the largest of which only supplied eighteen houses.[28]

Most of these private supplies were derived from underground springs, mountain streams and even disused coal levels. They all lacked sufficient means of storage, adequate protection against pollution, efficient arrangements for purification and satisfactory systems of distribution. The Llwynypia supply was distributed to short columns or standpipes with taps in the road, and the inhabitants of ten to twelve houses shared each tap.[29] Numerous complaints were received by the medical officer about the quality and quantity of the water supplied and, it was reported, 'owing to greater liability to pollution and to progressive loss of water from ground disturbance the difficulties encountered become accentuated from year to year'.[30] Plans to improve the supply in Clydach Vale under an Act of Parliament passed in 1920 were shelved on a number of occasions because of the economic difficulties of the Urban District Council, but by 1926 a tank with a capacity of a million gallons had been constructed and the necessary mains laid. This did not solve the problem, however, as householders had to connect their own houses to the mains and this proved too onerous a burden for most families. Most houses in Clydach Vale, therefore, continued to be supplied by the unsatisfactory supply of the colliery company, which continued to deteriorate.[31] Faced with reluctance

[24]   Rhondda UD, RMOH (1920), p. 74; (1925), p.109.
[25]   Rhondda UD, RMOH (1925), p. 113.
[26]   The whole of Cwmparc was supplied by the Ocean Coal Company; Rhondda UD, RMOH (1933), p. 77.
[27]   Rhondda UD, RMOH (1922), p. 78.
[28]   Rhondda UD, RMOH (1925), p. 114.
[29]   Ibid., p. 109.
[30]   Rhondda UD, RMOH (1922), p. 78.
[31]   Rhondda UD, RMOH (1926), p. 81; (1927), p. 82.

on the part of the owners to connect their houses to the council's new supply, the council finally served notices on owners which required them to connect their houses; failing this, they carried out the work themselves in default of the owners and then claimed back the costs. Around 400 houses were subsequently connected in 1929 and a further 600 the following year, while 281 houses in Llwynypia were also connected in 1930.[32] Almost a thousand houses in the urban district were still unconnected by 1930 but further orders issued by the council probably accounted for the majority of these during the following decade.[33]

While the various means by which water was controlled determined the sufficiency of supply, they also had a bearing on the quality and purity of water that was supplied. Legislative guidelines on water quality have, until recently, been few. The Waterworks Clauses Act of 1847 specified that any water supplied should be 'wholesome' without defining in any objective way what this meant.[34] Guidance as to bacteriological testing techniques and acceptable standards of drinking water quality was set out in a government report of 1934 and yet, although widely used by water authorities, this report was not mandatory and did not impose any legal requirements on water authorities.[35] Nevertheless, many of the larger water supply undertakings did employ a variety of screening and filtration devices aimed at ensuring a good quality supply. Mesh screens, slow sand filters and mechanical filters were used, with varying degrees of success, by many water authorities. As in other aspects of water supply, the financial power of the water provider partly determined the means of filtration employed. A gravity rapid filtration plant was erected at the Taf Fechan reservoir, for example, with a capacity of seven million gallons of water per day.[36] Yet some large concerns could be totally without means of ensuring high standards of water quality. Neither Swansea County Borough nor Merthyr County Borough screened or filtered its supplies until the mid 1930s. By 1937 the supply obtained from the Cray reservoir by the Swansea County Borough was chlorinated, in

---

[32] Rhondda UD, RMOH (1929), p. 80; (1930), pp. 89–90.
[33] Rhondda UD, RMOH (1930), pp. 90–1.
[34] J. F. Wright, 'The development of public water supplies in the Swansea area, 1837–1989' (unpubl. University of Wales Local History Diploma dissertation, 1991), 70; this was the sole legal requirement up until the 1970s.
[35] Ibid.
[36] British Waterworks Association, *British Waterworks Year Book and Directory* (1926), 94–100.

common with other supplies throughout Britain in the wake of the Croydon typhoid outbreak, while the supply from the Lliw reservoirs was chlorinated following an outbreak of dysenteric diarrhoea in 1937.[37]

Water supplies in other areas, dependent on smaller scale undertakings, were much less likely to be filtered. For example, in the urban district of Maesteg, which was supplied by streams and springs, the water was completely unfiltered despite the fact that many of the sources were open to contamination, while in Blaenavon it was a common occurrence for tadpoles, newts and other wildlife and matter to come through the taps of householders.[38] Public health officials were very concerned throughout the interwar period by this consumption of 'raw' water.[39]

The dangers posed by unfiltered water were determined by the nature of the supply. Referring to the Grwyne Fawr scheme, the Monmouthshire county medical officer stated that owing to the 'exceptional purity' of the water no filtration was necessary, although fine copper mesh screens were nevertheless installed immediately below the reservoir.[40] The Grwyne Fawr reservoir, situated at a great distance from urban communities, was clearly much less liable to contamination than supplies obtained from areas in close proximity to human habitation. In these latter cases supplies could only be safeguarded by the fencing off and supervision of catchment areas and reservoirs, and by frequent bacteriological examination.[41] At Llwynypia in the Rhondda, the dilapidation of fences surrounding the gathering grounds of the Cambrian Combine Company's private supply, together with the tendency of locked-out miners to enjoy the local hills, put this supply at risk during 1926.[42] The *bacillus coli* content of the Port Talbot Municipal Borough's supply was found to be 'dangerously high at times' due to faecal pollution by cattle at the gathering grounds.[43]

An important consideration with regard to water supplies that

[37]   Wright, 'Public water supplies in the Swansea area', 33; Swansea CB, RMOH (1937), pp. 79–80.

[38]   Maesteg UD, RMOH (1920), p. 6; Blaenavon UD, RMOH (1936), p. 9.

[39]   See for example Glamorgan CC, RMOH (1920), p. 34; (1923), p. 21; (1927), p. 24; Port Talbot MB, RMOH (1939), p. 13.

[40]   Monmouthshire CC, RMOH (1927), p. 16.

[41]   See for example Port Talbot MB, RMOH (1922), p. 37.

[42]   Rhondda UD, RMOH (1926), p. 82.

[43]   Port Talbot MB, RMOH (1927), p. 33.

had consequences for quality of life and even standards of health was the nature of the access that families had to water supplies. Although the vast majority of households received water within their own curtilage by the interwar period, some households were still dependent upon shared or communal supplies. This was most noticeable in rural communities but was not unknown in urban areas. In proportional terms the numbers were small. In the Neath Rural District 98 per cent of houses received a water supply within their own curtilage and the remaining 2 per cent were dependent on a public standpipe or pillar-tap supply.[44] A large number of houses was similarly dependent on pillar-tap supplies in the Port Talbot Municipal Borough, the majority of these concentrated in Cwmavon, although this number had been reduced to about 200 houses by 1930.[45] In the Rhondda, the 300 houses of Llwynypia Terrace, Llwynypia, depended on the Cambrian Combine Colliery Company and the occupants of every ten or twelve houses shared a standpipe.[46] Public health authorities successfully replaced all but a few of these communal supplies during the interwar period. The effect that such conversion must have had on the fifty-two house-holds of Fernhill Terrace that had previously been supplied by a single tap is scarcely imaginable.[47] As perhaps might be expected, the absence of internal supplies was more marked in rural areas. In the Monmouth Rural District, cottages without internal supplies were common and their inhabitants were forced to walk over a quarter of a mile to the nearest supply, while in the St Mellons district water either had to be carried in water carts or else rain-water was collected.[48]

The varied nature of water provision in south Wales was mirrored by the variety of means of sewage disposal utilized in the area. As with water supply, certain improvements were made so that sewerage systems no longer posed a serious threat to public health. In its examination of the area, the South Wales Regional Survey Committee, reporting in 1921, identified three different systems employed for sewage disposal.[49] First, trunk sewer systems had been

[44]   Neath RD, RMOH (1926), p. 18.
[45]   Port Talbot MB, RMOH (1925), pp. 28–9; (1930), p. 36.
[46]   Rhondda UD, RMOH (1925), p. 109.
[47]   Rhondda UD, RMOH (1934), p. 93.
[48]   Monmouth RD, RMOH (1932), p. 4; NLW, Welsh Board of Health collection, Box 62, R. Bruce Low, Untitled report on a sanitary survey of the St Mellons RD, 6 June 1928, p. 3.
[49]   NLW, E. L. Chappell papers, South Wales Regional Survey Committee, Notes for Report: section VIII, Engineering Services Sewerage.

built in many of the valleys and were adjudged to be the most effective means of disposal. Trunk sewers transferred sewage from an area within enclosed pipes whereas previously sewage had been discharged in its crude state into rivers and streams. Edwin Davies, the medical officer of Tredegar, commented that the trunk sewer that served his area reduced to a minimum the amount of 'objectionable matter' discharged into the Sirhowy river so that it was no longer a serious menace to the health of the district.[50] The Western Valley (Mon.) trunk sewer, completed in 1910, provided for the valleys of the River Ebbw and its tributaries, the Sirhowy and the Ebbw Fach, and served a potential population of 160,000 in the urban districts of Ebbw Vale, Nantyglo and Blaina, Abertillery, Abercarn, and Risca and portions of the Mynyddislwyn, Bedwellty and Tredegar urban districts and St Mellons Rural District. The Pontypridd and Rhondda trunk sewer served its respective areas and trunk sewers were similarly employed to serve the Ogmore and Afan valleys. The topography of the south Wales area naturally lent itself to this system of trunk sewers and other areas of south Wales adopted this means of disposal during the interwar period. By 1926 the Rhymney Valley main trunk sewer was completed and work continued into the 1930s to connect subsidiary sewers to it.[51] By 1933 subsidiary sewers in the urban districts of Rhymney, Bedwellty, Mynyddislwyn, Bedwas and Machen in Monmouthshire and Caerphilly and Gelligaer in Glamorgan were connected to the Rhymney Valley Sewerage Board trunk sewer.[52] A further trunk sewer scheme to serve the Afon Lwyd, or 'Eastern valley', of Monmouthshire had first been suggested to Parliament before the First World War but was rejected due to disagreements between the local authorities involved in the scheme.[53] A trunk sewer serving Llantarnam and Llanfrechfa Upper urban districts was completed in 1931 but the greater part of the Eastern valley was not served by a trunk sewer during the whole of the interwar period.[54]

[50]   Tredegar UD, RMOH (1925), p. 10.
[51]   Monmouthshire CC, RMOH (1926), p. 17.
[52]   Monmouthshire CC, RMOH (1933), p. 33.
[53]   Chappell, South Wales Regional Survey Committee, Sewerage, p. 2; for a history of the protracted negotiations to promote this scheme, see Monmouthshire CC, RMOH (1937), pp. 129–34.
[54]   Monmouthshire CC, RMOH (1931), p. 39; the Ministry of Health sanctioned a scheme in November 1937 but work had not begun when war broke out in 1939. By the late 1940s the county medical officer was still stressing the need for this work to be carried out; see Monmouthshire CC, RMOH (1937), p. 134 and (1945–47).

The second system utilized in south Wales was that of sewers connected to sewerage works that treated the sewage, by chemical or bacterial means, and then discharged the effluent into a nearby river or stream. Areas served by this type of system included the Merthyr and Aberdare districts, the neighbouring urban districts of Maesteg and Ogmore and Garw and the adjoining Penybont Rural District, and finally the hinterlands of Neath and Swansea.[55] Finally, many of the large coastal towns utilized a variation of the other systems and discharged sewage directly into the tidal waters of a river or into the sea. The problem with this method, it was stated, was that in many cases the outfalls into the sea were not situated at a sufficient distance from the towns and sewage tended to drift back towards the towns on the flow of the tide.

In the absence of any of these three systems of disposal, sewage was most often discharged directly into rivers and streams. In the Eastern valley of Monmouthshire, all sewage was discharged in its crude state into the Afon Lwyd, with the exception of one outfall at Panteg where the sewage was first treated and then released.[56] While the trunk sewer serving the Llantarnam and Llanfrechfa Upper areas did lessen the amount of crude sewage released into the river, the Afon Lwyd continued to pose serious health risks throughout the 1920s and 1930s.[57] The river constituted an open sewer from Blaenavon at the top of the valley to the point at which it entered the Usk at Newport.[58]

Sewerage systems employing long lengths of underground piping were generally efficient but were not without their problems. Chief among these were the effects of mining subsidence on the many miles of underground piping. This problem was obviated in some instances by the construction of sewerage pipes on brick pillars above ground, but for most districts on the coalfield subsidence was the cause of considerable damage and the source of much trouble and cost to the local authorities.[59] It was a major problem in the Rhondda valleys, for example, where numerous leaks resulted each

[55]   NLW, E. L. Chappell papers, South Wales Regional Survey Committee, Sewerage, pp. 1, 6–7.

[56]   Monmouthshire CC, RMOH (1922), p. 48.

[57]   Monmouthshire CC, RMOH (1929), p. 24.

[58]   Bruce Low, Report on the Sanitary circumstances of the Abersychan Urban District, p. 2.

[59]   Bruce Low, Report on the Sanitary Circumstances of the Maesteg Urban District, p. 20 (own pagination); Rhondda UD, RMOH (1925), p. 19; Nantyglo and Blaina UD, RMOH (1932), p. 10.

year.[60] Such leaks soaked into the ground and could seep into rivers and even water supplies. The medical officer of Brynmawr attempted to shift the blame for a typhoid[61] outbreak in his area in 1924 from the leaky condition of the sewer in the district to the habits of local people who, he claimed, were in the habit of throwing excrement onto the main road.[62] The Welsh Board of Health considered the Nantyglo and Blaina Urban District to be particularly liable to typhoid infection and gave the views of the Brynmawr officer short shrift. Outbreaks in the Nantyglo and Blaina area in the past had 'almost without exception' been traced to water infected by sewage leaking from the Brynmawr sewers.[63]

Subsidence had dire effects on the sewers of the Rhondda. By 1933 the subsidiary sewers in the mid-Rhondda area were said to have deteriorated to such an extent as to make them 'totally ineffective as channels for sewage' with the result that sewage had to be discharged into the river.[64] This was not the only problem faced by public health officials in the Rhondda. Hamish Richards has written how a considerable amount of excess capacity meant that the sewers in the Rhondda served the district admirably and that very little investment in the sewerage infrastructure was necessary between the years 1914 and 1960.[65] This was not the opinion of the medical officer of health who commented in 1923 that the main sewer of the district, 17 miles long and discharging into the sea, had served the area 'admirably' but, due to the rapid growth of population, the sewer capacity was now barely adequate even under normal conditions – 'any interference with the flow or an undue increase in the volume of the sewage causes the secondary or subsidiary sewers to be overcharged'.[66] The Rhondda sewers were

[60]   Rhondda UD, RMOH (1927), p. 72.

[61]   Typhoid is spread by bacteria shed in the stool of an infected person being ingested through contaminated food or water and is usually caused by a breakdown in the separation of sewage and water supplies; see Kiple, *The Cambridge World History of Human Disease*, pp. 1071–7.

[62]   NLW, Welsh Board of Health collection, Box 13Q, Minute sheet of conference with R. Bruce Low held on 2 December 1924, p. 2.

[63]   NLW, Welsh Board of Health collection, Box 58Q, Correspondence from Welsh Board of Health to Mr Infield (Ministry of Health?), 8 November 1927.

[64]   Rhondda UD, RMOH (1933), p. 68.

[65]   Hamish Richards, 'Investment in public health provision in the mining valleys of South Wales, 1860–1914', in Colin Baber and John Williams (eds), *Modern South Wales: Essays in Economic History* (Cardiff, 1986), pp. 130–1.

[66]   Rhondda UD, RMOH (1923), p. 79; for a similar complaint see Aberdare UD, RMOH (1924), p. 91.

so troublesome that the entire length of the main sewer from Treorchy to Trehafod had been enlarged or relaid by 1936. In the following few years, many of the main and subsidiary sewers were similarly renewed, most of the work financed by grants from the Commissioner of the Special Areas.[67] Wyndham Portal found that the Rhondda Urban District council, in common with other authorities, had a long list of sewerage work that they were unable to proceed with because sanction had been withheld by government departments.[68]

These were the three methods by which houses that were sewered discharged their waste. In addition, of course, there was a certain proportion of houses unconnected to any form of sewer system. Such houses depended on a variety of 'conservancy' systems, all of which were considered less satisfactory than sewers from a sanitary point of view. In his examination of housing in Victorian Britain, Martin Daunton has written how 'Sanitary history reveals a hierarchy of conveniences ranging from cess-pools, through middens, ash-closets and pail-closets, to water closets.'[69] Cess-pools and middens consisted of large, pervious receptacles that held more than one week's sewage.[70] As the nineteenth century ended, receptacles were made impervious and smaller so that in some cases the receptacle was reduced to a pail beneath the seat of the closet. At the top of the 'sanitary hierarchy' was the water closet, which itself had a number of forms. The variation in closets utilized within an area was determined by the by-laws in force in that particular area and by the improvements that a council was able or willing to make.[71]

Cesspools, privies, pail closets and dry earth closets were mainly vestiges of the nineteenth century and existed to a greater or lesser degree in just about most communities in south Wales during the interwar period,[72] but it was in the rural areas that these systems

[67] Rhondda UD, RMOH (1936–9).
[68] *Reports of the Investigation into the Industrial Conditions in Certain Depressed Areas* [Cmd. 4728], 1933–4, xiii, p. 169; Pontardawe RD, RMOH (1934), p. 8; Nantyglo and Blaina UD, RMOH (1935), p. 7.
[69] Daunton, *House and Home*, p. 248.
[70] The difference between the two was that in the case of middens ashes were mixed with the sewage to form a semi-solid mass while in cess-pools nothing was mixed with the excrement.
[71] Daunton, *House and Home*, pp. 248–9.
[72] In areas not served by a piped sewerage system new houses built during the interwar years had to be provided with conservancy type closets; see for example Port Talbot MB, RMOH (1922), p. 41; Magor RD, RMOH (1927), p. 5.

were most prevalent. The scattered, isolated nature of the rural communities meant that piped sewerage systems were prohibitively expensive and could only be extended to these areas in a very piece-meal fashion.[73] Urban communities in south Wales enjoyed much better facilities with regard to closet accommodation and sewerage systems than the rural areas and yet even here the legacies of the nineteenth century posed public health risks. It is evident that the vast majority of households were connected to sewers well before the interwar period. To take just a few examples, 91 per cent of all closets in the Gelligaer Urban District were connected to water-carriage sewerage systems by 1920 while the figures for the Rhondda and Tredegar were even more impressive – 99.5 per cent and 98.6 per cent respectively. In Aberdare 97.6 per cent of all closets were connected to sewers by 1924.[74] Throughout the interwar period, public health authorities were gradually able to bring about the replacement of pails and privies by connecting houses to sewerage systems. This was, of course, made easier by the trunk sewers and newly installed water services that had been made available. Connections to the Western Valley trunk sewer had been held up by the war but efforts were intensified in the early 1920s to convert privies and closets to the water-carriage system. Similarly, as the Rhymney Valley trunk sewer was completed, connections were made and closets converted. The county medical officer urged local authorities to press on urgently with the work but found that they were not as zealous as he would have liked and that householders were unable to carry out the work due to financial burdens.[75] Economic conditions retarded this work to some extent but progress was made throughout the interwar period.[76]

In Swansea, the borough council inherited a large number of insanitary closet types in 1918 when the borough boundary was extended to include the old-established communities of Treboeth, Llansamlet, Fforestfach and Bonymaen. This extension added over 5,000 pail closets and privies to the borough and an eleven-year

[73]   For a more detailed consideration of this issue in rural Monmouthshire, see Thompson, 'Social history of health', 210–11.

[74]   Gelligaer UD, RMOH (1920), p. 41; Rhondda UD, RMOH (1920), p. 63; Tredegar UD, RMOH (1920), p. 8; Aberdare UD, RMOH (1924), p. 91.

[75]   Monmouthshire CC, RMOH (1922), p. 47; (1923), p. 44.

[76]   Monmouthshire CC, RMOH (1920–39); Tredegar UD, RMOH (1929), p. 8. Locked-out miners in Ystradgynlais took advantage of the stoppage of 1926 to connect their houses to the local council's sewerage scheme; *Llais Llafur* (29 May 1926).

plan to erect sewers was drawn up to remedy the nuisance.[77] Implementation of this plan was postponed because of the high cost of materials and it was not until 1925 that the scheme was reactivated and progress made. Subsequently, sewers were extended to every part of the borough and insanitary closet types abolished.[78]

Conversion of insanitary closet types continued through the 1920s so that by 1929 the Monmouthshire county medical officer was able to assert that nearly the whole of the closet accommodation in the industrial areas was of the water-carriage type.[79] Nevertheless, problems remained. Many households remained without any closet accommodation whatsoever. About 600 old houses in Aberdare were without separate closet accommodation, while in Blaenavon 'large numbers of houses' lacked such accommodation.[80] At some places in Blaenavon only one closet was provided for the use of three families while at many places one closet served the needs of two houses. A Blaina resident, speaking to Mollie Tarrant, voiced the probable sentiments of a large number of householders at that time: 'No matter what else, every house should have its own lavatory. It's only healthy.'[81] Where such provision did not exist, it was stated, trouble was experienced in keeping the closet in a sanitary condition for, 'although used in common by members of two or more households, it appears to be no one's business to flush and cleanse, with the result that foul and dirty closets are not uncommon'.[82] Although a legacy of the nineteenth century, the inadequate provision in Blaenavon was not helped by the economic conditions of the interwar years; the medical officer noted that to enforce provision of a separate closet would cause severe hardship for house owners.[83] Large numbers of insanitary pail closets were also found in Hafodyrynys in the Abersychan district and Cwmavon near Port Talbot but most of these were replaced in the interwar period.[84]

[77] Swansea CB, RMOH (1920), pp. 29–30; (1922), pp. 32–3.

[78] Swansea CB, RMOH (1925–39).

[79] Monmouthshire CC, RMOH (1929), p. 26.

[80] Glamorgan CC, *Quarterly Report of the County Medical Officer to the Public Health and Housing Committee held on 29 February 1924*; Monmouthshire CC, RMOH (1929), p. 26.

[81] Calder and Sheridan, *Speak for Yourself*, p. 108.

[82] Monmouthshire CC, RMOH (1929), p. 26.

[83] Blaenavon UD, RMOH (1933), p. 8.

[84] Monmouthshire CC, RMOH (1927), p. 20; Abersychan UD, RMOH (1931), p. 15; Port Talbot UD, RMOH (1923), p. 50; (1926), p. 35; (1926), p. 35; (1933), p. 66.

If the water supply and sewerage systems of south Wales improved during these decades, the same could not be said for standards of air quality. The industries of the area were chiefly to blame for the dire standards of air quality found in south Wales. The coal industry continually produced a supply of coal dust – the 'dust epidemic' as Bert Coombes characterized it[85] – which was a constant source of irritation. Dust sullied clothes on washing lines, made the domestic burden of keeping a house clean more onerous than it already was and generally tarnished the everyday environment of south Wales.[86] Proximity to a pithead, a railway line or the docks was an important factor, and the large extent to which housing in the mining communities of south Wales was clustered around the collieries was relevant, 'giving rise to much uncleanliness and discomfort'.[87] In congested areas such as the Rhondda, where houses had been built in close proximity to the collieries, this difficulty was 'a serious one and causes much annoyance'. In contrast, T. J. Bell Thomas, the medical officer of Maesteg, was able to comment in 1930 that 'Although a colliery district the inhabited areas [of Maesteg] are much cleaner than many other mining districts, the collieries being well away from the populated areas, which is unusual in the valleys of South Wales.'[88] Topography, the timing and nature of the expansion of the coal industry in a particular area and the extent to which housing development could be controlled all played a part in determining the proximity of housing to the collieries.

An examination of the Rhondda Urban District provides many insights into the significance of air pollution in coalmining communities.[89] Throughout the interwar period the council received complaints from residents about coal dust blown from collieries, aerial ropeways, railway sidings and tips, and the grit produced by mechanical stokers at colliery pitheads.[90] It was found that clothes could not be dried outside when the wind blew in a certain direction for fear of being immediately sullied and rooms rapidly covered in a

---

[85] B. L. Coombes, *Miners Day* (Harmondsworth, 1945), pp. 52–3.
[86] See for example Brian Luxton, *In our own words, in our own pictures: People's History to Commemorate the Barry Docks Centenary* (Barry, 1989), p. 32, testimony of Leonard Davies.
[87] Ministry of Health, *Report of the South Wales Regional Survey Committee*, p. 64.
[88] Maesteg UD, RMOH (1930), p. 9.
[89] The following is obtained from Glamorgan Record Office, Rhondda UDC, Correspondence and papers relating to air pollution.
[90] See for example Rhondda UD, RMOH (1932), pp. 93–4.

film of fine coal dust if windows were left open. Indeed, coal dust was forcing itself into houses through the gaps in window- and door-frames. In response to such complaints the medical officer monitored the nuisance and attempted to remedy the problem through negotiation. This conciliatory approach meant that pollution continued for some time even while under the observation of the public health authorities, and abatement only came about at the whim of colliery managers or by a change in working practice. Some colliery managers played on economic worries to avoid incurring the expense of lessening pollution.[91]

More generally, coal fires within the home produced dust and grit both within the home environment and in the wider community. Nearly every town, iron and steel works and many collieries possessed gas works or coke ovens from which a wide variety of by-products were obtained but which also released dust and sulphurous fumes into the atmosphere.[92] However, it was perhaps the metallurgical industries of the region that had the greatest detrimental effect on air quality. Swansea in particular had long been infamous for the scale and nature of air pollution produced by its various metal industries and problems continued into the interwar period.[93] The Swansea County Borough Council received many complaints from the residents of the Llansamlet Ward and investigation by the medical officer of health found that crops on nearby farms were left withered by the fumes of the spelter (zinc) works situated at Landore. Many people, including the medical officer himself, believed that the fumes were a predisposing cause of respiratory diseases.[94] In an investigation into the problem just before the First World War a fellow medical officer, examining a horse that was alleged to have died as a result of poisoning by fumes, found that the internal organs of the horse showed presence of lead, arsenic and zinc. No such post-mortem examination could be carried out on the people of the area although the medical officer felt that he could not rule out the possibility of similar metallic poisoning.[95]

[91] Glamorgan Record Office, Rhondda UDC, Correspondence from General Manager, Cory Brothers & Co. Ltd, to Dr J. D. Jenkins, MOH, Rhondda UDC, 12 May 1931.

[92] E. M. Bridges, *Healing the Scars: Derelict Land in Wales* (Llandysul, 1988), p.18.

[93] See Clapp, *Environmental History*, p. 27; R. Rees, 'The south Wales copper-smoke dispute, 1833–95', *Welsh History Review*, 10, 4 (1981), 480–96; Morton, *In Search of Wales*, p. 223.

[94] Swansea CB, RMOH (1924), p. 56.

[95] Ibid., pp. 53–6.

Although air quality was generally poor in interwar south Wales, it seems likely that it improved to some extent in some localities during the interwar period. Certainly the standard of air quality improved as mines and works shut down during the Depression. Port Talbot Municipal Borough Council had received no complaints during 1926, for the first time, and the town had been free from its usual 'pall of smoke' due to its various furnaces having been partly or wholly closed down during the year.[96] Furthermore, the recording of atmospheric pollution in Cardiff suggests that the amount of soluble and insoluble matter in the atmosphere was declining in the years 1926 to 1938.[97] In addition, the Smoke Abatement by-law of 1926 encouraged medical officers to investigate polluting nuisances and to take measures to abate them, although the effectiveness of this by-law was mitigated by the weak powers it had at its disposal and its permissive nature. Nevertheless, although there were improvements in some areas in the quality of air that people breathed, it seems likely that there was still much room for improvement by the outbreak of the Second World War.[98]

Apart from these sanitary aspects of the environment, daily life brought the people of south Wales into contact with other areas of the environment which posed a risk to health. For example, Tom Richards, the MP for West Monmouthshire and secretary of the South Wales Miners' Federation, described roads in the mining districts as 'grossly insanitary'.[99] This description is confirmed by evidence contained in the annual reports of the local medical officers of health. The urban district of Maesteg provides an example of an authority that energetically and effectively dealt with the conditioning of its roads. The report of its medical officer for 1920 was able to record that, despite some opposition, the Private Street Works Act was now being applied in the district, and that work was in progress. 'The streets concerned are being made pleasant to walk through, instead of remaining tortuous to passengers and an eyesore to every one concerned.'[100] Progress was such that by 1923

---

[96]   Port Talbot MB, RMOH (1926), p. 45.
[97]   Cardiff CB, RMOH (1926), p. 72; (1938), p. 121.
[98]   Neil L. Tranter, *British Population in the Twentieth Century* (London, 1996), p. 80; Tranter asserts that 'Of all the principal determinants of environmental quality only the quality of the urban air supply failed to improve in the course of the interwar period.'
[99]   T. Richards, 'The improvement of colliery districts', *Welsh Housing and Development Association Yearbook* (1917), 76–80.
[100]   Maesteg UD, RMOH (1920), p. 9.

the medical officer was able to comment that 'I feel that the substitution of clean and convenient footpaths, where formerly mud and stagnant pools existed, is an improvement which directly affects the health of the district and the standard of local sanitation'.[101]

Despite this apparent zeal in tackling the condition of the roads in this district, it seems that even these efforts failed to eradicate the nuisance completely. Dr Bruce Low noted how 'Some of the back lanes are a quagmire and require making up', although he admitted that the council had in recent years given this matter their attention with the result that the situation was very much better than it had been previously.[102] In Swansea, the high costs of materials and the restricted financial resources of the council meant that road works were not being carried out in the early 1920s. By the time the economic situation allowed private street works to be recommenced in 1924 there were over 150 front streets (measuring 15 miles) and over 100 back streets (5 miles) that required surfacing.[103]

If the condition of roads was at times poor in districts such as Maesteg, where a proactive policy was followed, and Swansea, with its relative prosperity and greater financial capability, it was decidedly worse in areas where councils had neither the desire nor the wherewithal to tackle the problem. In the urban district of Nantyglo and Blaina, where a large amount of unemployment was evident even from the immediate post-war years, the medical officer was forced to admit that:

> The present condition of the roads in the Nantyglo area calls for comment. The dust is a nuisance and a danger to the public. It causes infantile diarrhoea, unhealthy tonsils, with all its complications, eye trouble, etc. Tar spraying at long intervals does not seem to be sufficient treatment for roads subject to such heavy traffic. There are some holes 4 to 6 inches deep. The surface is undulating, something like a hair wave. I hope it will not be allowed to become 'permanent'.[104]

Similarly, in the equally depressed community of Blaenavon the reconditioning of access roads and back lanes was listed as a task needing urgent attention.[105] As local authorities struggled to deal

---

[101] Ibid. (1923), p. 4 (own pagination).
[102] Bruce Low, 'Report on the sanitary circumstances of the Maesteg Urban District', pp. 24–5.
[103] Swansea CB, RMOH (1924), p. 52.
[104] Nantyglo and Blaina UD, RMOH (1925), p. 6.
[105] Blaenavon UD, RMOH (1935), pp. 4–5.

with this problem in these years it is noticeable how it was the financially hard-pressed districts that took longer to deal with the nuisance. Less depressed communities were largely able to resolve the problem during the 1920s, while districts such as Nantyglo and Blaina, and Blaenavon had still to tackle the problem in the late 1930s. The Rhondda medical officer was still calling for the improvement of the streets and lanes of the district in 1934.[106]

While unformed and unmade streets did serve to encourage the accumulation of refuse and rubbish, it seems clear that reconditioning roads counted for little if the system of scavenging house refuse was inefficient. At Maesteg, Dr Bruce Low found that 'all sorts of tins, old boxes, tubs and pails are used, which often leak or are otherwise unsatisfactory. Very few houses use proper sanitary dust bins; the result of this is that the streets are fouled and the back streets and lanes become littered with old paper, tins, ashes and organic matter.'[107] This seems to have been a problem throughout south Wales and even the medical officer of relatively prosperous Cardiff was driven to call for the provision of sanitary dustbins in the city, stating that barely 20 per cent of the households were appropriately equipped.[108] For various reasons, the efforts of local authorities to scavenge their districts failed to eradicate the nuisance caused by the accumulation of refuse. Scavenging was done in two ways: either the council carried it out by direct labour using its own workmen or else a contract system was employed. In most districts a combination of the two methods was used although the contract system came increasingly under criticism. Bruce Low found that in the Neath Rural District the lowest tender was always accepted irrespective of any other factors that should have been considered, 'such as honesty or business capability of the contractor', and so the system was grossly ineffective.[109]

Contractors often employed a horse and cart to carry out their work and only visited houses at intermittent periods, whereas the councils, where they were able, used motorized lorries and collected refuse more regularly and thoroughly. Increasingly during the

[106]   Rhondda UD, RMOH (1934), p. 16.
[107]   Bruce Low, 'Report on the sanitary circumstances of the Maesteg Urban District', pp. 23–4.
[108]   Cardiff CB, RMOH (1929), p. 7.
[109]   Bruce Low, Untitled report on the sanitary circumstances of the Neath Rural District, p. 5.

interwar period, motorized lorries were replacing the horse and cart as the means by which refuse was collected. By the early 1930s most of the scavenging done in the county of Monmouth, for example, was carried out by motor lorry. This meant that scavenging could be done more regularly and also that refuse tips could be located at greater distances from houses.[110]

Owing to the irregular nature of refuse collection when carried out under the contract system, it was observed that householders frequently tipped their refuse in backlanes, in rivers or streams or on to unauthorized dumps – 'heaps of refuse [are] left upon roadsides in all directions' recorded the medical officer of the Neath Rural District.[111] A similar problem was experienced in Nantyglo and Blaina and the medical officer there wondered if it was due to cuts in council expenditure on scavenging. In the period 1925–8 expenditure had been cut almost by half and collection was made on alternate days as opposed to daily, as had happened previously. This cutting down of scavenging was done on the instructions of the Ministry of Health and was one of the conditions imposed on the district council in connection with a loan it had applied for, and without which it could not continue its administration.[112]

Various sources suggest that this problem of haphazard dumping of refuse was increasing during the war years and in the 1920s. The medical officer of Gelligaer stated that it was a recent phenomenon and suggested that it might have been due to 'difficulties occasioned by [the] war'. He also stated that it had 'become very nearly a custom'.[113] In Rhymney, it was found in 1929 that 'whereas years ago many of the spaces and gardens round houses were prettily cultivated gardens, they are now merely rubbish heaps littered with old tins and where very often kitchen slops and potato peeling and tea leaves are dumped'.[114] It seems clear that this was a problem that was increasing in some areas during the 1920s, suggesting not that householders cared little for their environment and dumped haphazardly, but that systems of scavenging had suffered as a result

[110] Monmouthshire CC, RMOH (1930–4).

[111] Neath RD, RMOH (1925), p. 25.

[112] Bruce Low, Untitled document on the sanitary administration of Nantyglo and Blaina UD, p. 3.

[113] Gelligaer UD, RMOH (1920), p. 72.

[114] NLW, Welsh Board of Health collection, Box 70Q, R. Bruce Low, Untitled report on the sanitary circumstances of the Rhymney Urban District, 30 January 1929, p. 4 (own pagination).

of cuts in expenditure. The unsatisfactory nature of the contract system meant that the Ministry of Health constantly advised local authorities to carry out the scavenging of their districts by direct labour. Gradually, this came to be done in most areas.[115]

The environment of south Wales was scarred and tainted by the winning of coal. Most obvious were the huge tips of colliery refuse that so dominated the landscape and which brought innumerable problems. These 'monuments to Industrialism' were initially deposited in the valleys themselves, but they later came increasingly to be dumped on the hillsides and mountains above the valley communities.[116] One such pyramid-shaped tip situated on the hillside above Tylorstown was apparently so large that it was visible from Somerset, 30 miles across the Bristol Channel.[117] Landslides and slips were common occurrences and caused damage to houses and roads, while rivers filled with slurry and subsequently flooded. Inundation during wet weather was a commonplace experience in the steep-sided valley communities creating innumerable problems. Houses were flooded and damaged, debris blocked roads, drains were choked and sewers became overcharged.[118] Councils did carry out some work to ameliorate the problems caused by flooding but it seems likely that this continued to be a problem well into the period after the Second World War.[119]

One aspect of the public environment in which there was marked improvement during the interwar years was in the provision of recreational and leisure amenities. Most industrial districts of south Wales lacked sufficient recreational facilities at the start of the period, while amenities specifically for children were considered by many to be one of the most pressing needs. The sight of young children 'wallowing during their play in the dusty, narrow thoroughfares' of Ebbw Vale moved a *Merthyr Express* reader to call for playgrounds to be erected around the town. The conditions in which they played constituted 'a crime against their health'.[120]

The Save the Children Fund attempted to highlight the dire need

---

[115] See for example Rhondda UD, RMOH (1931), p. 79; (1932), p. 70; (1937), p. 87.

[116] Richards, 'Improvement of colliery districts', p. 78.

[117] B. Naylor, *Quakers in the Rhondda 1926–1986* (Chepstow, 1986), p. 14.

[118] Rhondda UD, RMOH (1925), p. 22.

[119] For examples see Rhondda UD, RMOH (1937), p. 84; Nantyglo and Blaina UD, RMOH (1930), p. 10; it was only after the Aberfan tragedy of 1966 that problems of drainage and unstable coal-tips were given systematic consideration.

[120] *Merthyr Express* (12 July 1924), 3.

through its journal, describing how in Tonypandy, where there were no playgrounds, two children had been killed and three more injured by a slide in 1932 while playing on a nearby slag tip. In Tonypandy, at least, a playground was provided by the staff of the International Labour Office, while in other localities such facilities were being provided for by the Miners' Welfare Fund.[121] However, it seems clear that too often during the interwar period the coal-tip, the sewage-polluted river and the litter-strewn back lanes were the places of play of the children of south Wales.

Throughout the coalfield, groups of men and women were spurred on by the lack of leisure facilities in their towns and villages to make conscious efforts to improve their environment.[122] Such efforts were aided by the Miners' Welfare Fund, set up by the Mining Industry Act of 1920. This Fund was derived from a levy of one penny per ton on the output of every coal-mine, to be paid by the coalowners, and was intended 'to provide the miner and his family with fuller opportunities for recreation both of body and mind, with a brighter social life, and generally with a healthier and sweeter environment than the nature of his occupation can otherwise offer to him'.[123] In the first place the Fund was able to contribute to efforts to improve the health of miners and their families in a very direct way. Large grants were made to the convalescent homes, such as that at Talygarn, to branches of the St John's Ambulance Association, and to hospitals which treated miners. In addition, the Fund was instrumental in the provision of pithead baths during the interwar period and by 1938 was able to point to the thirty-two baths in operation and the nine under construction, together affording accommodation for 53,688 men, as evidence of the beneficial effect it was having on the quality of life in Welsh communities.[124] Almost £1 million had been expended in the construction of pithead baths.[125]

The most popular function of the Fund, at least as far as the men of south Wales were concerned, was the money spent on

[121] 'Children of unemployed Welsh miners', *The World's Children*, 12, 11 (1932), 164–7.

[122] See for example *Second Report of the Commissioner for the Special Areas* [Cmd. 5090], 1935–6, xiii, pp. 76–9.

[123] Miners' Welfare Fund, *First Report of the Committee Appointed by the Board of Trade to Allocate the Fund, 1921–22* (London, 1923), p. 6.

[124] On pithead baths see Evans and Jones, '"A blessing for the miner's wife"', 5–28; see also B. L. Coombes's comparison of Resolven and Glynneath in his *Miners Day*, pp. 106–7.

[125] Miners' Welfare Fund, *First Report*, p. 92.

recreational amenities. Three hundred schemes were financed in the period up to December 1938 in south Wales at a cost of £1.25million. These schemes ranged from the provision or extension of indoor activities in the form of workmen's institutes or welfare halls to the construction of outdoor amenities such as parks, children's playgrounds and recreation grounds. The extent to which grants made by this Fund could transform an area was demonstrated by the annual reports of the medical officer for Maesteg. In his report of 1920 the medical officer stated that the area was without 'recognised Parks, Recreation Grounds, and Swimming Baths, which would afford healthier recreation than Cinemas and Billiard Halls, however desirable the latter forms of amusement might be'.[126] By 1930 the medical officer was able to report that in recent years:

> much headway has been made with our social conveniences. Within the district we have the Miners' Welfare Grounds at the lower end of the valley, which consist of a children's playground, swimming bath, tennis courts, football and cricket field, and a bowling green with a commodious pavilion. In the central district we have the new park, which was opened in 1924 and which when completed will also have a children's playground, cricket and football fields, tennis courts, a bowling green, and flower sections.[127]

Work was also in progress on a similar park to serve the Caerau district.

During the mid and late 1930s the Commissioner for the Special Areas was instrumental in aiding efforts to improve facilities. Grants were provided to help purchase tools, materials, working-clothes and midday meals for volunteers engaged in work on recreational schemes initiated by the unemployed. Up to 1936 twelve recreation grounds, fourteen children's playgrounds and paddling pools, eleven football or cricket grounds, four tennis courts, two bowling greens, one putting green and an ornamental fishpond had been granted financial assistance.[128]

Chapter 4 has shown that working-class homes in interwar south Wales were often characterized by unhealthy conditions and it is evident that the region was also characterized by an unwholesome

---

[126] Maesteg UD, RMOH (1920), p. 4.
[127] Maesteg UD, RMOH (1930), p. 9.
[128] *Third Report of the Commissioner for the Special Areas* [Cmd. 5303], 1935–6, xii, p. 131.

public environment. While some improvements did take place in aspects of the public environment and sanitary infrastructure, it is also evident that other aspects of the environment deteriorated. Major improvements to the water supply came to fruition in the interwar period and large numbers of households were connected to a reliable, wholesome supply of fresh water for the first time. Similarly, sewerage systems were extended and improved in many parts of south Wales and many houses were connected to water-carriage sewerage systems for the first time. However, economic depression served to retard this work to some extent and fewer improvements were carried out than might have been anticipated in more favourable economic conditions. Councils were often unable to carry out essential public health work and householders generally lacked the means to connect their houses to the new water supplies and sewerage systems.

Some improvements were made to methods of scavenging in south Wales and to the leisure facilities available to the population but standards of air quality continued to be appalling. Thus, improvements were made to the environment of south Wales during the interwar period and a large proportion of the population found their lives and health chances improved as a result. However, the region continued to be characterized by unwholesome and insanitary conditions when compared with the rest of England and Wales.

VI

THE MIXED ECONOMY OF MEDICAL SERVICES

Recent work on the history of welfare has emphasized the 'mixed economy' of welfare providers and the 'moving frontier' over time between voluntary and statutory providers. In contrast to an older historiographical tradition that emphasized the 'crowding out' of other providers of welfare by the increasing responsibility of the state, this more recent work is a useful reminder that the state was not the only, nor indeed the main, provider of welfare and medical services during much of the twentieth century.[1] Medical historians, on the other hand, have long been aware that alternative medical systems and practitioners coexisted in competition with the orthodox, legally sanctioned system of medicine in a 'medical marketplace'; but, as has been noted by a number of historians, studies of twentieth-century medicine have tended to focus on the delivery of medical services by local government and the central state, and have only recently began to examine the 'mixed economy' of medical and welfare services in the twentieth century.[2] An examination of the range of providers of medical services in interwar south Wales allows us to understand what people did when they became ill and the services they utilized when deciding that medical aid was necessary.

This examination of medical services must be set in the context of the study as a whole in order to assess these services' effectiveness and their role in shaping the demographic landscape of interwar south Wales.[3] Until recently, the effectiveness of medicine and its

---

[1]   Geoffrey Finlayson, 'A moving frontier: voluntarism and the state in British social welfare, 1911–1949', *Twentieth Century British History*, 1, 2 (1990), 183–206; *idem, Citizen, State, and Social Welfare in Britain, 1830–1990* (Oxford, 1994); David Gladstone, *The Twentieth-Century Welfare State* (London, 1999), pp. 4–5. As Pat Thane noted, when her *Foundations of the Welfare State* was first published in 1982, it concentrated on the state as the primary provider of welfare but had to be revised to take account of this recognition of the 'mixed economy' of welfare when it was republished in 1996; Pat Thane, *Foundations of the Welfare State* (London, 1996), p. 4.

[2]   Jane Lewis, 'Providers, "consumers", the state and the delivery of health-care services in twentieth-century Britain', in A. Wear (ed.), *Medicine in Society: Historical Essays* (Cambridge, 1992), p. 317; Berridge, *Health and Society since 1939*, p. 1.

[3]   Attention is given to certain welfare and health services in Chapters 7 and 8.

success in prolonging and improving human life were unquestioned. The massive decline in mortality and improvements in life expectancy and quality of life were attributed to progress in medical science and the application of these advances through increasingly comprehensive medical services.[4] More recently, however, historians have questioned the influence of medicine on the demographic transition of the modern period. Most noticeably, the writings of Thomas McKeown challenged the view that developments in medical science were the cause of the 'modern rise of population'.[5] He argued that curative medicine was responsible for only a very small part of the decline in mortality during the late nineteenth and early twentieth centuries, and only began to make a difference in the latter half of the twentieth century. After eliminating other possible explanations, McKeown attributed the massive fall in mortality to improvements in living standards and, in particular, improvements in the nutritional standards of the population, which, he asserted, accounted for about half of the total decrease in mortality. Such arguments were controversial and provoked prolonged debate and detailed criticism.[6] It is, therefore, necessary to outline what medical services were available to the population of interwar south Wales and, second, to assess their influence on standards of health and mortality patterns.

On becoming ill and deciding that action was required, sufferers were faced with a wide variety of medical services and practitioners. Medical anthropologists have often employed a schema that divides a society's medical services into three parts. Each of these three

---

[4]   Brieger, 'Historiography of medicine', 24; Virgina Berridge, 'Health and medicine', in F. M. L. Thompson (ed.), *The Cambridge Social History of Britain, 1750–1950*, vol. 3, *Social Agencies and Institutions* (Cambridge, 1990), pp. 171–3; examples of this celebratory, positivist tendency in a Welsh context include J. H. L. Mabbitt, *The Health Services of Glamorgan* (Cowbridge, 1977), pp. 12–19; John Cule (ed.), *Wales and Medicine* (Llandysul, 1975).

[5]   Thomas McKeown, *The Modern Rise of Population* (London, 1976); *idem*, *The Role of Medicine: Dream, Mirage or Nemesis?* (Princeton, 1979).

[6]   Many of the contributions to this debate were published in *Population Studies*. Particularly important contributions include Simon Szreter, 'The importance of social intervention in Britain's mortality decline, *c.*1850–1914: a reinterpretation of the role of public health', *Social History of Medicine*, 1 (1988), 1–37; R. I. Woods, P. A. Watterson and J. H. Woodward, 'The causes of rapid infant mortality decline in England and Wales, 1861–1921', part I, *Population Studies*, 42, 3 (1988), 343–66; part II, *Population Studies*, 43, 1 (1989), 113–32; the essays collected in the following volumes also engage with the McKeownite thesis: A. Brändström and L.-G. Tedebrand (eds), *Society and Health during the Demographic Transition* (Stockholm, 1988); R. Schofield, D. Reher and A. Bideau (eds), *The Decline of Mortality in Europe* (Oxford, 1991).

overlapping sectors of medical care – the 'popular', the 'folk' and the 'professional' – has its own way of explaining and treating disease.[7] The first sector of a society's health system is the 'popular' sector. This is the lay, non-professional, non-specialist domain where illness is first recognized and defined, and health care activities first initiated.[8] This is the largest medical sector of any society and, according to some estimates, deals with between 70 and 90 per cent of all illness incidents.[9] At times of illness, the first port of call for advice and treatment was, and indeed still is, the family, and this was the main arena of this sector.[10] The woman or women within a family, or else a female relative or neighbour, provided medical treatment and nursing care in working-class families.[11] Lay knowledge and treatment were invariably passed down from mother to daughter but women also consulted close friends and neighbours and shared favourite cures with each other.[12] Gossip and conversation played a vital role in the sharing and support networks that underpinned life in many working-class districts and served as a conduit for various forms of useful information, including medical advice and treatments.[13]

Systems of 'family', or 'domestic', medicine occupied an integral position in working-class strategies to maintain health and treat illness. Barbara Hardy of Swansea remembered how 'Daily life was stiff with superstition', much of it concerned with health:

> If you put too much vinegar on your food . . . it would thin your blood. Too much salt would dry it up. If you ate too much of anything, you would die of eating diabetes. If you fidgeted or shuffled in your chair at meals, you had worms or St Vitus's dance.[14]

'Superstitious' fears of the type remembered by Hardy were usually on behalf of children who were thought to be vulnerable

---

[7] Arthur K. Kleinman, *Patients and Healers in the Context of Culture* (London, 1980), pp. 50–60; Cecil Helman, *Culture, Health and Illness: An Introduction for Health Professionals* (London, 1984), pp. 43–64.

[8] Kleinman, *Patients and Healers*, p. 43; Helman, *Culture, Health and Illness*, p. 50.

[9] Helman, *Culture, Health and Illness*, p. 50.

[10] Margaret Pelling, 'Unofficial and unorthodox medicine', in Irvine Loudon (ed.), *The Oxford Illustrated History of Western Medicine* (Oxford, 1997), p. 271.

[11] Jones, *Health and Society in Twentieth Century Britain*, p. 59.

[12] Roberts, *A Woman's Place*, p. 191.

[13] Melanie Tebbutt, 'Women's talk? Gossip and "women's words" in working-class communities, 1880–1939', in Andrew Davies and Steven Fielding (eds), *Workers' Worlds: Cultures and Communities in Manchester and Salford, 1880–1939* (Manchester, 1992), pp. 49, 54.

[14] Barbara Hardy, *Swansea Girl: A Memoir* (London, 1994), p. 34.

throughout the year, 'especially if they were thin, fat, nervy or pale'. Parents were 'obsessed' with the dangers of childhood constipation. Responding to these fears parents utilized preventive treatments and dosed their children with all manner of tonics, potions and medicines. In Hardy's case it was brimstone and treacle, Californian syrup of figs or 'that most loathsome of all . . . medicines', senna.[15]

It was not only children who were treated in this way. People of all ages resorted to a great variety of domestic treatments in their efforts to prevent sickness and cure illness. Ron Berry of Blaenycwm in the Rhondda Fawr valley remembered the large range of domestic *materia medica* used to battle sickness in his home:

> we fought against sickness with goose grease, hot salt in socks, poultices, warmed flannels, Sloan's liniment, zinc ointment, vinegar and brown paper, the squeezed juice of *Mind your own business* grown in a tin on the windowsill for earache, senna pods, wintergreen oil, liquid paraffin, Epsom salts, bicarb., Vaseline, cloves, elderflower tea, *Syrup of Figs*, olive oil, borax powder, eucalyptus oil.[16]

Patent medicines were also easily acquired and newspapers contained numerous advertisements extolling the virtues of various medicines.[17] Seidlitz powders, Fennings Fever Cure, Ipecacuanha Wine, Parishes Food, Zambuk, Virol, Cod Liver Oil and Malt were just some of the patent medicines that allowed people to treat themselves.[18] The elaborate, alien-sounding names of these products were meant to be part of the attraction. Walter Haydn Davies noted how salesmen plying these products in the marketplaces of Dowlais and Pontypridd went to great lengths to emphasize the novelty and exotic nature of their products:

> Often salesmen donned cap and gown to give a note of academic distinction to their sales talk. They often had a diagram of the human body, with the circulatory system traced in pillar-box red . . . These persons called themselves Professors, and if they were dark-skinned – the darker the better – the

---

[15] Ibid., pp. 34–5; see also J. Grenfell-Hill (ed.), *Growing up in Wales 1895–1939* (Llandysul, 1996), 40; Eyles and O'Sullivan, *In the Shadows of the Steelworks*, p. 53.

[16] Ron Berry, *History is What you Live* (Llandysul, 1998), p. 35.

[17] To such an extent that patent medicines were sometimes known as 'tabloid medicines'; *Report as to the Practice of Medicine and Surgery by Unqualified Persons in the United Kingdom* [Cd. 5422], 1910, XLIII, p. 45.

[18] Twamley, *Cardiff and Me*, p. 43.

more gullible were more ready to buy, hoping that whatever they bought would contain some Eastern magic.[19]

The second sector of a medical system consists of the 'folk' *folk* sector, in which certain individuals specialize in forms of healing that are outside the official, orthodox system of medicine.[20] This sector includes a wide range of practitioners and was surprisingly large in interwar south Wales. A government inquiry carried out just before the First World War found that certain types of unofficial practitioners were very prevalent in south Wales. For example, the people of the mining valleys, in common with other mining districts and the slate quarrying communities of north Wales, were strong believers in the efficacy of the techniques of bonesetters.[21] These (usually male) practitioners attempted to give relief to stiff joints, dislocations, sprains and fractures by the manipulation of limbs or the body. Belief in these men was said to be implicit and bonesetters were regarded as medical practitioners in their own right. Something of their status and position in south Wales can be gauged from the fact that two bonesetters, William Price of Merthyr and Albert Whittle of Aberdare, advertised their services in a local directory.[22] Bonesetters held a privileged position among practitioners in south Wales and were even accepted, albeit with qualifications, by the medical establishment. Bonesetters were later accepted into the medical profession as chiropractors and osteopaths, and it is indicative, for example, that D. Rocyn Jones, the Monmouthshire county medical officer, was the descendant of three generations of bonesetters and had a brother who continued the family tradition during the interwar period.[23]

The inquiry of 1910 also noted that herbalists were very popular *herbalist* in Wales and this continued to be the case during the interwar period despite a decline in the number of practitioners.[24] Medical

---

[19] W. H. Davies, *Blithe Ones* (Port Talbot, 1979), p. 61.

[20] Helman, *Culture, Health and Illness*, p. 46; Kleinman, *Patients and Healers*, pp. 59–60.

[21] On bonesetters, see Roger Cooter, 'Bones of contention? Orthodox medicine and the mystery of the bone-setters craft', in Bynum and Porter, *Medical Fringe and Medical Orthodoxy*, pp. 158–73.

[22] *Kelly's Directory of Monmouthshire and South Wales* (1926), p. 1261.

[23] Thomas Jones, *Rhymney Memories* (Newtown, 1938), pp. 63–5.

[24] P. S. Brown has demonstrated how the numbers of herbalists in south Wales rose dramatically in the period 1871 to 1921 and then fell sharply in the interwar years and has suggested that the numbers mirrored the region's economic fortunes; see his 'The vicissitudes of herbalism in late nineteenth- and early twentieth-century Britain', *Medical History*, 29, 1 (1985), 71–92.

herbalism was characterized by the desire that medicine should be as democratic and open as possible and by the belief that ordinary people treating themselves with simple herbal remedies could break the monopoly of the medical establishment. Democratic, self-improving and providential, medical botany flourished in those communities where that culture was strongest and where dissenting religion was able to challenge the established church for adherents.[25] Health and faith did not derive from doctors or priests but lay within the power of the individual.[26] Ranging themselves against the sectional, monopolistic interests of the medical establishment, herbalists presented their skills and knowledge as a means by which ordinary people could become their own doctors and treat themselves without recourse to the 'poisonous' and 'evil' polypharmacy of orthodox medicine. 'I believe in Medical liberty' declared Dr John Rees Yemm.[27] Furthermore, natural, health-giving herbal treatments were infinitely preferable to the unnatural methods practised by qualified doctors and were, in any case, more effective.

Most vocal among south Wales herbalists was the Revd Thomas Gwernogle Evans of Neath. In 1922 he published a pamphlet on medical botany, costing 1s 6d, encouraging readers to administer to their own health and illnesses.[28] 'Keep it on your table, alongside of the Bible', he advised his readers, 'consult the both continually for the highest welfare of your body and soul'.[29] Stating that he had no quarrel with the medical profession, Evans nevertheless attacked it for its 'poisonous drug system', the unnecessary operations it carried out, and the elitism and egotism of the profession that only allowed qualified practitioners to be recognized – 'Degrees and diplomas will not cure diseases' he asserted.[30] In Evans's opinion, the means

[25]   Ursula Miley and John V. Pickstone, 'Medical botany around 1850: American medicine in industrial Britain', in Roger Cooter (ed.), *Studies in the History of Alternative Medicine* (London, 1988), pp.140–54; John V. Pickstone, 'Establishment and dissent in nineteenth-century medicine: an exploration of some correspondence and connections between religious and medical belief systems in early industrial England', in W. J. Sheils (ed.), *The Church and Healing* (Oxford, 1982), pp. 165–89; Roy Porter, *The Greatest Benefit to Mankind: A Medical History of Humanity from Antiquity to the Present* (London, 1997), pp. 283–4, 389–96.

[26]   Roy Porter, 'Religion and medicine', in Bynum and Porter, *Companion Encyclopedia of Medicine*, p. 1461.

[27]   NLW, MS 306B, T. D. Gwernogle Evans, 'Llysieuwyr (Herbalists) Hen, a Newydd, Yng Nghymru', Eisteddfod Genedlaethol Llanelly, 1930, 98.

[28]   T. D. Gwernogle Evans, *The Cup of Health* (Cardiff, 1922).

[29]   Ibid., p. 14.

[30]   Ibid., p. 9.

to maintain health and battle illness were present in the herbs and plants that had been provided by God.[31] Plants were heaven-sent preventives and treatments that were in harmony with nature and could therefore maintain or restore equilibrium.

Herbalists that practised in south Wales during the interwar period ranged from highly educated, 'professional' practitioners to self-educated lay practitioners. Dr John Rees Yemm is characteristic of this first type. Yemm first became interested in herbalism through the works of Nicholas Culpeper, an English herbalist of the seventeenth century, when his father became ill. Later acquainting himself with the works of other notable herbalists, Yemm embarked on a prolonged course of professional training in herbalism. In 1921 he sat and passed the examinations of the National Association of Medical Herbalists (NAMH), embarked on a lecture tour of Lancashire and, in 1926, was elected to the council of the NAMH. Yemm then took courses in physiotherapy and naturopathy in Chicago and received a doctorate in the latter from the National College of Naturopathy in Iowa.[32] He built up an extensive practice in the Ammanford area and, at the same time, promoted the interests of organized herbalism through his editorship of the journal *Medical Herbalist*, the official organ of the NAMH, which he held from its creation in 1925 to 1936.[33] This côterie of herbalists in south Wales, and the wider movement of which it was a part, saw itself as a highly skilled profession and aspired to official recognition. Constantly criticizing the state-protected monopoly of orthodox medicine, the NAMH lobbied the government to grant it professional status.[34] A fund was started to build a college where herbalists could be trained and professional qualifications conferred.

At the other end of the spectrum were the 'unqualified', non-professional herbalists to be found in most communities in south Wales who were either the inheritors of family traditions of herb-lore or who had educated themselves in the methods and treatments of herbalism. Most families used some form of herbal remedy even if it was only elderflower wine, nettle tea or some sort of poultice. Despite this widespread lay knowledge, certain persons

[31]   Evans co-authored a series of articles on herbalism that were published in *Medical Herbalist* entitled 'The garden of the Lord'.
[32]   Evans, 'Llysieuwyr (Herbalists) Hen, a Newydd, Yng Nghymru', pp. 96–7.
[33]   Ibid., p. 98; *Medical Herbalist* (Dec. 1936).
[34]   Brown, 'Vicissitudes of herbalism', 81–8.

knowledgeable in the use of herbs became practitioners in their communities and were consulted by sufferers in the same way as any other medical practitioner.[35] An example of this type of herbalist was 'Granny Marsh' of Griffithstown, Pontypool, who grew her own herbs in her garden, charged nothing for the various ointments she administered for fear that they would lose their efficacy, and who passed secret remedies to her daughter so that they could continue to be used.[36] Despite the aspirations of the 'professional' herbalists, they often felt an affinity with these folk practitioners. An article in the *Medical Herbalist* by W. J. Gwyddonwy Evans praised 'Gwen of Berthlwyd', a herbalist in the Swansea valley, for her knowledge of physiology and pathology, and for her excellent diagnostic skills.[37] Herbalists in interwar south Wales did not confine themselves to medical herbalism but saw themselves as eclectic practitioners of a wide variety of the systems of 'naturopathy'. The herbalist J. F. Bridgman of Neath, for example, received a great deal of work as a urine-caster while John Yemm claimed to be skilled in 'Osteopathy, Chiropractic, Eclecticism, Biochemic, Hydrotherapy, Physio-Medicalism, scientific herbalism'.[38]

Apart from these various classes of practitioner who aspired to some form of professional and legal recognition, there existed in south Wales a great variety of alternative practitioners who stood outside the legal and professional establishment and who were strongly attacked and condemned by orthodox practitioners. Despite this scorn and opposition, many of the unofficial folk practitioners were enormously popular among a large proportion of the population. For example, many Welsh people placed a great deal of faith in 'Water Casters' or 'Water Doctors' and, once having obtained a reputation as such, practitioners could build an 'immense practice, people coming from miles around sending him specimens of urine, from which he professes to diagnose their

[35] For example see Webb, *From Caerau to the Southern Cross*, pp. 35–6.

[36] L. Duncombe, D. Page, D. Stokes and S. Wilcox (eds), *Under the Doctor* (Pontypool, 1995), pp. 41–4. 'Secret' remedies were commonly passed down through families; for example see Davies, *Story of my Life*, p. 230.

[37] W. J. Gwyddonwy Evans, 'The oldest Welsh herbalist', *Medical Herbalist*, 10, 10 (May 1935), 186–7.

[38] Evans, 'Llysieuwyr (Herbalists) Hen, a Newydd, Yng Nghymru', p. 97. Bridgman was the sixth generation of a Lancashire family of herbalists and his brother, T. E. Bridgman, was also a herbalist, in Swansea. Upon J. F. Bridgman's death his practice went to his son; *Neath Guardian* (6 January 1939), 6.

ailments'.[39] J. F. Bridgman of Neath was said to be extremely busy
in his practice.[40] Urine-casting, or uroscopy, was a diagnostic proced-
ure which dated from antiquity but which had been attacked during
the sixteenth and seventeenth centuries as irrational and magical,
and had undergone decline as a respectable medical practice.[41] And
yet the practice continued to be popular among lay people, especially in the more remote parts of the country. Urine-casters either
treated their patients themselves or else referred them to another
practitioner after identifying their ailments and they were the only
purely diagnostic practitioners outside orthodox medicine in Wales
during the interwar period.[42]

The medical establishment was even more vehemently opposed
to other unofficial practitioners, as the practice of 'torri'r llech'
demonstrates. This practice dated from at least the eighteenth
century and was intended as a cure for rickets or for 'all cases of
backwardness from whatever cause'.[43] It involved an 'operation'
that consisted of making an incision into a certain part of a child's
ear. Carried out with a razor blade during the waxing of the moon,
the process was usually performed by a woman who had been
instructed in the custom by her mother. The operation had to be
carried out three times on a child before success could be assured.
Originating in Cardiganshire and Pembrokeshire, the custom
spread to urban areas of south Wales through the migration of
people to the industrialized south. Doctors who came across the
custom condemned it as a 'barbarous practice' and a 'fetish',
appealing only to the ignorant and the superstitious, and were
concerned with the risk of septic poisoning. The practice of 'torri'r
llech' was characterized by many aspects common to other forms of
folk medicine. For example, the importance of carrying out the
'operation' at a particular time in the moon's phase points to a

[39] *Report as to the Practice of Medicine and Surgery by Unqualified Persons in the United Kingdom*,
5–6.
[40] Evans, 'Llysieuwyr (Herbalists) Hen, a Newydd, Yng Nghymru', p. 95.
[41] Roy Porter, '"I think ye both quacks": the controversy between Dr Theodor
Myersbach and Dr John Coakley Lettsom', in Bynum and Porter, *Medical Fringe and Medical
Orthodoxy*, p. 58.
[42] On the position of diagnosticians in other cultures see David Landy (ed.), *Culture,
Disease and Healing: Studies in Medical Anthropology* (London, 1977), pp. 161–2.
[43] On 'torri'r llech' see *Western Mail* (20 April 1921), 3; (21 April 1921), 5; *Llanelly Star*
(11 March 1933), 1, 6; (18 March 1933), 1; J. C. Davies, *Folk-lore of West and Mid-Wales*
(Aberystwyth, 1911), p. 286; T. Gwynn Jones, *Welsh Folklore and Folk Custom* (London, 1930), p.
144. *Torri* – to cut; *llech* – rickets.

holistic conception of the body that placed it at the centre of the universe. The links between the moon and the blood were thought to be strong.[44]

Another controversial and criticized system of medicine in south Wales was spiritualism, a system of healing that depended on the assistance of the spirits of the dead. Spiritualists asserted that there was no such reality as somatic disease – all sickness was in the mind and so spiritualism, or 'mind healing', would dispel the 'illusions' of illness. W. J. Lewis, the medical officer of Pontardawe, found that in his district in the immediate post-war years this type of treatment was on the increase. 'All standards are in the melting pot', he commented, 'every canon repudiated. Sports and spirits are usurping the place of purpose in our lives.' Lewis attributed this increase to the uncertain economic conditions of the early 1920s and the prospect of an even more uncertain future but it is clear that spiritualism increased in popularity following the losses of the First World War as relatives attempted to communicate with family members who lost their lives in the war.[45] Uncertainty, worry and distress were manifesting themselves in ailments, and spiritualism can, in part, be seen as a reaction to contemporary concerns. Many commented that spiritualists were primarily patronized by women.[46] It seems evident that the pressures faced by the women of the mining communities during the course of their everyday lives were manifesting themselves in mental and psychosomatic problems. This is not to argue that the illnesses and ailments that afflicted women were 'all in the mind' or merely psychosomatic, only that the constant strains of many women's lives affected their sense of well-being and that they often sought relief in spiritualism.

Thus, there existed a wide variety of unofficial medical practitioners in interwar south Wales who competed with the medical establishment to meet the medical needs of the population. The efficacy of these practitioners and their treatments varied. It is hard to imagine that the techniques of urine-casters were of any use to ill people, and the practices of 'torri'r llech' and spiritualism can similarly be dismissed as curative treatments. Bone-setting and

[44] Françoise Loux, 'Folk medicine', in Bynum and Porter, *Companion Encyclopedia of the History of Medicine*, pp. 665–7.

[45] On spiritualism in this period, see Jennifer Hazelgrove, *Spiritualism and British Society between the Wars* (Manchester, 2000).

[46] Armbruster, 'Social determination of ideologies', 123; Grenfill-Hill, *Growing up in Wales*, p. 167.

herbalism, on the other hand, cannot be completely dismissed and brought some relief to patients. Lay knowledge and self-treatment, with their emphasis on preventive measures and the management of the regimen of the patient, were probably of some use in preventing illness. This lay knowledge was based on the management of the 'six non-naturals' of food and drink, retention and evacuation, environment, sleep, exercise and state of mind, and was, in this sense at least, not dissimilar to orthodox, scientific medicine.[47] The treatments and cures that derived from lay knowledge were probably much less successful in effecting cures and there is no reason to believe that lay knowledge in south Wales was significantly different or superior in its curative capacities than lay knowledge elsewhere in Britain.

The third and last sector of a medical system is the professional sector, which comprises the organized, legally sanctioned healing professions.[48] By the twentieth century, this sector was considerable in size and very powerful in its ability to influence governments and determine social policy.[49] In the first place, it is important to note that south Wales was a relatively disadvantaged region in terms of medical resources despite the massive need that existed. The fact that such a large proportion of the population was engaged in metallurgical industries and coalmining had profound consequences for standards of health and the precise nature of illness and sickness to be found in the region. Coalmining, in particular, was an extremely dangerous and hazardous occupation that caused a large amount of injury and disease. In addition, the South Wales Coalfield, because of the geology of the coal measures and the character of the coal, was one of the most unhealthy and injurious coalfields in Britain, characterized by a greater incidence of accidents and a greater degree of industrial disease than other coalfields or industrial districts.[50] In such an environment, it might be argued,

---

[47]   L. J. Rather, 'The "six things non-natural": a note on the origins and fate of a doctrine and a phrase', *Clio Medica*, 3, 4 (1968), 337.

[48]   Helman, *Culture, Health and Illness*, pp. 50–3; Kleinman, *Patients and Healers*, pp. 53–9.

[49]   Useful surveys of medicine and health services in the interwar period include Steven Cherry, *Medical Services and the Hospitals in Britain, 1860–1939* (Cambridge, 1996); Berridge, 'Health and medicine'.

[50]   N. Woodward, 'Why did south Wales miners have high mortality? Evidence from the mid-twentieth century', *Welsh History Review*, 20, 1 (2000), 116–41; Francis and Smith, *The Fed*, pp. 438–41; J. Benson, *British Coalminers in the Nineteenth Century: A Social History* (Dublin, 1980), pp. 37–47.

Table 6.1. Number of doctors in south Wales and England and Wales as a whole, 1921

	No. of doctors	Population per doctor
England and Wales	22,965	1,650
Glamorgan AC	592	2,116
Monmouthshire AC	188	2,398
Cardiff CB	75	2,669
Newport CB	63	1,466
Swansea CB	72	2,188
Merthyr Tydfil CB	22	3,642
Aberdare UD	15	3,667
Rhondda UD	63	2,583
Mountain Ash UD	19	2,278
Abertillery UD	13	2,985
Tredegar UD	6	4,185

Source: Census of England and Wales, 1921.

there was a massive demand for doctors and yet, because of the character of medical practice before the creation of the National Health Service in 1948, and because of the overwhelmingly working-class character of the population in south Wales, the region experienced a shortage of doctors relative to other parts of Britain. Table 6.1 demonstrates the number of doctors in certain districts of south Wales and the ratio of population to doctors.

These statistics are crude in that they assume that the doctors serving the population of a particular urban district also lived in that district. It is entirely possible, of course, that doctors lived outside the local authority districts in which they practised. However, despite the problems inherent in these statistics, they give an indication of the relative shortage of medical practitioners in south Wales, and in particular the industrial districts where the demand for their services was so high. The massive workloads caused by these high patient-to-doctor ratios, and the social isolation experienced by doctors who practised in industrial districts, could result in stress, ill health and even substance abuse on the part of doctors.[51]

[51] See for example James Mullin, *The Story of a Toiler's Life* (London, 1921), pp. 151, 152, 160; Francis Maylett Smith, *The Surgery at Aberffrwd: Some Encounters of a Colliery Doctor Seventy Years Ago* (Hythe, Kent, 1981), p. 88; Anne Digby, *The Evolution of British General Practice, 1850–1948* (Oxford, 1999), p. 281.

Apart from the number of doctors available to the population, it is also important to inquire into the ways in which these primary medical services were organized, that is, how ordinary people gained access to general practitioner services. Before the creation of the National Health Service (NHS) in 1948, working-class people obtained medical attendance and care by a variety of means. First, working-class patients were able to consult a doctor as a private patient.[52] A private consultation was relatively expensive for working-class families and further care or treatment could impose unbearable burdens on their budgets. Moreover, the increasingly scientific and technical nature of medicine in the early twentieth century meant that medical care was becoming more expensive and even placed a burden on the budgets of middle-class families.

If the fees of doctors were too onerous, working-class or poor families were able to draw on the medical services offered under the Poor Law, although these were stigmatizing to recipients and tended to discourage people from using them. In addition to these methods of obtaining medical attendance there was a variety of insurance systems of medical provision, whereby a weekly payment bought rights to medical attendance and medicines. Notable among working-class efforts to provide medical attendance were the works' clubs where workers arranged with their employer for an agreed sum to be deducted from their pay and for a doctor to be employed through the resulting fund. These works' clubs, which existed throughout Britain and in many industries, achieved their most developed state in the industrial areas of south Wales.[53] Known more commonly in south Wales as 'medical aid societies', these organizations provided sick benefits and, more importantly, medical attendance and drugs for the workmen and their dependants in return for a payment of about 2d or 3d in each pound of the workers' wages. Workers contributed when they were healthy and in employment, and benefited during times of illness.

Initially begun as works' clubs in the late nineteenth and early twentieth centuries, many of the more active societies by the

[52]   See David G. Green, *Working-Class Patients and the Medical Establishment: Self Help in Britain from the Mid-Nineteenth Century to 1948* (Aldershot, 1985).

[53]   Steven Thompson, 'A proletarian public sphere: working-class self-provision of medical services and care in South Wales, *c.*1900–1948', in Anne Borsay (ed.), *Medicine in Wales, c.1800–2000: Public Service or Private Commodity?* (Cardiff, 2003), pp. 86–107; Ray Earwicker, 'Miners' medical services before the First World War: the South Wales Coalfield', *Llafur*, 3, 2 (1981), 39–52.

interwar period had evolved to become sophisticated organizations providing medical attendance and a host of other services to the whole community in which they were situated. Higher revenues meant a better developed and more comprehensive service and so it was common for committees to approach and welcome additional groups of workers to their schemes and make them as universal as possible.[54] A typical example of these larger, more inclusive societies was the Tredegar Medical Aid Society. Begun in 1874 by a section of the miners and steelworkers of the town, the society gradually developed into a much more ambitious and comprehensive scheme so that by the 1920s about 95 per cent of the population of the town was covered for medical treatment by the society. The miners and steelworkers paid according to a poundage system by deductions of 2d in each pound of their weekly wages, while so-called 'town subscribers' paid 18s a year directly to the society.[55] Similarly, the Ebbw Vale Workmen's Medical Society provided medical attendance and benefit for 24,000 people by 1920.[56] Thus, although eligibility was based on the payment of a subscription, these funds and societies established by a section of the workforce in many cases became a public service as efforts were made to make them accessible to large proportions of the population. In contrast to the system of medical care created under the National Insurance scheme, many club practices in south Wales also made provision for the wives and children of workers. Furthermore, aged workmen and widows were able to call on the Tredegar society's services at no charge.[57]

This mutuality was evident during the interwar years when public meetings were held to ask certain workmen to increase their contributions to aid societies through the difficult economic period[58] and meetings of the unemployed were also held to discuss their relationship with the societies. Five meetings of the unemployed in different parts of Maesteg were held in February 1931, for example, to discover their response to a proposed

[54]   Thompson, 'Proletarian public sphere'.

[55]   *Picture Post* (27 April 1946), 20–1; Finch, *Memoirs of a Bedwellty MP*, pp. 33–5; Green, *Working-Class Patients and the Medical Establishment*, p. 174.

[56]   A. Gray-Jones, *A History of Ebbw Vale* (Risca, 1970), p. 245; the population of the Ebbw Vale Urban District was enumerated as 35,381 by the census of 1921.

[57]   Earwicker, 'Miners' medical services', 41.

[58]   See for example South Wales Coalfield Collection, Bedlinog Medical Committee minutes, 30 September 1924 and 1 October 1924; see also Gwent Record Office, Tredegar Workingmen's Medical Aid Society, General Purposes Committee minutes, 13 July 1921.

Unemployment Scheme offered by the Maesteg Medical Fund. In the event, all meetings were 'Unanimously in favour' of the proposed scheme which required a fee of 2d per week from unemployed families.[59] In these ways the medical aid societies and cottage hospitals of south Wales were an articulation not only of an individualized notion of self-help but also of a collectivized mutuality that made the sick and the ill a charge on the whole community. It was even suggested that the Mountain Ash and Penrhiwceiber Hospital should be renamed 'The Temple of Equal Chance'.[60]

Although the 1911 National Health Insurance Act curtailed the expansion of these medical aid societies, it did not completely emasculate them. Small improvements continued to be made so that by the interwar period the schemes of south Wales were among the most sophisticated and highly developed health services in the whole of Britain. To take Tredegar as an example once more, by the 1920s the society offered its members the services of five doctors, one surgeon, two pharmacists, a physiotherapist, a dentist, and a district nurse. For an additional 4d a week members were insured against the cost of hospital treatment, and a car was provided to the railway station where a first-class ticket was made available to reach the hospital.[61] Glasses could be obtained for 2s 6d, while false teeth were sold at less than cost price. Artificial limbs, injections, patent foods, drugs, X-rays and even wigs were free to members.[62] Similarly, the Llanelli and District Medical Service

[59]   South Wales Coalfield Collection, Maesteg Medical Fund Committee minutes, 17 Jan. and 28 Feb. 1931.

[60]   Mountain Ash and Penrhiwceiber Hospital, *Thirteenth Annual Report and Financial Statement* (1937), 15.

[61]   Many medical aid societies subscribed to hospitals in Cardiff, Swansea, Bristol and even London to allow their members access to specialist medical services not available in the smaller hospitals of the valleys. Medical aid societies do not seem to have existed in the coastal towns of south Wales, or at least were not as well developed as those in the inland valleys. The workers in the coastal towns contributed to hospital contributory schemes so as to gain access to hospital medical services. On hospital contributory schemes, see Steven Cherry, 'Beyond national health insurance: the voluntary hospitals and hospital contributory schemes: a regional study', *Social History of Medicine*, 5, 3 (1992), 455–82; T. G. Davies, *Deeds Not Words: A History of the Swansea General and Eye Hospital, 1817–1948* (Cardiff, 1988); T. A. Jones, 'The Royal Gwent Hospital (Workmen's Fund)', in *Newport Encyclopedia: Coronation Year and Royal Visit Souvenir* (Newport, 1937), p. 134. In this last case the Workmen's Hospital Fund provided 60% of the hospital's income in the years preceding the advent of the NHS; T. B. Jones and W. J. T. Collins, *History of the Royal Gwent Hospital* (Newport, 1948), pp. 54–60.

[62]   *Picture Post* (27 April 1946), 20–1; Green, *Working-Class Patients and the Medical Establishment*, p. 172.

offered its members general practitioner service, opthalmic, ear, nose, throat and general surgery services and defrayed the cost of special drugs.[63] Therefore, working-class people in south Wales successfully created robust, democratically controlled, mutualistic organizations that provided a range of medical services to a significant proportion of the population.

However, the quality of doctors in south Wales varied enormously. South Wales did not offer doctors the opportunity of practices with large numbers of wealthy, fee-paying, middle-class patients but was instead characterized by large practices with overwhelmingly working-class patients. There was a preponderance of doctors in regions such as the south-east of England, and London especially, where doctors were assured of a large number of relatively affluent patients in genteel surroundings. Many doctors did not consider south Wales an attractive option for medical practice and preferred to look for more profitable locations. On the other hand, employment in the large, well-organized medical aid societies could mean relatively high wages and some young doctors, fresh from medical college, looked to medical practice in industrial districts in order to earn a lump sum with which to purchase an established practice in a more affluent middle-class district. Some doctors were ideologically inclined to work in working-class districts while others were members of medical families who had practised in south Wales for generations. In consequence, the standard of medical practitioners to be found in south Wales varied enormously. Upon filling his first medical post in south Wales in 1922 the doctor, and later novelist, A. J. Cronin found that:

> in recent years Tregenny had seen an irregular coming and going of raw youngsters fresh from college, older practitioners unaware of what they had 'let themselves in for', licensed apothecaries with quasi-medical degrees, and, worst of all, a draggled succession of 'dead beats', doctors who had failed elsewhere, fallen into disrepute, or even been struck off the register for professional misconduct.[64]

Moreover, in the same way that south Wales did not attract many general practitioners it similarly did not attract many specialists

---

[63]   Political and Economic Planning (PEP), *Report on the British Health Services* (London, 1937), p. 151.

[64]   A. J. Cronin, *Adventures in Two Worlds* (London, 1952), p. 125; for similar comments, see Smith, *The Surgery at Aberffrwd*, p. 88.

and, as a result, general practitioners in south Wales were faced with a much wider set of responsibilities than their counterparts elsewhere. Florance O'Sullivan, a doctor who practised at Cwm, Ebbw Vale, observed that since there were so few specialists in the valleys of south Wales general practitioners were forced to attempt any emergency surgery, such as appendectomies or tonsillectomies, which they carried out, as he comments, 'with varying degrees of success'.[65] Similarly, there were very few qualified dentists in south Wales and doctors were forced to perform dental work as best they could.[66]

On the other hand, many doctors devoted their lives to service within working-class, industrial communities and were, for many people, respected and distinguished members of the community.[67] The doctor was, to some people at least, 'the king of life and death', a 'God-like man'.[68] Hard-working, dedicated doctors were liked and respected for their kindness and generosity, and, more importantly, for the sympathetic way in which they treated their patients. They served their communities not only in a medical capacity but also more generally in the wider community, whether in cultural, musical, political, social or other terms. The 'miner-writer' Bert Coombes, for example, maintained that, while there were doctors who were 'brutal and overbearing' in manner, these were only a minority and that for the most part 'no praise could be overdone' for the majority of doctors in mining regions. Likening them to 'guardian angels', Coombes emphasized the massive workloads, the social isolation doctors faced in colliery districts and the thankless nature of their work. The colliery doctor, Coombes opined, acted as 'confessor, clerk and general advisor to his people'.[69]

Another factor which mitigated the influence that doctors were able to have on the health of the population was the paucity of effective therapeutic weapons in a doctor's arsenal. This was because up until the 1930s, there was little that general practitioners could do to save lives from infectious or degenerative diseases that

---

[65]   F. O'Sullivan, *Return to Wales* (Tenby, 1974), p. 50.

[66]   Baker, 'Yan Boogie', pp. 120, 141–2; Bill Phillips, *A Kid from Splott* (Cardiff, 1985), pp. 34–5; Smith, *The Surgery at Aberffrwd*, p. 76.

[67]   See the reminiscences in Duncombe et al., *Under the Doctor*, pp. 17–20.

[68]   C. B. Edwards, '"It was like this": personal recollections of Garndiffaith in the 1930s', part II, *Gwent Local History*, 77 (1994), 44.

[69]   Coombes, *Miners Day*, pp. 124–5; for a further insight by the same author, see Coombes, *Those Clouded Hills*, p. 54.

had already been contracted by patients.[70] Salvarsan was an effective treatment for syphilis which was available from 1910, while
insulin was used in the management of diabetes after 1922.[71]
Immunization did protect individuals from certain diseases, such as
smallpox and diphtheria, but there was little that could be done to
cure other bacterial diseases until the development and use of
sulphonamides from the late 1930s and antibiotics from the 1940s.
The development of sulphonamides was an important break-
through in the fight against streptococcal infections, and while its
most noticeable influence was in reducing puerperal mortality it
was also used to treat whooping cough, measles, scarlet fever and
other infections, although with varying degrees of success.[72]
Similarly, sulphapyridine was developed from the sulpha drugs in
1938 and was effective in the treatment of lobar pneumonia.
However, effective immunization against these various infections
was not achieved until after the Second World War.

The treatment of tuberculosis in Wales was, in many ways, very
well developed as a result of the efforts of the Welsh National
Memorial Association established in 1910, but, as Linda Bryder has
shown, there is little reason to believe that the association had a
significant effect on the level of tuberculosis mortality and
morbidity in Wales.[73] In the first place, in common with tuberculosis services elsewhere, the association placed an emphasis on
individual behaviour rather than on social and economic factors
and so could not hope to lessen significantly the effects of poverty,
substandard diet and inadequate housing on patterns of tuberculosis morbidity and mortality in Wales.[74] The institutional treatment
of tuberculosis sufferers that characterized official approaches to
the problem in the early twentieth century was largely ineffective

---

[70]   Even members of the medical profession were doubtful of the efficacy of many of the
drugs they prescribed. A. J. Cronin's *The Citadel* (London, 1937) can be read as an attack on
the conservative nature of orthodox medicine and, in particular, the 'medicine swillers' who
believed that the remedy for every ailment could be found in the pharmacopoeia; see esp.
pp. 22–3, 28, 40–1, 133.

[71]   Cherry, *Medical Services and the Hospitals in Britain*, p. 19; Berridge, 'Health and medicine', p. 234.

[72]   Porter, *Greatest Benefit*, pp. 453–4; McKeown, *Role of Medicine*, pp. 50–2.

[73]   Linda Bryder, 'The King Edward VII Welsh National Memorial Association and its
policy towards tuberculosis, 1910–48', *Welsh History Review*, 13, 2 (1986), 194–216.

[74]   Ibid., 199.

because sufferers returned to the living conditions in which they had first contracted the disease.

Secondly, tuberculosis physicians and surgeons increasingly turned to surgical treatments during the 1930s as a result of the failure of these conservative methods, but there is no evidence that these surgical procedures were any more successful in preventing death or effecting cures.[75] Moreover, many councillors during the 1930s argued that local authorities were granting a disproportionate amount of their public health expenditure to the association and a larger proportion than their English counterparts. While tuberculosis only accounted for a small proportion of total deaths, it seemed incongruous that as much as half of the total expenditure of local public health authorities was granted to the association.[76] Tuberculosis was not effectively treated until the development of streptomycin and chemotherapy in the 1940s. Bacillus Calmette-Guerin (BCG) immunization was available from 1924 but was not widely used in Britain until the 1950s.[77] Despite the robust and comprehensive nature of working-class medical aid societies, variation in the skills and abilities of doctors, and a lack of effective therapeutic weapons against disease meant that medicine was only of limited value in the battle against sickness, disease and mortality in interwar south Wales.[78]

While the extent and quality of primary services in interwar south Wales were in certain respects inferior to those in other parts of Britain, the regional inequalities in the quality and extent of secondary services were even greater. This again was a result of the social and economic character of south Wales. In the period before the creation of the National Health Service, hospitals and other medical institutions and services were provided through philanthropic effort and, later and to a greater degree, by local authorities. Therefore, the financial capabilities of localities and local authorities determined the nature and scale of medical provision in an area, and working-class areas or regions were poorly provided with medical services. The philanthropic provision of hospital services in the nineteenth century left an important legacy of hospitals in twentieth-century south Wales as it did in other parts of Britain.

[75] Ibid., 200–2.
[76] Ibid., 207.
[77] Porter, *Greatest Benefit*, p. 442; McKeown, *Role of Medicine*, p. 50.
[78] For a similar point see Earwicker, 'Miners' medical services', 49.

Older, larger hospitals existed at Swansea (opened in 1817), Cardiff (1837), Newport (1860) and Merthyr Tydfil (1888). These had been provided through philanthropic activity in the nineteenth century and had been expanded in the period after their creation so that, by the interwar period, they were relatively large hospitals, at least in Welsh terms, equipped with a wide range of services and equipment.[79]

The extraordinary development of the coal industry in the late Victorian and Edwardian periods necessitated the development of hospital services for the burgeoning population of the industrial valleys of south Wales. A large number of general, cottage and accident hospitals were opened within a very short space of time: at Port Talbot in 1893, Porth and Barry in 1895, Mountain Ash in 1896, Ferndale in 1900, Ebbw Vale in 1901, Pontypool in 1903, Tredegar and Rhymney in 1904, Aberbargoed in 1909, Abertysswg in 1910, Blaina and Pontypridd in 1911, Oakdale in 1915, Maesteg and Aberavon in 1916, and at Aberdare and Caerphilly in 1917. During the interwar period, further hospitals were built at Abertillery in 1922, Mountain Ash and Pentwyn in the Rhondda Fawr valley in 1924, Clydach in 1925, Treherbert and Blaenavon in 1927, Port Talbot in 1932 and Llwynypia in 1935. Workers' contributions, donations from industrialists and landowners, and the more general philanthropic giving of the wider public in each community financed the erection of these hospitals, although it should be noted that the first of these sources provided the majority of funding. They ranged in size from general hospitals such as the Aberdare General Hospital with 96 beds and Merthyr Tydfil General Hospital with 115 beds to smaller hospitals such as the Abertysswg Workmen's Cottage Hospital with 14 beds and Ebbw Vale Workmen's Cottage hospital with 16 beds.[80]

[79] A. Trevor Jones, J. A. Nixon and R. M. F. Picken, *Hospital Survey: The Hospital Services of South Wales and Monmouthshire* (London, 1945); Jones and Collins, *History of the Royal Gwent Hospital*; Mabbitt, *The Health Services of Glamorgan*; Davies, *Deeds Not Words*; A. Lewis, 'The Story of Merthyr General Hospital', *Merthyr Historian*, 4 (1989), 104–30; Neil Evans, '"The First Charity in Wales": Cardiff Infirmary and South Wales Society, 1837–1914', *Welsh History Review*, 9, 3 (1979), 319–46.

[80] This was the number of beds in 1938; see Trevor Jones, Nixon and Picken, *Hospital Survey*, pp. 55, 57, 60; on hospital provision see also Steven Thompson, 'To relieve the sufferings of humanity, irrespective of party, politics or creed: conflict, consensus and voluntary hospital provision in Edwardian south Wales', *Social History of Medicine*, 16, 2 (2003), 247–62; *idem*, 'Hospital provision, charity and public responsibility in Edwardian Pontypridd', *Llafur*, 8, 3 (2002), 53–65.

Table 6.2. Hospital beds in England and 'South Wales', 1938

Type of hospital beds	Beds per 1,000 population, 1938	
	'South Wales'	England
Acute	2.16	3.32
Chronic	1.11	1.28
Maternity	0.18	0.27
Infectious disease	0.66	1.00
Tuberculosis	0.76	0.71
Total	4.87	6.58

Source: Martin Powell, 'How adequate was hospital provision before the NHS?', *Local Population Studies*, 48 (1992), 26. 'South Wales' = Breconshire, Cardiganshire, Carmarthenshire, Glamorgan, Monmouthshire, Pembrokeshire and Radnor.

This list of hospitals appears impressive but a closer analysis reveals that south Wales was a 'deprived region' in terms of hospital provision, both quantitatively and qualitatively.[81] Martin Powell, using the South Wales Hospital Survey carried out as part of a wider survey of hospital services in England and Wales, has demonstrated that hospital services in south Wales fell far short of the standards achieved in other regions of England and Wales. Powell showed how south Wales compared unfavourably with the other nine survey regions in England and Wales in all the criteria used to examine provision (see Table 6.2). In terms of the number of hospital beds per capita, south Wales was the most disadvantaged of the regions surveyed and, while it compared favourably to England as a whole in terms of tuberculosis beds, it was insufficiently supplied with beds for acute, chronic, maternity and infectious disease cases. Moreover, the institutions in south Wales were unsatisfactory by virtue of their small size, their age and their structural condition.[82] Therefore, south Wales was a 'deprived region' in terms of hospital provision and this supports the conclusion that, in

[81] Martin Powell, 'How adequate was hospital provision before the NHS? An examination of the 1945 South Wales Hospital Survey', *Local Population Studies*, 48 (1992), 31; see also *idem*, 'Hospital provision before the National Health Service: a geographical study of the 1945 hospital surveys', *Social History of Medicine*, 5, 3 (1992), 483–504; *idem*, 'The geography of English hospital provision in the 1930s', *Journal of Historical Geography*, 18, 3 (1992), 307–16; *idem*, 'Did politics matter? Municipal public health expenditure in the 1930s', *Urban History*, 22, 3 (1995), 360–79.
[82] Powell, 'How adequate was hospital provision before the NHS?'; Trevor Jones, Nixon and Picken, *Hospital Survey, passim*.

the period before the creation of the NHS, the geographical distribution of health care resources varied inversely with need.[83]

Faced with such a wide variety of practitioners and medical systems it is important to inquire who sufferers consulted and in what circumstances. It is not enough to describe and evaluate the various systems of medicine; we also need to know the extent to which sick individuals utilized the various practitioners and systems available to them and the circumstances in which they did so. What were the conventions and processes leading from sickness to response? What factors governed the choice of therapeutic action? How did ordinary people view the skills and techniques of the various practitioners available to them?[84] The answers to these questions can only be very tentative due to the scarcity of the sources. First, in most families every effort was made to treat an illness at home using domestic remedies. Sufferers typically followed a 'hierarchy of resort' that ranged from self-medication to consultation of other family members, usually the mother or wife, to consultation of neighbours or members of the community. Most communities possessed a person, usually a woman, who, though unqualified and unskilled, was consulted by friends and neighbours in times of illness.[85] A good example of this type of practitioner was 'Mrs Scott' of 'Aberffrwd' as described by Francis Maylett Smith. If anyone in 'Gwynfa Terrace' became ill, Mrs Scott, famous for her linseed poultices, was called. Once diagnosed by Mrs Scott sufferers saw no need to consult a doctor.[86] While these unofficial practitioners were cheaper than doctors,[87] it was also the case that their treatments were preferred. 'Mrs Pugh Zambuck', renowned throughout Bedlinog for her skill in treating boils and abscesses with poultices, was, to many people, infinitely preferable to the local doctor's ready lance.[88]

Certain practitioners gained a reputation as especially skilled in treating particular ailments. Mrs Scott was apparently adept at

---

[83] Julian Tudor Hart, 'The inverse care law', *The Lancet* (27 February 1971), 405–12; Jones, *Health and Society*, p. 174.

[84] Porter, 'Patient's view', 187.

[85] Such figures constituted the 'wise women ' and 'cunning men' of modern society; see Keith Thomas, *Religion and the Decline of Magic* (Harmondsworth, 1973), pp. 209–51.

[86] Smith, *The Surgery at Aberffrwd*, pp. 84–5.

[87] See for example Twamley, *Cardiff and Me Sixty Years Ago*, p. 43; Webb, *From Caerau to the Southern Cross*, p. 35.

[88] W. H. Davies, *Ups and Downs* (Swansea, 1975), p. 161; 'Zambuck' was the name of a patent medicine for skin complaints widely advertised in newspapers.

treating 'inflammation' while 'Granny Marsh' was famous for her various cure-all ointments.[89] It was said that the only thing that 'Granny Marsh' would not treat was ulcers and sufferers were sent straight to the hospital.[90] 'Quack-Quack' was renowned in Bedlinog for his various tonics intended to restore vitality and vigour, and he also formulated an embrocation greatly favoured by rheumatic miners.[91]

A doctor would only be called if it was 'absolutely necessary' and if the illness was 'serious'.[92] Just what this meant differed from one family to the next. The parents of Florence Amor of Cardiff were apparently terrified of infectious diseases and called the doctor in every instance of infectious disease, while Gwyneth Evans of Merthyr remembered how cases of diphtheria were 'expertly and quietly' nursed at home so as to avoid admittance to an isolation hospital.[93] Other families consulted the pharmacist for advice on treating infectious diseases.[94] Families differed in their ability to afford doctor's fees and also in the estimation of their own abilities, the seriousness they attached to an illness and the ailments they believed warranted the attentions of a doctor. One respondent in the popular history of medical care, *Under the Doctor*, remembered that when his or her brother broke his leg, their father set the leg between two pieces of wood and used crutches made from the branches of a tree – 'there was no money for the doctor you see, and even if there was this was not one of the things the doctor was consulted about'.[95]

Many practitioners were antipathetic towards other systems of medicine and often conceived of their own system of medicine as being diametrically opposed to that of other practitioners. Their patients, however, were much more ambivalent and less dogmatic. A patient of 'Granny Marsh', the herbalist from Griffithstown, suffering a septic wound to his hand, attended the doctor's surgery

[89]   Smith, *The Surgery at Aberffrwd*, p. 84; Duncombe et al., *Under the Doctor*, pp. 41–4; Grenfell-Hill, *Growing up in Wales*, p. 93.

[90]   Duncombe et al., *Under the Doctor*, p. 42.

[91]   Davies, *Blithe Ones*, pp. 58–62.

[92]   Anne Eyles's mother only called the doctor when domestic remedies had failed: *In the Shadow of the Steelworks*, p. 53. This was probably typical.

[93]   Grenfell-Hill, *Growing up in Wales*, p. 67; G. E. Evans, 'Reminiscences of the 1920s and early 1930s', Afon Tâf History Research Group, *Recollections of Merthyr's Past* (Newport, 1979), 52.

[94]   Duncombe et al., *Under the Doctor*, p. 33.

[95]   Ibid., p. 32.

weekly to obtain a sick note before seeing 'Granny Marsh' for treatment.[96] Sufferers used bonesetters for certain complaints and injuries while at the same time consulting a doctor for other illnesses.[97] The men of the Nixon's Collieries medical fund, for example, expressed the hope that they could employ a bonesetter with the money contributed from their weekly pay-packets in addition to the orthodox practitioner they were already paying for.[98] Similarly, despite the vehemence of the response of official medicine to the practice of 'torri'r llech', the two systems were not, in the perceptions of patients, mutually exclusive or antagonistic. In the Ammanford area some mothers took their ailing children to both the local doctor and the 'torri'r llech' practitioner and, complained one doctor, in the event of a cure were prone to give credit to the unofficial practitioner rather than the orthodox treatment.[99]

Other patients attended herbalists as a result of their experiences at the hands of orthodox practitioners. An inquest into the death of a Llantwit Major woman in 1927 found that the woman had had an operation for breast cancer eighteen months previously, but since this had not been successful she had refused the services of the doctor and had been consulting a 'spiritual healer' who had treated her with a poultice of herbs and castor oil. Her doctor had urged another operation but the woman refused.[100] Similarly, families often preferred to treat themselves because of disagreements over past treatment by doctors.[101] In other instances, women consulted herbalists to obtain abortifacients that they could not obtain from orthodox practitioners.[102] In short, patients were not in the least bit dogmatic in their responses to illness. Sometimes attending a number of practitioners at the same time, sometimes for the same ailment, patients made their choice of therapeutic action based on their conception of their illness and its causation, and their estimation of the skill of various practitioners. From the sufferer's point of

---

[96]   Ibid., p. 41.

[97]   *Report as to the Practice of Medicine and Surgery by Unqualified Persons*, p. 8.

[98]   *Aberdare Leader* (29 March 1913), 4.

[99]   *Western Mail* (21 April 1921), 5. A correspondent to the *Western Mail* pointed out 'that when Nature effects a cure it is the doctor who invariably gets the credit, so this kind of statement cuts both ways' (22 April 1921), 8.

[100]   *Western Mail* (16 June 1927), 12.

[101]   For examples see Webb, *From Caerau to the Southern Cross*, pp. 12–13, 28–9.

[102]   For example see *Caerphilly Journal* (18 September 1920), 1.

view, folk medicine and official medicine were just two options available in the medical marketplace.[103]

Thus, in any study of health and mortality in the twentieth century it is not enough to consider the nature and extent of orthodox medical services alone. Studies of medicine from below remind us that sick individuals did not immediately, or even eventually, seek professional medical advice or assistance when they became ill. Rather, advice and assistance were obtained from a large range of individuals whose understanding of the body and illness, and whose methods and therapeutics, differed often quite markedly. We need to be wary of claims made by the medical profession that scientific medicine was more effective in preventing illness and curing disease because it seems likely that it was not until the mid to late 1930s that effective treatments were developed and made available for many ailments. In the context of this study, it seems unlikely that therapeutic treatments had a significant influence on the patterns of mortality in interwar south Wales. Doctors and other practitioners lacked the means to prevent illness or effect cures. Furthermore, medical services in south Wales were quantitatively and qualitatively inferior to those in most parts of Britain in the interwar period and if they did have an influence on standards of health and levels of mortality in interwar south Wales, it was only to intensify the regional inequalities.

---

[103] Cooter, *Studies in the History of Alternative Medicine*, p. x; Loux, 'Folk medicine', p. 665.

VII

'THE SMELL OF DEATH WAS EVERYWHERE'[1]: MORTALITY

This chapter examines mortality in interwar south Wales. It focuses upon general mortality levels but also disaggregates the general death rates in order to present a more detailed picture of the mortality landscape. The death rates are disaggregated according to sex, age-group, social class and cause of death. An important aspect of the methodology employed in this study of mortality is to set the aggregate England and Wales mortality rates against those of south Wales. Average England and Wales death rates do not refer to any particular group of the population and, by their very nature, are abstract values: they refer to diverse groups of people, characterized by social, economic and cultural differences. Their validity for comparisons with districts in south Wales might therefore be questioned. And yet, any population study of mortality must necessarily employ averages to make meaningful and comprehensible generalisations.

Although this chapter is primarily descriptive, it attempts to analyse some of the more interesting points that arise where these are particularly revealing about the mortality experiences of interwar south Wales. For, as Samuel Preston has argued, 'descriptive studies [have] implications for causal interpretations, because variation in death rates over time, space, or social group cast light on the part played by various underlying factors'.[2]

MORTALITY: GENERAL

Table 7.1 sets out the crude death rates[3] for the main administrative areas of south Wales together with the England and Wales average.

---

[1] White and Williams, *Struggle or Starve*, p. 129.
[2] Preston, 'Population studies of mortality', 529.
[3] 'Crude' death rates refer to rates calculated from the number of deaths and population figures; they have not been 'standardized' to take account of differences in the sex and age structure of different populations.

Table 7.1. Crude death rates in the major administrative areas of south Wales and England and Wales, 1920–39 (deaths per 1,000 population)

	England and Wales	Glam. AC	Mon. AC	Cardiff CB	Merthyr Tydfil CB	Swansea CB	Newport CB
1920	12.4	11.9	11.9	11.3	14.1	12.6	12.4
1921	12.1	11.2	11.3	11.6	12.7	11.9	11.1
1922	12.7	12.1	11.4	13.2	14.2	13.5	12.6
1923	11.6	10.5	10.4	12.0	12.1	12.2	10.7
1924	12.2	10.9	10.6	12.1	12.3	12.6	11.3
1925	12.1	11.2	10.6	12.8	12.7	12.4	11.9
1926	11.6	10.5	9.4	10.8	12.0	11.8	10.5
1927	12.3	11.1	11.0	12.6	12.9	13.5	12.5
1928	11.7	11.5	10.9	11.7	12.6	12.6	11.2
1929	13.4	11.0	11.3	12.9	14.2	13.5	12.6
1930	11.4	10.7	10.2	11.4	12.5	12.8	11.0
1931	12.3	12.1	12.0	12.8	14.2	12.6	13.1
1932	12.0	11.9	11.1	12.5	13.7	13.2	11.9
1933	12.3	12.7	11.5	13.5	13.9	14.5	13.2
1934	11.8	11.7	11.7	12.3	13.9	12.9	12.1
1935	11.7	12.0	11.5	12.3	14.7	12.9	12.4
1936	12.1	12.2	12.2	12.6	13.9	14.1	12.1
1937	12.4	12.9	12.6	12.6	14.3	13.9	12.8
1938	11.6	12.6	12.1	11.9	15.7	13.2	12.1
1939	12.1	13.1	12.8	13.7	14.5	12.4	12.9

Crude death rates were highest in the borough of Merthyr Tydfil where the rate did not fall below 12 deaths per 1,000 population during the interwar period and were consistently above the England and Wales rates. More interestingly, the crude death rates in the two administrative counties and, to a lesser extent, the boroughs of Cardiff, Swansea and Newport seem to suggest a rise in mortality. In the administrative county of Glamorgan, for example, the average death rate rose from 11.3 deaths per 1,000 persons in 1920–4 to 12.6 in 1935–9 while in Monmouthshire it increased from 11.2 to 12.5 in the same periods.[4] Furthermore, the crude death rates for these six areas appear to have increased relative to the aggregate rate for England and Wales so that from a

[4]   Ministry of Health investigators noted in 1934 that the death rate in south Wales, in contrast to that in other depressed areas, was increasing; National Archives, London, MH 79/337, Undated and unsigned summary of reports into malnutrition among unemployed, pp. 2–3.

relatively advantageous position in the early 1920s (with the exception of Merthyr) south Wales by the later 1930s had become a relatively unhealthy region which experienced greater levels of mortality than the England and Wales average.[5]

However, the mortality rates (as set out in Table 7.1 and Appendices 7.1 and 7.2) suffer from being 'crude' indices of mortality and fail to account for the age and sex composition of the population of each district. The mortality level of a population is partly determined by its age-structure and an older population consequently suffers higher levels of mortality than a younger population. This is significant for coalfield regions such as south Wales which traditionally attracted relatively young immigrants and which experienced high fertility rates. For this reason the mortality indices need to be 'standardized' to take account of these factors.[6] Standardized mortality rates for the main administrative units are set out as Figures 7.1 and 7.2.

These graphs demonstrate the unreliability of crude rates since they show that when the age-structures of the populations are taken into account mortality was consistently higher in all the major administrative divisions of south Wales than the England and Wales average. The rate for Monmouthshire did momentarily fall below that of England and Wales, in 1925 and 1926, but mortality was generally greater in the major administrative districts of south Wales than the England and Wales average throughout the interwar period. Merthyr Tydfil again emerges as the area with the highest level of mortality.

The standardized mortality rates for interwar south Wales demonstrate that mortality was not increasing as the crude rates suggested. In the case of the two administrative counties and the borough of Merthyr Tydfil it is evident that mortality rates remained stationary during the interwar period, which meant that, in relation to the England and Wales aggregate, these areas were even more unfavourably positioned by the end of the interwar period than they had been in the early 1920s. The county boroughs

---

[5] See Appendix 7.1.

[6] Death rates in south Wales have been standardized by the direct method according to the males and females in the age-groups 0–4, 5–14, 15–24, 25–44, 45–64 and over 65 in England and Wales as enumerated by the census of 1901. See Appendix 7.3. On standardization, see Roland Pressat, *Demographic Analysis: Methods, Results, Applications* (London, 1972), pp. 101–6; A. H. Pollard, F. Yusuf and G. N. Pollard, *Demographic Techniques* (Oxford, 1981), pp. 70–4.

Figure 7.1. Standardized death rates for England and Wales and the administrative counties of Glamorgan and Monmouthshire, 1921–39

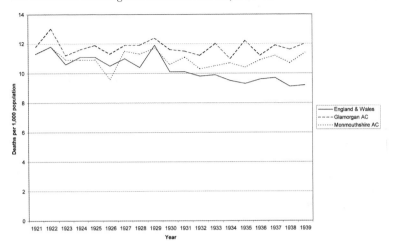

Figure 7.2. Standardized death rates for England and Wales and the county boroughs of Cardiff, Merthyr Tydfil, Swansea and Newport, 1921–39

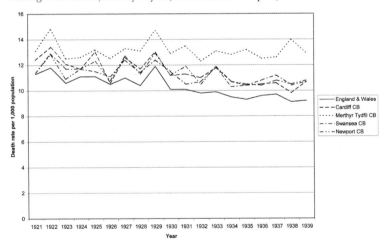

of Cardiff, Newport and Swansea, although experiencing higher levels of mortality than the England and Wales average, nevertheless shared in the decrease in mortality and, while they experienced levels of mortality similar to those of the rest of south Wales in the early 1920s (of between 12 and 14 deaths per 1,000 population), they were in a relatively more advantageous position by the late 1930s when mortality had decreased to below 12 deaths per 1,000 population.

As has been noted, a major methodological problem encountered in the use of crude rates is that the rates do not take account of intercensal changes in the age-structure of the population. Due to the fall in the birth rate and the emigration of large numbers of young people from south Wales during the interwar period, the average age of the population increased, and the area thus experienced higher mortality risks, thereby making it appear that mortality increased. While the direct method of standardization employed in this study takes differences in age-structure between populations into account, it cannot account for intercensal changes in age-structure in the same district. By assuming that the proportions of population in the six age-groups remained the same as enumerated by the previous census, the population estimates used to calculate annual standardized rates have inevitably failed to take changing age-structure into account. However, because the calculation of the standardized death rates by the direct method includes age-specific deaths in a way that the crude rates do not, the standardized rates more closely approximate to the actual level of mortality than do the crude rates.[7] In order to calculate standardized rates that take changing age-structure into account, it would have been necessary to ascertain the age-structure of a population in each year, but clearly annual censuses of the population were not practical. It is possible that, if changing age-structure could be assessed more accurately, the standardized rates might show an even greater improvement in mortality.

Standardized death rates calculated by the direct method are calculated from age-specific deaths. Unfortunately, deaths in each sex- and age-group in south Wales were published only for the two administrative counties and the four county boroughs. No such detailed figures were published for the other districts of south Wales and standardized rates cannot be calculated by the direct method for

---

[7] However, the age-specific rates are themselves dependent on less than exact population estimates calculated from annual population estimates and the age-specific proportions enumerated by the previous census. Nevertheless, the standardized rates take into account the changing age-structure of deaths and therefore partly correct the errors produced by changing age-structure.

smaller administrative units.[8] For this reason, the indirect method has been utilized to standardize death rates in the urban and rural districts of south Wales. This indirect method calculates the number of deaths that would have occurred in a population (expected or standard deaths) had it experienced the same age- and sex-specific death rates as a standard population, in this case England and Wales.[9] The difference between the 'expected deaths' and the 'actual deaths' that a population experienced can then be used to calculate a standardized rate.[10] Quinquennial averages for the periods 1920–4 and 1935–9 are illustrated in Figures 7.3 and 7.4.

Figure 7.3 demonstrates how the districts of Maesteg, Glyncorrwg, Rhondda, Aberdare, Mountain Ash, Pontypridd, Merthyr Tydfil, Caerphilly, Rhymney, Bedwellty, Bedwas and Machen, Pontypool and Blaenavon experienced mortality rates exceeding 110 (England and Wales = 100). These were all, of course, industrial, and predominantly mining, districts. Neath and Cardiff similarly experienced high mortality. The lowest mortality was found in the rural districts of eastern Monmouthshire and the Gower peninsula. Figure 7.4 demonstrates even more clearly how the highest mortality rates were experienced by the mining communities of the Rhondda, Cynon, Taff and Rhymney valleys while the agricultural districts of eastern Monmouthshire stood in a much more favourable position.

However, the indirect method of standardization, whilst able to make death rates for different populations comparable, suffers from the same problem as the crude rates in that it does not take changing age-structure into account. Since the age-specific death rates for England and Wales are applied to the populations of each district, the indirect method of standardization takes some account of changing age-structure in England and Wales but does not account for a changing age-structure in the district to which the resulting standardized rate refers. The apparent increase in

---

[8]   Many medical officers published the number of deaths in each age-group in their annual reports but did not disaggregate them according to sex. The direct method is, in any case, unsuitable in the case of many districts because of the small populations and low numbers of age- and sex-specific deaths in each year.

[9]   The sex- and age-specific death rates for any population can be used but the England and Wales rates for each year are used so as to compare the experience in south Wales with the average for England and Wales.

[10] Standardized death rates by this method, averaged for the four quinquennia, have been set out in Appendix 7.4

Figure 7.3. Standardized death rates for local authority districts in south Wales, 1920–24 (England and Wales =100)

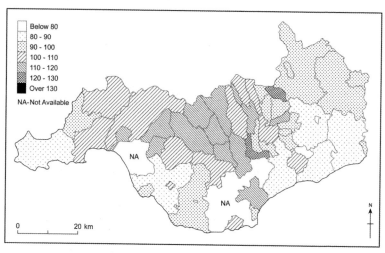

Note: For key to figures 7.3 and 7.4, see Maps 1 and 2.

mortality during the interwar years as shown by the standardized rates calculated by the indirect method, and illustrated by the difference between Figures 7.3 and 7.4, was the result of an ageing of the population rather than any increased mortality risk. This is clearly a major methodological problem since the question of the extent to which the apparent increases in crude mortality were the result of higher mortality or an ageing population is an important one. Throughout the interwar period the annual reports of the medical officer for Glamorgan County Council repeatedly made the point that the crude death rate was increasing due to these demographic reasons. In 1933, for example, the medical officer commented:

> The slight increase in the death rate is to be expected. The higher relative proportion of elderly people in the County population is due to (a) increased average duration of life, (b) migration of younger folk to centres with better prospects of employment, (c) a smaller birth rate.[11]

---

[11]   Glamorgan CC, RMOH (1933), p. 21; for similar comments see esp. Glamorgan CC, RMOH (1929), p. 9; (1931), p. 20; (1932), p. 21; (1936), p. 2; Caerphilly UD, RMOH (1936), p. 11.

Figure 7.4. Standardized death rates for local authority districts in south Wales, 1935–39 (England and Wales = 100)

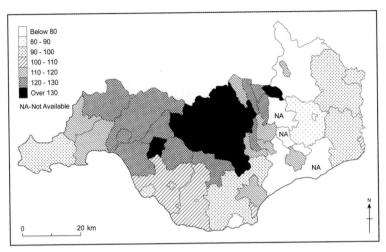

It is possible to examine a number of sources to evaluate the impression that rising mortality rates were due to the ageing of the population in south Wales. As the Glamorgan medical officer pointed out, the birth rate declined each year and a greater proportion of deaths occurred in older age-groups. In the Rhondda Urban District, for example, the number of deaths in the under 5 years age-group fell dramatically from 830 in 1920 (35 per cent of all deaths in that year) to 160 (9.3 per cent) in 1939 while the number of deaths in the over 65 age-group rose from 367 in 1920 (16 per cent) to 768 in 1939 (44.8 per cent). South Wales experienced a transformation in its mortality regime in the interwar period. Figures 7.5 and 7.6 demonstrate the dramatic changes in age-specific mortality in the administrative county of Glamorgan from 1920–2 to 1937–9. The changing age profile of mortality is clear and was, to a lesser or greater degree, a characteristic of the rest of south Wales during the interwar period.

A more distinctive aspect of the changing demographic structure of the region was the effect of the high level of out-migration from the area during this period, though it is difficult to assess this factor. No detailed or accurate figures exist to determine the ages of those who left south Wales or the type of person who migrated and, in any case, the large proportions of emigrants who returned after a

Figure 7.5. Proportion of deaths in different age-groups, Glamorgan Administrative County, 1920–22

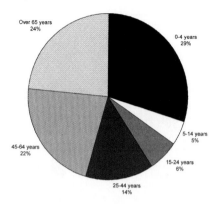

Figure 7.6. Proportion of deaths in different age-groups, Glamorgan Administrative County, 1937–39

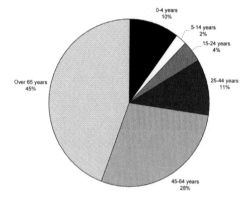

short period further complicate this matter.[12] Some idea can be gained from a study made of Welsh migrants to Oxford during the period 1928 to 1937. It was found that 19.1 per cent of these migrants had left Wales between the ages of 16 and 19, a further 39.4 per cent between the ages of 20 and 24 and around 80 per cent of the total had left when aged below 35.[13] Furthermore, it was

[12]   As an example of this tendency see Jennings, *Brynmawr*, p. 145.

[13]   Peter Scott, 'The state, internal migration, and growth of new industrial communities in inter-war Britain', *English Historical Review*, 115, 461 (2000), 342; see also the findings of H. W. Singer described in Chapter 1.

often commented that it was the more energetic and productive members of the community who emigrated from south Wales during the interwar decades, leaving behind less healthy individuals who inevitably experienced greater mortality and inflated mortality levels. Certain officials in the Ministry of Health, for example, believed that emigration may have been responsible for higher death rates.[14]

Using census figures, it is possible to gain some idea of the changing age-structure of south Wales.[15] It is also possible, by utilizing the figures provided by the National Register taken on 29 September 1939, to gain some idea of these changes during the 1930s when the extent of emigration was at its greatest. Although districts in south Wales experienced greater proportional decreases in the numbers of young people in the population and greater proportional increases in the older age-groups than the England and Wales average, south Wales nevertheless continued to possess a relatively young population by the end of the interwar period. This was true even in the most depressed districts of south Wales. In Gelligaer, for example, 43.5 per cent of the population was below 25 years of age in 1939 as opposed to 36 per cent of the England and Wales population.

Therefore, the apparent increases in crude mortality in south Wales can be attributed to the considerable changes in the age-structure of the population and the faster rate of change experienced in the region than in England and Wales as a whole, despite the fact that south Wales continued to support a relatively young population by the end of the interwar period. This confirms what the standardized death rates suggest. In addition, the selective nature of migration probably had some effect on overall levels of mortality but its precise impact is impossible to assess. The changes in the age-structure were a significant demographic feature of the interwar period and one that had major implications for the mortality landscape of south Wales. As is shown below, it was a significant factor in the transition from a high mortality society

[14] National Archives, London, MH55/629, J. Pearse, T. W. Wade, O. Evans and J. E. Underwood, 'Inquiry into conditions affecting health through unemployment in South Wales and Monmouthshire', pp. 1–3.

[15] The following analysis is based on statistics derived from Census of England and Wales, 1921 and 1931; and *National Register, United Kingdom and the Isle of Man, Statistics of Population on 29 September 1939* (London, 1944); some of this data is set out in Thompson, 'Social history of health', 416–18.

characterized by acute, communicable diseases to a lower mortality pattern featuring higher levels of chronic, 'degenerative' illnesses associated with older age-groups.

While this analysis provides a number of useful insights, it represents average experiences for large areas. In order to refine further the analysis of mortality it is necessary to disaggregate mortality experiences and examine how different groups of the population experienced differing levels of mortality.

SEX-SPECIFIC MORTALITY

Crude sex-specific death rates have been calculated for each of the administrative districts in south Wales using annual sex-specific deaths and annual population estimates.[16] Standardized sex-specific death rates by the direct method have been similarly calculated for the main administrative units and standardized rates by the indirect method have been calculated for all the administrative units.[17] As might be expected, the districts with the highest total death rates also experienced the highest male and female death rates.[18] The male and female mortality rates in any one area were clearly connected and areas with high male mortality generally had high levels of female mortality, and vice versa. This is to be expected since the factors that determined male mortality in an area also had an influence on the level of female mortality.

The question of the degree to which the factors which influenced both male and female mortality in any area were the same is difficult to answer. Men and women had different working environments; inhabited different public environments; varied in the success with which they satisfied the demands they made on the family budget and, more importantly, the food resources of the

[16] See Thompson, 'Social history of health', 419–24.

[17] Ibid., 428–33. Crude rates can be used to study mortality in an area because they represent mortality experiences in an easily understandable and recognizable form; standardized rates by the direct method are used to compare large areas and take some account of changing age-structure; and standardized rates by the indirect method can be used to compare male or female mortality between smaller districts and take some account of the different age-structures.

[18] This seems an obvious point but it is by no means inevitable. A high total death rate in a district might have been due to excess male *or* excess female mortality rather than high male *and* high female mortality.

household; made differing demands on the health services utilized by a family; and, of course, differed biologically. For example, male mortality in a mining district might have been determined by working conditions in the coal industry while female mortality was likely to be determined more by housing conditions and cultural factors that influenced the amount and quality of food consumed by a miner's wife. And yet despite these different experiences it seems reasonable to assume that the male and female death rates in any one district were influenced by many of the same determinants. Factors such as water quality and the efficacy of sewerage systems had a broadly similar influence on male and female mortality.

A further important point about sex-specific death rates is that south Wales experienced an excess of male mortality over female mortality. In most societies in the modern, developed world male mortality exceeds female mortality and in all age-groups. Various social and biological factors explain this phenomenon.[19] Throughout the interwar period, crude male mortality rates for England and Wales varied between 112 per cent and 116 per cent of the corresponding female rates. The experience in south Wales differed to some extent. In the administrative county of Glamorgan the crude male death rate remained in excess of the female rate until the early 1930s to the same extent as the England and Wales rates, but from the mid to late 1930s the male rate diverged even more markedly from the female rate, so that in the period 1935–9 the male rate was 122.5 per cent of the female rate. The male excess in Monmouthshire and Merthyr was generally less than the England and Wales excess. In Cardiff and Swansea the male excess was relatively high. The male rate in Cardiff varied from about 115 per cent to 135 per cent of the female rate.

In absolute terms, the crude and standardized sex-specific death rates show that it was the areas that experienced the highest mortality that also experienced the highest male and female mortality. This is to be expected (although is not inevitable) since the male and female rates combine to form the total rate. However, the proportion of each total rate that is made up by the male or female rates varies from district to district. As the crude sex-specific mortality data demonstrate, it was in urban districts such as Barry,

[19]   See Bernard Benjamin, *Population Statistics: A Review of UK Sources* (Aldershot, 1989), pp. 41–3; Winter, 'Decline of mortality', pp. 104–5.

Penarth, Porthcawl, Abergavenny and Pontypool that the male excess over female mortality was at its highest. The reasons for this varied. In the case of Barry, male mortality was generally higher than the Glamorgan administrative county average while female mortality was generally lower and this was not due to differences in the sex-specific age-structure. It would seem that the working environment of Barry males in the docks was especially deleterious to their health since the differences between male and female mortality cannot be attributed to the standard of life allowed by dockworkers' wages; female mortality would have been higher had this been the case.

In the cases of Penarth, Porthcawl and Abergavenny it is evident that the migration of the young males of these towns into the mining districts in search of work left an older male population which experienced higher levels of mortality and thereby inflated the male death rate.[20] However, the standardized rates for these three towns show that, while male mortality was at or below the level of mortality of England and Wales as a whole, female mortality was often even further below the England and Wales rate. In these districts, something other than the age-structures and a general tendency toward lower female mortality was causing female mortality to be lower than male mortality. The districts where the male excess mortality was at its lowest were typically the industrialized districts of the coalfield. Was this due to higher female mortality in these districts and lower male death rates or was it due to differences in the sex-specific age-structure?

If the standardized male and female rates for the Rhondda and Porthcawl are compared, it is clear that the relatively high crude male mortality in Porthcawl was the result of an older male population since the standardized male rates were lower than the England and Wales average. In the Rhondda, the standardized male mortality was significantly in excess of the England and Wales rate. With regard to female mortality, the standardized death rate in Porthcawl was lower than the England and Wales average, considerably so in the 1920s, but in the Rhondda female mortality was in excess of the corresponding England and Wales rate to a greater degree than the male standardized rate. In towns similar to

[20]   See Census of England and Wales, 1921, Glamorgan, p. 30; ibid., Monmouthshire, p. 27, which show how the male population in the 15–39 age range was significantly smaller than the female population in the same age range.

Table 7.2. Standardized male death rates in selected industrial areas, 1920–39

	1920–4	1925–9	1930–4	1935–9
Aberdare UD	103.3	112.0	116.3	132.9
Gelligaer UD	99.3	111.0	119.1	130.3
Merthyr Tydfil CB	114.9	116.5	120.4	130.3
Mountain Ash UD	109.9	111.4	119.5	129.4
Rhondda UD	110.9	114.4	118.4	131.3
Bedwellty UD	112.7	108.4	123.9	125.9
Blaenavon UD	116.2	104.7	113.9	133.2

Source: Annual reports of the medical officers of health of the individual districts and *Registrar-General's Statistical Review of England and Wales*, 1920–39; this data is collated in Thompson, 'Social history of health', 430–3. It must be remembered that the standardized male and female death rates used in the tables are not comparable within a particular district but only to the England and Wales sex-specific rates. Therefore, the male rates in the tables are comparable to the England and Wales male death rate and the female rates are comparable to the England and Wales female death rate (England and Wales = 100).

Table 7.3. Standardized female death rates in selected industrial areas, 1920–39

	1920–4	1925–9	1930–4	1935–9
Aberdare UD	121.1	121.5	132.4	140.1
Gelligaer UD	119.1	122.3	127.6	140.3
Merthyr Tydfil CB	122.4	127.0	141.7	144.4
Mountain Ash UD	113.8	121.1	126.3	138.6
Rhondda UD	119.8	125.8	134.1	140.5
Bedwellty UD	118.8	110.0	137.9	135.8
Blaenavon UD	132.5	119.0	135.9	144.2

Source: See Table 7.2.

Porthcawl which experienced low excess male mortality, such as Penarth and Abergavenny, male and female mortality approximated to each other at a level just below the England and Wales average. In mining districts such as the Rhondda valleys, on the other hand, female mortality, standardized for differences in age-structure, exceeded the England and Wales female mortality to a greater degree than male mortality exceeded the corresponding male death rates for England and Wales. Tables 7.2 and 7.3 demonstrate the high excess female mortality in mining districts.

Thus, while male and female mortality in the industrialized areas exceeded the England and Wales averages, and male and female mortality in the rural districts and coastal resorts, the excess was greater for female mortality than for male mortality. Excess female mortality over the England and Wales average was greater than excess male mortality. The girls and women of the industrial districts of south Wales suffered from living in these areas to a greater degree than the boys and men. This contrasts with male and female mortality in Cardiff, Swansea and Newport which exceeded the corresponding male and female England and Wales averages to the same extent. Clearly, there was something about the coalmining communities that had a greater effect on female mortality than on male mortality.

AGE-SPECIFIC MORTALITY

While mortality varies according to sex, it also varies according to age. Generally, mortality is highest at the extremes of age. The risks of mortality are high immediately following birth and fall rapidly so that the risk of mortality is relatively low during infancy and childhood. Occupational influences on health during adolescence cause mortality to rise, and various biological and social influences mean that mortality continues to rise in an uninterrupted pattern as age advances. At older ages, levels of mortality approach, and surpass, the high levels experienced by the youngest age-groups in the population.[21] For the purposes of this study, age-specific mortality has been calculated for the six main administrative units of south Wales and for England and Wales. Age-specific rates for smaller units of administration, such as the urban and rural districts, have not been calculated because of the small numbers of deaths and persons in any age-group in many districts in a particular year and the difficulty of obtaining statistics for age-specific deaths disaggregated according to sex. The age-groups used in this study are 0–4 years, 5–14, 15–24, 25–44, 45–64 and over 65 years. Ideally, a larger number of age-groups would have been used but it was not always possible to obtain comparable statistics or continuous series from the sources. The six age-groups used are sufficient to encapsulate the experiences of the major generational groupings of the population at any one time.

[21] Benjamin, *Population Sources*, p. 41; Pressat, *Demographic Analysis*, p. 78
[22] See Thompson, 'Social history of health', 434–44.

Close examination of the age-specific death rates and the description of the method of their calculation reveal a methodological problem.[22] Since the calculation of the rates has been on the basis of the proportions of population in an age-group, as enumerated by the census, the age-specific rates are dependent on the age-structure of the population in any district remaining the same as in the previous census. As an example, the proportions of the Glamorgan administrative county male population enumerated by the 1921 census (that is, 11 per cent in the 0–4 age-group, 21.9 per cent in the 5–14 age-group, etc.) have been applied to the annual population estimates for Glamorgan for the rest of the 1920s without taking into account how the age-structures might have changed during the intercensal years.

The age-structure remained roughly similar in the years immediately following the census but was more prone to change as time passed so that the population estimates for each age-group in the late 1920s and late 1930s are likely to be less accurate than in the early part of each decade. It is evident that this problem has a greater effect on the rates at the extremes of age. The fall in birth rates that occurred in the interwar years meant that the proportion of the population in the 0–4 age-group decreased quite rapidly. This produces an underestimated death rate later in each of the two decades as the falling number of deaths in the 0–4 age-group is applied to an exaggerated population estimate based on the proportion in that age-group at the last census. Similarly, the falling birth rate, the emigration of young adults and the ageing of the population mean that the proportion of the population in the over 65 age-group increased rapidly. In this case, the high rates evident in the latter half of each decade are produced by an increased number at risk, and dying, being applied to an underestimated population estimate. It follows that the rates are least reliable for those districts, such as Merthyr Tydfil, which experienced the largest decreases in the birth rate and the highest levels of emigration of young adults, since these areas saw the greatest changes in age-structure. The rates for the middle age-groups are less likely to be affected by changes in age-structure because of the greater range in ages and the larger number of persons in each group. For these methodological reasons, average age-specific death rates have been calculated for the quinquennia 1921–5 and 1931–5. It is in these periods that population estimates calculated from the proportions in each age-group as enumerated by the last census are most reliable and the following analysis is based on these averages.

It is evident that death rates in all age-groups for England and Wales as a whole fell during the interwar period.[23] The decrease was greatest in the 0–4 age-group whose death rates fell by about a third and, therefore, improvements in life expectancy in the interwar years were primarily the result of lessened mortality at the youngest ages. The situation in south Wales differed from this in many important respects. The fall in mortality in the youngest age-group was considerable. In most cases its mortality fell by about a third. The Monmouthshire Administrative County was typical in that the male death rate in the 0–4 age-group fell from 28.6 deaths per 1,000 males in 1921–5 to 20.8 in 1931–5, while the female rate fell from 23 in the first period to 17.3 in the latter. Despite the fact that death rates in this age-group fell in all areas of south Wales during the interwar years, it is evident that the decrease in all six areas surveyed was less than for England and Wales as a whole.

The trends are much more complicated for the 5–14 age-group. The administrative county of Monmouthshire experienced an increase in male mortality, as did the county boroughs of Cardiff, Merthyr and Newport, while a small decrease in mortality was experienced by Glamorgan and Swansea boroughs. In all cases, female mortality in this age-group decreased or remained constant. The decreases in this age-group were proportionately smaller than those in the 0–4 age-group. In the 15–24 age-group, male mortality generally decreased, although Monmouthshire and Merthyr experienced small increases. Significantly, female mortality increased in the administrative counties of Glamorgan and Monmouthshire and in Merthyr. In the case of Merthyr, the increase was substantial and the death rate rose from 4.14 deaths per 1,000 females in 1921–5 to 5.26 in 1931–5. Perhaps even more significant than these increases were the absolute levels of mortality in this age-group. The England and Wales rates demonstrate the tendency for male mortality to exceed female mortality in this age-group. A male rate of 3.14 deaths per 1,000 males in 1921–5 corresponded with a female rate of 2.84, while in the 1931–5 period the male rate stood at 2.7 and the female rate at 2.38. In south Wales, male mortality exceeded female mortality by much less and was even exceeded by

23   See Thompson, 'Social history of health', 434–44.

female mortality in some districts. In the two administrative counties, Newport in the former period and Merthyr in the latter period, female mortality exceeded male mortality in absolute terms, while the more prosperous boroughs of Cardiff and Swansea experienced excess male mortality, a pattern approximating to that of England and Wales.

In the 25–44 age-group the two administrative counties experienced only very small changes in mortality. Cardiff, Swansea, Newport and, to a lesser extent, Merthyr experienced more significant decreases in mortality. More importantly, the two administrative counties and Merthyr experienced female mortality equal to, or exceeding, male mortality in this age-group whereas Cardiff, Newport and Swansea more closely resembled the England and Wales pattern of excess male mortality. In the 45–65 age-group excess male mortality was often quite significant in the more prosperous areas but was limited in the more depressed areas. The area with the smallest differential in male and female mortality in this age-group was Merthyr; the explanation is that, whereas the male mortality there approximated to male mortality in other areas, the female mortality was much higher than elsewhere and almost approached the level of male mortality. The largest differentials were in the more prosperous county boroughs of Cardiff, Newport and Swansea where female mortality in this age-group was only about 70 per cent of male mortality.

In the oldest age-group (65 years and over) the England and Wales rates demonstrate excess male mortality and a slight fall in mortality for both sexes during the interwar years. Again, south Wales differed markedly from this trend. In each area, male mortality exceeded female mortality, although again the differentials were greatest in the more prosperous boroughs of Cardiff and Swansea, and least in the depressed areas. In Newport, the differential was even greater than the England and Wales average and female mortality stood at just over 80 per cent of male mortality. More importantly, in every case, with the exception of the male rate in Newport and the female rate in Cardiff, mortality in this age-group in south Wales increased from 1921–5 to 1931–5; this was probably as a result of greater numbers of people living to ages beyond 65.

In the context of south Wales, it is evident that, with the exception of the male death rates in the 25–44 and 45–64 age-groups,

death rates in each sex- and age-group were highest in Merthyr
Tydfil. This emphasizes the relative disadvantages faced by all the
citizens of Merthyr. Interestingly, male mortality in the 25–44 and
45–64 age-groups was higher in the boroughs of Cardiff and
Swansea than in relatively unhealthy and economically depressed
Merthyr. Neither Cardiff nor Swansea displayed excess mortality in
other age-groups for either sex, but in the male 25–44 and 45–64
age groups, it was especially marked in Cardiff.[24]

If these age- and sex-specific death rates for the areas of south
Wales are expressed as a percentage of the equivalent rates for
England and Wales then it is evident that not only did south Wales
experience higher levels of mortality than the England and Wales
average (which has already been established by the general death
rates) but that in many cases the excess mortality in south Wales was
considerable. It was greatest in the 15–24 age-group and for females
in particular. The lowest level of female mortality in this age-group
in south Wales was still 120.4 per cent of the England and Wales
rate (in the case of Swansea in 1921–5). In all areas, the excess
mortality of women in south Wales over women in England and
Wales as a whole in this age-group rose during the interwar years,
and in the case of Merthyr was a staggering 221 per cent of the
England and Wales rate in 1931–5.

Not only was mortality greater in south Wales than elsewhere but
the gap between south Wales and England and Wales increased
during the interwar period. Of the seventy-two sex- and age-groups
resulting from the disaggregation of death rates for the six administrative areas in the periods 1921–5 and 1931–5, only ten improved
their position relative to the England and Wales rate from 1921–5
to 1931–5 and these were primarily in the boroughs of Cardiff,
Newport and Swansea. The population of south Wales, while
sharing in the improvements in mortality experienced elsewhere,
did not enjoy these improvements to the same extent. This means
that, relative to the people of other parts of England and Wales, the
population of south Wales became less healthy during the interwar
years as indeed was demonstrated by the total death rates.

High female mortality in the 15–44 age-groups was a noted
mortality pattern of other 'depressed areas' during the interwar
period. An article published in the *New Statesman and Nation* in 1935
noted how female mortality in the depressed areas exceeded female

---

[24]   The reasons for this are examined in the section below on causes of death.

Table 7.4. Excess male and female mortality in 'depressed areas' over 'rest of the country', 1934

Age-group	% excess of deaths in 'depressed areas' over 'rest of the country', 1934	
	Male	Female
0–14	30	30
15–44	16	24
45–64	16	21
65 and over	16	21
Total	18	23

Source: New Statesman and Nation (23 November 1935), 759; the article did not define 'depressed areas' and the 'rest of the country'.

mortality in the 'rest of the country' to a greater extent than male mortality in the depressed areas exceeded male mortality in the 'rest of the country'.

The article maintained that this pattern of mortality was a result of the economic depression but it seems, to some extent, that it was typical of areas characterized by old, heavy industries in times of prosperity and not just a product of the industrial depression. E. Lewis-Faning, in his criticism of the *New Statesman* article, stated that it was not enough to show that death rates in the depressed areas were higher than elsewhere but that they were higher in the depressed areas in the interwar period than they had been before the First World War.[25] As far as south Wales is concerned, Dot Jones has shown how female mortality in these age-groups was relatively high in the Rhondda valleys for many decades before the First World War and that this was a consequence of the nature of women's lives in industrial society.[26] This evidence seems to suggest that the high female mortality in these age-groups was not solely a consequence of economic depression in the interwar period but a characteristic feature of the mortality landscapes of these industrial communities during the late nineteenth and early twentieth centuries.[27]

[25]   Ministry of Health, *Reports on Public Health and Medical Subjects*, 86: E. Lewis-Faning, *A Study of the Trend of Mortality Rates in Urban Communities of England and Wales, with Special Reference to 'Distressed Areas'* (London, 1938), p. 4.

[26]   Jones, 'Counting the cost of coal'.

[27]   Similarly, Michael Anderson, 'The social implications of demographic change', in F. M. L. Thompson (ed.), *The Cambridge Social History of Britain, 1750–1950* (Cambridge,

How should this pattern of female mortality be explained? Dot Jones makes the point that this was a 'traditional' pattern of mortality 'characteristic of pre-industrial communities', a point with which Winter would presumably agree since he notes that the rising sex differential in mortality in Britain during the twentieth century was not shared by other countries which industrialized later and where mortality differentials were less favourable to women.[28] The implication is that industrialization served to increase excess male mortality and that relatively high female mortality in these age-groups was a characteristic of pre-industrial societies or un-developed regions. This seems to contradict the experience of communities in south Wales in the late nineteenth and early twen-tieth centuries and the depressed areas of the interwar period. These, the most industrialized regions of Britain, experienced rela-tively high female mortality, and even, at times, an excess of female mortality over male mortality, in the adult age-groups. This was an integral feature of their mortality landscapes that cannot be explained as some sort of aberration more akin to pre-industrial or developing societies.[29] Rather, the low status of women in these communities and the gendered effects of the interwar depression were reflected in the sex-specific patterns of mortality.[30]

The analysis of these age-specific death rates formed an import-ant part of E. Lewis-Faning's rebuttal of claims that economic depression caused death rates to increase.[31] Lewis-Faning's study

1990), vol. 2, p. 18, points out that excess female mortality in ages up to about 35 character-ized the mortality patterns of rural areas and mining districts in the period to 1914.

[28]   Jones, 'Counting the cost of coal', p. 126; Winter, 'Decline of mortality', p. 104; these authors seem to have relied on Sheila Ryan Johansson, 'Sex and death in Victorian England: an examination of age- and sex-specific death rates, 1840–1910', in Martha Vicinus (ed.), *A Widening Sphere: Changing Roles of Victorian Women* (London, 1977), 163–82, and George J. Stolnitz, 'A century of international mortality trends: II', *Population Studies*, 10, 1 (1956–7), 17–42, respectively.

[29]   Johansson, 'Sex and death in Victorian England', p. 166, argues that although England was the world's first and only industrial society by 1840, it nevertheless displayed a 'traditional', rather than 'modern', mortality pattern. Johansson defines a traditional mortality pattern as 'one in which both males and females have relatively low and relatively equal expectations of life at birth. In addition, in many traditional societies females in certain age groups sometimes have higher death rates than males.' This seems a rather Whiggish interpretation of changing mortality patterns and one that forces mortality patterns into preconceived ideas of 'traditional' and 'modern' societies.

[30]   D. A. Coleman and John Salt, *The British Population: Patterns, Trends, and Processes* (Oxford, 1992), p. 39.

[31]   Lewis-Faning was a member of the Medical Research Council's statistical staff and his report was published by the Ministry of Health. His findings have been drawn upon by a

grouped the county boroughs of Merthyr and Newport together as
representing a 'coal mining and steel smelting' area of south Wales.
Considering the nature of these two towns and their differing
fortunes during the interwar period, this seems a strange aggregation to make if the purpose was to assess the consequences of
industrial depression on mortality patterns, as Lewis-Faning
claimed. Newport was not even scheduled as a 'Special Area' by the
Act of 1934.

It is evident from the age-specific mortality rates that Newport
experienced lower mortality than Merthyr at most ages, often
considerably so, and that Lewis-Faning's aggregation of the two
boroughs served to underestimate the level of mortality in
depressed regions of south Wales such as Merthyr. As has been
demonstrated above, Newport experienced more favourable levels
of mortality than did other depressed areas of south Wales and so
its combination with Merthyr served to mask some of the excess
mortality in depressed areas.[32] Furthermore, Lewis-Faning's
method of calculating mortality rates, whereby he aggregated the
numbers of deaths and the population figures before calculating the
death rates, meant that the larger population of Newport and its
relatively smaller number of deaths had a disproportionately
greater influence on his combined rates than did the Merthyr
mortality levels. Therefore, Lewis-Faning's study, intended to show
the nature of mortality in depressed areas, created a false impression of mortality in the depressed areas of south Wales. If it had
been his intention to examine the general level of mortality in the
south Wales region, then the combination of an area with higher
than average mortality and a district with a lower level of mortality
(in a south Wales context) – the combination of Merthyr and
Newport – would have been defensible. But since the express intention of the study was to examine the effects of economic
Depression on mortality in the depressed regions, Lewis-Faning's
methodology, at least as far as south Wales was concerned, was
badly flawed and served to underestimate the true effects of the
depression on mortality levels in south Wales.[33] This is another

popular textbook, Peter Dewey, *War and Progress: Britain, 1914–1945* (London, 1997), p. 271,
and therefore need to be critically assessed.

[32]   Lewis-Faning's own study shows that Newport had a lower level of mortality than
other areas of south Wales and the aggregate mortality for 'South Wales'; Lewis-Faning, *Study
of the Trend of Mortality Rates*, pp. 6–7.

[33]   Dr G. C. M. M'Gonigle, medical officer of Stockton-on-Tees, pointed out that Lewis-

instance of an official report conveying an overly optimistic picture
of mortality in the depressed areas.

CAUSES OF DEATH

This analysis of mortality patterns in interwar south Wales can be
further refined to take account of causes of death.[34] Crude cause-
specific death rates have been calculated for interwar south Wales
for the main causes of death.[35] Figures 7.7 and 7.8 illustrate the
proportions of deaths by various causes in Monmouthshire administrative county in the quinquennia 1920–4 and 1935–9.

In common with the rest of Britain, south Wales experienced a
decrease in mortality from communicable infectious diseases during
the interwar period. Although deaths from diphtheria, scarlet fever,
whooping cough and measles contributed only a small part of the
total mortality in the early 1920s (6 per cent in the case of
Monmouthshire), mortality from these causes continued to decline
during the interwar period so that they accounted for an almost
negligible proportion of deaths in the late 1930s (1 per cent in
Monmouthshire). These great killers of nineteenth-century childhood had become relatively insignificant by the interwar period in
terms of overall mortality rates. In absolute terms, however, deaths
from these infections were sufficiently numerous to loom large in
people's lives and since deaths from infectious disease were concentrated in the very youngest portion of the population the impact
seemed that much greater.[36] The forty-three diphtheria deaths in
Merthyr in 1934, for example, would have had a much greater
emotional impact on the community than an equivalent number of
deaths from heart disease in older age-groups.[37]

Faning used geographical counties as units and that these masked regional differences within
counties. Some parts of these counties were more prosperous than others and even in the
most depressed districts there were individuals in employment; *Medical Officer* (17 December
1938), quoted in J. Hadfield, 'Health in the industrial North-East, 1919–39' (unpublished
University of Sheffield Ph.D. thesis, 1977), 192–3.

[34] For a consideration of the methodological problems inherent in the use of cause of
death statistics, see Thompson, 'Social history of health', 294.

[35] The following analysis of cause-specific mortality is based upon statistics collated in
Thompson, 'Social history of health', 445–71.

[36] Numerous working-class autobiographies contain reminiscences of people visiting
childhood friends who died from infectious diseases.

[37] For a more detailed consideration of infectious disease mortality, see Thompson,
'Social history of health', 296–9.

Figure 7.7. Proportion of deaths from various causes, Monmouthshire Administrative County, 1920–4.

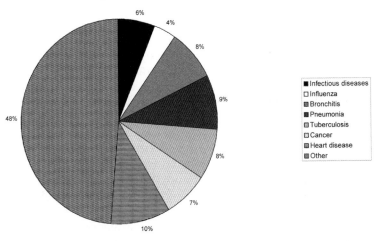

Note: 'Infectious diseases' consist of measles, whooping cough, scarlet fever and diptheria.

Figure 7.8. Proportion of deaths from various causes, Monmouthshire Administrative County, 1935–9

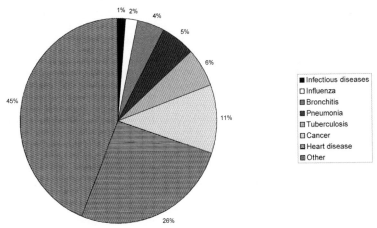

Respiratory diseases accounted for a large proportion of deaths in interwar south Wales, though here too death rates decreased. As Figures 7.7 and 7.8 demonstrate, respiratory diseases caused 25 per cent of all deaths in the administrative county of Monmouth in the period 1920–4, although this fell to 15 per cent by 1935–9. Bronchitis mortality, in particular, displays a very strong positive correlation with social class, and both infection and mortality were often caused by a breakdown in immunological resistance as a result of nutritional deficiency or another illness.[38] South Wales generally experienced higher levels of bronchitis mortality than the England and Wales average. In the two administrative counties, death rates were generally lower than this average in the early 1920s but increasingly exceeded the England and Wales aggregate rates during the 1930s. The rates for Merthyr exceeded the England and Wales rate by an increasing margin during the course of the interwar period and this means that although mortality in these districts was decreasing during the interwar period it was doing so more slowly than the England and Wales average. The county boroughs of Cardiff and Swansea, on the other hand, though experiencing higher levels of mortality seem to have improved their position relative to the England and Wales rate. Newport experienced lower levels of mortality than the other districts of south Wales and the England and Wales average. As far as pneumonia mortality is concerned, south Wales, with the exception of Merthyr, experienced lower levels of mortality than England and Wales, while south Wales generally experienced higher levels of mortality from 'other respiratory diseases'.

A number of historians have noted the high correlation between respiratory mortality, especially as a result of bronchitis, and atmospheric pollution.[39] This is especially significant for interwar south Wales where pollution of the atmosphere by industry was chronic and where few improvements occurred at this time. In addition, while the quality of the macro-environment was important in respiratory disease mortality, so too was the nature of the micro-environment within the home. Medical officers continually bemoaned the tendency of families to block up windows, fire-grates and flues thereby preventing the flow of air through the house.[40]

---

[38] *Registrar-General's Decennial Supplement* (1921), p. xiv, shows that mortality of all occupied and retired males aged 20 to 65 in Class V was almost seven times the mortality experience of Class I in the period 1921 to 1923; Alex J. Mercer, *Disease, Mortality and Population in Transition* (Leicester, 1990), p. 108; Jacalyn Duffin, 'Pneumonia', in Kiple, *Cambridge World History of Human Disease*, pp. 938–9.

[39] Mercer, *Disease, Mortality and Population in Transition*, p. 108; I. M. Buchanan, 'Infant mortality in British coal mining communities, 1880–1911' (unpubl. University of London Ph.D. thesis, 1983), 74–5; Duffin, 'Pneumonia', p. 939.

[40] See for example Mountain Ash UD, RMOH (1925), p. 17.

Furthermore, the tendency in the terraced housing of south Wales was for all cleaning and cooking processes to be carried out in the kitchen using a coal fire. Since this was the room in which families spent most of their time, the stuffy atmosphere would have further predisposed individuals to respiratory disease. The Pontardawe medical officer was concerned by mothers who nursed sick infants 'in the kitchen with closed doors and windows, close to the fire, fearfully overclothed'.[41]

Due to the nature of the disease, patterns of tuberculosis mortality reveal more about the nature of a society than do other causes of death and have been used by historical demographers as an indicator of the socio-economic condition of communities. Pulmonary tuberculosis rates in south Wales varied considerably. In contrast to other causes of death, it was Cardiff County Borough which experienced the highest levels of tuberculosis mortality and these rates invariably amounted to roughly 150 per cent of the England and Wales rate. The two administrative counties experienced favourable mortality rates relative to the aggregate England and Wales rate during the 1920s but seem to have fallen increasingly behind by the 1930s. Monmouthshire appears to have experienced no improvement in pulmonary tuberculosis mortality during the interwar period although it experienced a low rate during the 1920s and continued to experience the lowest rate of the six administrative areas by the late 1930s. The four county boroughs suffered higher mortality rates than the England and Wales average and also higher rates than the two administrative counties. Cardiff and Newport, in particular, experienced relatively high mortality rates (see Figure 7.9).

This pattern of high pulmonary tuberculosis in Cardiff and lower mortality in the mining districts stands in stark contrast to other measures of mortality. It suggests that the relationship between tuberculosis mortality and economic conditions is not a simple or uncomplicated one. This is further demonstrated by Figure 7.10 which illustrates the regional variation in tuberculosis mortality in south Wales. The geographical pattern of tuberculosis mortality displays many of the same characteristics as the patterns of total mortality. High levels of mortality were experienced in the communities of the Rhondda, Cynon, Taff and Rhymney valleys and, to a lesser extent, the upper Sirhowy and Ebbw valleys, while lower levels

[41]   Pontardawe RD, RMOH (1930), pp. 13–14.

Figure 7.9. Pulmonary tuberculosis death rates in south Wales and England and Wales as a whole, 1921–39

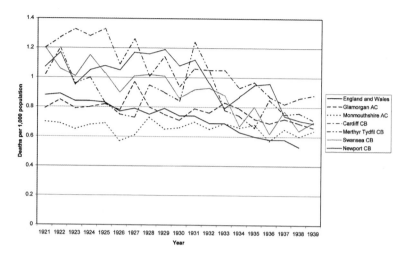

Figure 7.10. Average annual death rates from tuberculosis (all forms) in south Wales, 1930–6

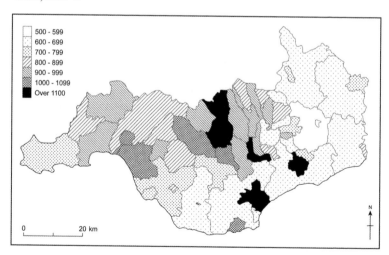

Source: Report of the Committee on the Anti-Tuberculosis Service in Wales and Monmouthshire (London, 1939), 258–60; the average rate for Wales as a whole was 958 deaths per million; for key, see Map 1.

were experienced in the more agricultural areas of the vale of Glamorgan and eastern Monmouthshire. What is also interesting about Figure 7.10 is the high mortality it reveals in coastal towns such as Cardiff, Newport, Barry, Port Talbot, Neath and Swansea.

This was a matter of concern to the medical officers of Cardiff who struggled to explain the reasons for the high pulmonary tuberculosis mortality in the borough during the interwar period. As the medical officer Ralph Picken pointed out in 1925, the relatively high rate in Cardiff during the 1920s was a result of the slower rate of decrease in the tuberculosis death rate in Cardiff in previous decades in comparison with the rates for other towns and cities and for England and Wales as a whole, rather than any overall increase in tuberculosis mortality.[42] The pulmonary tuberculosis death rate had only decreased by 9.6 per cent in Cardiff in the period 1916 to 1925 compared to 28.6 per cent in Manchester and 31 per cent in Liverpool, so that Cardiff had the highest death rate among towns of comparable size by the mid 1920s.[43] Attempts to explain this focused on Cardiff's seafaring population. Of the 2,333 males found to be suffering from pulmonary tuberculosis during the period 1924 to 1934, 445 (or 19.1 per cent) were seamen.[44]

The patterns of tuberculosis mortality in the coalfield communities of the inland valleys differed from those of the coastal towns. First, respiratory tuberculosis mortality increased in certain coalfield communities during the interwar period (see Figure 7.11). The increase in respiratory tuberculosis mortality during the late 1920s and early 1930s is clear and it is evident that Merthyr and the Rhondda valleys were out of step with the improvements that occurred in England and Wales as a whole.[45]

Clues as to the reasons for the specific patterns in different districts of south Wales can be found in cause-specific death rates disaggregated according to sex and age. Figures 7.12 and 7.13 illustrate the pulmonary tuberculosis death rates for different districts of south Wales and compare them to England and Wales as a whole.

[42]   Cardiff CB, RMOH (1925), p. 7; see also (1934), p. 57.
[43]   Cardiff CB, RMOH (1925), p. 7; see also *Western Mail* (31 August 1926); *South Wales News* (31 Aug. 1926).
[44]   Cardiff CB, RMOH (1934), p. 51; for a more detailed examination of the influence of foreign seamen on tuberculosis death rates in Cardiff, see Thompson, 'Social history of health', 303–4.
[45]   The urban districts of Barry, Pontypridd and Mountain Ash similarly experienced increases in respiratory tuberculosis mortality during the interwar period while other mining districts of south Wales experienced little or no change in mortality.

Figure 7.11. Respiratory tuberculosis mortality in the Rhondda Urban District, Merthyr Tydfil County Borough and England and Wales as a whole, 1920–38

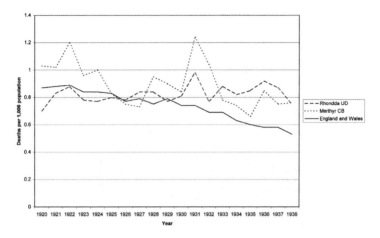

The usual tendency was for female tuberculosis mortality to exceed male mortality during childhood and early adulthood but for male mortality to exceed female mortality after about the age of 30.[46] In Cardiff and, to a lesser extent, Swansea, excess mortality was more evident in the male adult age-groups, and in particular the 25–44 and 45–64 age-groups. This excess pulmonary tuberculosis mortality was the cause of the high overall death rates in these age-groups in Cardiff and Swansea. In Merthyr and the Rhondda, on the other hand, excess mortality was most marked for females aged 15–44. In the 15–24 age-group, female mortality from pulmonary mortality in Merthyr in 1931–2 was 275 per cent of the England and Wales rate, and it was only slightly less in the Rhondda Urban District.

It is reasonable to assume that high male tuberculosis mortality in Cardiff and Swansea was not the result of housing conditions (which would have shown up in excess female, rather than excess male, mortality) nor due to economic depression (in view of the gendered experiences of poverty). The reasons for such high male mortality might be found in the nature of the work that engaged such large proportions of the male populations of these towns.[47] As

[46]   W. D. Johnston, 'Tuberculosis', in Kiple, *Cambridge World History of Human Disease*, p. 1060.
[47]   Census of England and Wales, 1921, Glamorgan, pp. 52–4, 64–5; Monmouthshire, pp. 40–1.

Figure 7.12. Sex- and age-specific mortality from pulmonary tuberculosis, Cardiff and Swansea County Boroughs and England and Wales, 1931–3

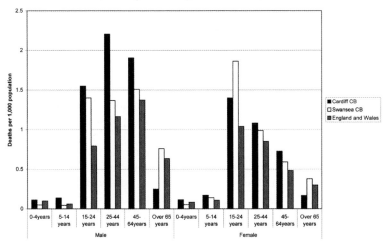

Figure 7.13. Sex- and age-specific mortality from pulmonary tuberculosis, Merthyr Tydfil County Borough, Rhondda Urban District and England and Wales, 1931–3

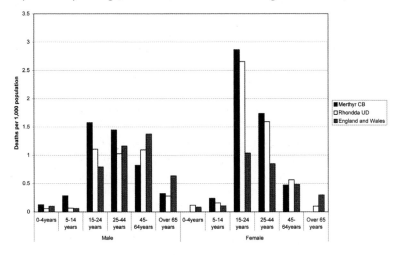

Figure 7.12 reveals, it was males of working age, in particular, who suffered excess tuberculosis mortality and not males generally. Males under the age of 15 and over 65 experienced comparable or lower levels of mortality than the England and Wales averages.

Therefore, the high male adult tuberculosis mortality levels in the coastal towns of south Wales can be attributed to the working conditions of seamen and dock labourers.[48]

The causes of excess female tuberculosis mortality in Merthyr and the Rhondda in the 15–44 age-group seems likely to have been a combination of the working conditions of women in the home and the cultural practices that ensured that the male 'breadwinner' obtained the greater part of the household's available food resources, together with the economic factors of the interwar period. This last point needs qualification for, as has been demonstrated, women in these age-groups in south Wales experienced high levels of mortality in the period before the First World War, while excess female mortality in these age-groups in England and Wales in the nineteenth century was primarily caused by pulmonary tuberculosis.[49] However, women's responsibility for the household budget meant that it was easier for a housewife to sacrifice her own food consumption in order to balance the budget than it was to devise an alternative strategy, and this was a factor of greater significance in the interwar depression than previously.

Mortality from pulmonary tuberculosis for females aged 15–24 and 25–44 in Merthyr was greater in 1931–3 than in 1921–3 and this can perhaps be attributed to the economic fortunes of the borough in the intervening decade.[50] While death rates from this cause increased for males in Merthyr aged 5–14 and 15–24, the increases for females aged 15–24 and 25–44 were even greater. Mortality in the 15–24 age-group in the Rhondda was over twice as high for females as it was for males and a number of factors might have contributed to this. First, constant childbearing imposed considerable strains on women's bodies which made them more susceptible to the effects of the disease, and this was of significance in the mining districts with their high fertility rates and low ages at which women were married.[51] However, teenage girls experienced

---

[48]   Anderson, 'Social implications of demographic change', p. 23, maintains that the high levels of respiratory tuberculosis mortality of these two occupational groups was due more to social factors rather than to working conditions, although Anderson does not expand on this point.

[49]   Jones, 'Counting the cost of coal', pp. 124–8; Edward Shorter, *A History of Women's Bodies* (London, 1983), p. 232; Johansson, 'Sex and death in Victorian England', pp. 169–70.

[50]   For further evidence of increases in tuberculosis death rates in south Wales, see Linda Bryder, *Below the Magic Mountain: A Social History of Tuberculosis in Twentieth Century Britain* (Oxford, 1988), pp. 114–16, 124.

[51]   Ibid., pp. 99–100; Johnston, 'Tuberculosis', p. 1060.

higher levels of tuberculosis mortality than their male counterparts and this was not due to the effects of pregnancy. The onset of puberty contributed to the peak in female mortality at this age since metabolic changes in the bodies of teenage girls increased the need for protein and when protein is unavailable resistance to infection decreases.[52] The effects of menstruation would also have depleted the nutritional status of teenage girls and it is significant that high levels of anaemia were found among girls attending secondary and continuation schools in the Rhondda in the 1930s.[53]

These biological factors were exacerbated by a cultural practice that favoured the nutrition of boys and young men of this age over girls and young women. It is possible that the earning power of boys of this age needed to be safeguarded and boys who contributed to the household income were more likely to be able to satisfy their food requirements.[54] It is also possible that girls and young women from valley communities contracted tuberculosis while in service and returned home to die and thereby inflated the death rate, but it is difficult to measure the extent of this phenomenon. Lastly, girls and women were more likely to nurse sick members of the family and this increased the likelihood that they would contract tuberculosis.

Despite these contributory social and biological factors, the economic conditions of the interwar depression are likely to be the major cause of the increase in female tuberculosis mortality in Merthyr and probably in other depressed areas of south Wales. An investigation carried out by senior Ministry of Health officials in 1934 described the increasing mortality among young adults in south Wales as 'striking' and, while failing to explain this increase, concluded that unemployment could not be ruled out as a factor.[55] Subsequent official inquiries also found evidence of increases in tuberculosis death rates in the depressed communities of south Wales.[56] Public statements, however, were confined to observations

[52]   Johnston, 'Tuberculosis', p. 1060.
[53]   Rhondda UD, RSMO (1936), pp. xliv–xlv; (1937), p. lii.
[54]   Gillian Cronjé, 'Tuberculosis and mortality decline in England and Wales, 1851–1910', in Robert Woods and John Hugh Woodward (eds), *Urban Disease and Mortality in Nineteenth-Century England* (London, 1984), p. 89; Anderson, 'Social implications of demographic change', p. 19. The Rhondda medical officer noted inadequate nutrition as a causative factor in the mortality of girls and young women from respiratory tuberculosis; Rhondda UD, RMOH (1937), p. 155.
[55]   National Archives, London, MH79/336, J. Pearse, J. Alison Glover, A. P. Hughes Gibb and T. W. Wade, 'Inquiry into the present conditions as regards the effects of continued unemployment on health in certain distressed areas', 3 July 1934, pp. 2–4.
[56]   Bryder, *Below the Magic Mountain*, p. 116.

that unemployment could not be causing premature death because tuberculosis mortality in England and Wales as a whole was declining and that the total rates in certain districts of south Wales were decreasing.[57] Some medical officers in south Wales opposed this official, optimistic interpretation. Ralph Picken, the medical officer of Cardiff County Borough, described tuberculosis mortality as 'that sure measure of extreme hardship', while J. Glyn Cox demonstrated how tuberculosis mortality in Barry rose during the 1920s and peaked during the trough of the Depression in the early 1930s.[58]

Further insights into the gendered experience of tuberculosis mortality and the influence of occupation can be found in the *Registrar-General's Decennial Supplements*. The *Decennial Supplement* referring to the years 1921–3 demonstrated that coal miners, though experiencing higher levels of overall mortality relative to occupied males in England and Wales as a whole, nevertheless experienced lower than average tuberculosis death rates. Furthermore, in the context of British miners as a whole, the 'hewers and getters' class of miners in Glamorgan and Monmouthshire experienced more favourable pulmonary tuberculosis rates than their colleagues in other coalfields, as did the 'other underground workers' of Monmouthshire.[59] Dockworkers, on the other hand, while experiencing higher levels of mortality than other working males, suffered considerably higher pulmonary tuberculosis rates.

The extent to which this pattern of tuberculosis mortality can be attributed to working conditions rather than wider social factors may be partly gauged by the findings of the Registrar-General's subsequent *Decennial Supplement*, for the period 1930–2, which also surveyed the mortality patterns of married females according to their husbands' occupations. It found that, while the overall level of mortality and the level of pulmonary tuberculosis mortality of miners had increased in relation to those of all males during the intervening period, miners continued to experience relatively low

---

[57]   *Annual Report of the Chief Medical Officer of the Ministry of Health* (1932), p. 17; Ministry of Health, *Report of an Investigation in the Coalfield of South Wales and Monmouth*, p. 5.

[58]   Cardiff CB, RMOH (1930), p. 7; Glyn Cox, *Report of an Investigation into the Incidence of Tuberculosis*, pp. 32–3; see also Rhondda UD, RMOH (1931), p. 57; Nantyglo and Blaina UD, RMOH (1925), p. 4.

[59]   *The Registrar-General's Decennial Supplement, England and Wales, 1921: Part II. Occupational Mortality, Fertility, and Infant Mortality* (London, 1927), pp. lv–lvii, lx–lxiv.

Table 7.5. Standardized death rates of males in coalmining and dock work from all causes and pulmonary tuberculosis, England and Wales 1921–3 (all occupied and retired males aged 20–65 = 1000).

Occupation	Standardized mortality from	
	all causes	pulmonary tuberculosis
All occupied and retired males	1000	1000
Coal miners – hewers and getters	938	686
Coal miners – other underground workers	1203	847
Coal miners – workers above ground	1183	978
Stevedores	1619	2232
Coalboat loaders and dischargers	1231	1018
Other dock labourers	1532	1903

Source: The Registrar-General's Decennial Supplement, England and Wales, 1921: Part II. Occupational Mortality, Fertility, and Infant Mortality (London, 1927), pp. xxii–cxxiv.

levels of pulmonary tuberculosis.[60] Their wives, on the other hand, experienced relatively high levels of pulmonary tuberculosis mortality in comparison with the wives of other workers. Dockworkers continued to experience relatively high levels by 1930–2. However, the number of deaths from this cause among their wives was not sufficient to produce statistically significant death rates and so no rates were published in the *Decennial Supplement*.

Thus, it seems that the high tuberculosis mortality in Cardiff and Swansea, and perhaps in other coastal towns in south Wales, was a result of the high male death rates, which were caused by the working conditions experienced in the docks and by the living conditions of seamen at sea. The coalmining communities of the valleys, on the other hand, experienced higher than average female mortality in the young adult age-groups because of the specific circumstances of women's lives rather than because of factors such as the nature of the environment in coalmining communities or the standard of life allowed by a collier's income. The working environment experienced each day by a miner's wife, the cultural practice that allocated a greater proportion of the household's resources to the males and children of the household, and the onerous burden

[60]   *The Registrar-General's Decennial Supplement, England and Wales, 1931: Part IIa. Occupational Mortality* (London, 1938), pp. 329, 333, 337–8; this data is collated in Thompson, 'Social history of health', 474.

that constant childbearing and work in the home imposed on a woman's body all served to increase female pulmonary tuberculosis mortality.

A significant aspect of twentieth-century mortality patterns is the transition from a vital regime characterized by acute communicable diseases to a lower mortality pattern which featured higher levels of chronic 'degenerative' illnesses associated with older age-groups. Increasingly during the interwar period, medical officers noted the increasing cancer death rates and began to face the problem of cancer mortality. Cancer death rates in south Wales, in common with those in England and Wales, increased during the interwar period and this cause of death accounted for about a tenth of all deaths at that time.[61] However, cancer mortality was lower in south Wales than in England and Wales and this was not due to the younger age-profile of the population in south Wales. Standardized cancer death rates for south Wales were generally lower than the England and Wales rate and mortality in the region was greater in the relatively prosperous boroughs of Cardiff and Swansea than in the mining districts represented by the administrative counties and Merthyr County Borough.

It is with some justification, therefore, that cancer has been described as a 'disease of affluence'. The same cannot be said for mortality from heart disease. Mortality from this cause more than trebled in south Wales during the interwar period but for most of the period remained below the England and Wales average.[62] However, standardized death rates show that, when age-structure is taken into account, certain districts of south Wales experienced greater heart disease mortality by 1931–3 than the England and Wales average.[63] The level of heart disease mortality in south Wales, with the exception of Newport, was less than, or approximated to, the England and Wales average in 1921–3 but exceeded it in all districts by the later period.

Dr Bruce Low, a medical officer of the Welsh Board of Health, carried out a simple investigation of mortality in Maesteg in 1926.

[61] Thompson, 'Social history of health', 445–71.
[62] Ibid.
[63] Ibid., 473.

He noted that the significant feature of mortality there was the large number of deaths from 'largely preventable' causes, such as tuberculosis, childbirth, heart disease and injury or violence, experienced by young adults. 'It is safe to conclude', he commented, 'that too many people are dying in or before the prime of life'.

Low pointed out that the sanitary administration of the district was satisfactory and that acute infectious diseases, which had occupied the attention of public health authorities for so long, no longer accounted for as many deaths as in the past. The water supply and sanitary arrangements, although not ideal, had been improved in recent years but, Low pointed out, 'these measures do not apparently stop people dying from Tuberculosis and Cancer',

> nor does the sanitary administration afford them the provision of sufficient nourishment and healthy surroundings in their homes and the amenities of life which go a long way to keeping them in good health. There is reason to believe proper housing and the payment of adequate wages are at present time two of the most important factors which determine the health of people . . . Food, fresh air and the removal of the people from dirt, squalor and poverty are the pressing needs of the population of Maesteg, which may be taken as a type of many mining and industrial districts of Wales.[64]

This report on Maesteg, never intended for publication, was a great deal more candid than the published opinions of many public health officials. In its recognition of the social determinants of mortality, it is a critique of orthodox public health policy at that time and might have been an attempt by a senior official to change the methods utilized by public health authorities. At a time when official explanations of mortality focused more on personal behaviour than on social inequality, Low's interpretation was exceptional.

As the economic depression worsened, official claims that unemployment had not affected mortality levels were increasingly based on total death rates. While it is impossible to obtain separate mortality statistics for the unemployed, if the mortality rates are disaggregated, it is possible to observe that for certain sections of the population mortality rates increased in relation to certain causes of death, in a period when they decreased elsewhere in England and Wales. As has been shown by this and other studies, government officials were aware that this was happening but gave no

---

[64] Bruce Low, 'Report of the sanitary circumstances of the Maesteg Urban District', pp. 10–19.

indication of it in their public statements.[65] More generally, it is evident that the economic depression of the interwar period retarded improvements in the levels of mortality in south Wales that were being experienced elsewhere, leaving south Wales a relatively disadvantaged region by the end of the period.

---

[65]   Webster, 'Healthy or hungry thirties?', 110–29.

VIII

INFANT MORTALITY

> The Infant Mortality Rate ... gives probably the best index of the social
> welfare and sanitary administration of any district.
>
> (Dr J. Thomas, Medical Officer of Health)[1]

The idea that the infant mortality rate is a useful indicator of the
economic prosperity and sanitary conditions of a community had
become commonplace in nineteenth-century Britain, and the infant
mortality rate has been used by historians ever since as a sensitive
index of the health status of a population. As C. H. Lee has stated:

> Infant mortality has been widely accepted as an important and significant
> indicator of health achievement, because infancy has always been one of the
> most vulnerable periods of human life, and because the scale of infant
> mortality has important consequences. Furthermore, infant mortality has
> been shown to be associated, in various studies, with a number of important
> economic and social indicators, such as income per head, equality of income
> distribution, and material deprivation.[2]

Edward Stockwell has described the infant mortality rate as 'the
most sensitive indicator of the overall health status of any population group' and has even gone so far as to suggest that infant
mortality is 'a much more accurate indicator of the level of socio-
economic well-being of a people than its per capita gross national
product or any other of the more conventional indices of economic
development'.[3]

Perhaps not surprisingly, attention focused on infant mortality
during the interwar depression. Expert opinion on the matter was
divided as some medical officers echoed the official view that unemployment did not have an adverse effect on mortality, while other
medical officers posited a causal relationship between unemployment and infant mortality. Typical of the first group of medical
officers was Dr E. Colston Williams, the medical officer for

[1] Gelligaer UD, RMOH (1920), p. 66.
[2] C. H. Lee, 'Regional inequalities in infant mortality in Britain, 1861–1971: patterns
and hypotheses', *Population Studies*, 45, 1 (1991), 55.
[3] E. G. Stockwell, 'Infant mortality', in Kiple, *Cambridge World History of Human Disease*,
pp. 224, 226.

Glamorgan, who maintained throughout the interwar period that unemployment did not have a detrimental effect on mortality levels. In 1928, for example, he argued that: 'It is remarkable that hard times are not more clearly reflected in statistics, the probable explanation, however, is that public and private assistance have substantially helped in preventing much sickness and death.'[4] When the statistics did take a turn for the worse, as in 1931, Williams commented: 'Not so good as last year, but remarkable when considered as the health statistics of bad times'.[5] The nearest that Williams came to recognizing a causal relationship between unemployment and infant mortality was in 1932 when he commented that 'bad times are not without effect on both mother and child'.[6]

Other medical officers were adamant that unemployment did indeed have a detrimental effect on levels of infant mortality. The medical officers of Maesteg and of Nantyglo and Blaina both commented in 1934 that infant deaths were more numerous in homes where the father was unemployed. 'It may be that the undernourishment of the expectant mother and the harassing conditions of the home have contributed to this factor', reasoned the Nantyglo and Blaina medical officer.[7] The medical officer of Penybont Rural District was more definite in his estimation of the precise consequences of unemployment:

> Where the weekly amount going into the house is a small one, and where it is impossible to make ends meet, the nursing or expectant mother is the first to suffer, and in consequence the child is deprived of that nourishment which is essential to its well-being.[8]

In a British context it is evident that south Wales experienced high levels of infant mortality during the interwar period.[9] As Table

[4]   Glamorgan CC, RMOH (1928), p. 2.
[5]   Glamorgan CC, RMOH (1931), p. 2.
[6]   Glamorgan CC, RMOH (1929), p. 10. The *Western Mail* was keen to publicize such statements; see for example 10 July 1925, 5.
[7]   Maesteg UD, RMOH (1934), p. 9; Nantyglo and Blaina UD, RMOH (1934), p. 16; see also Rhondda UD, RMOH (1925), p. 37.
[8]   Penybont RD, RMOH (1928), p. 5; also (1927), p. 6; (1931), p. 3.
[9]   Lee, 'Regional inequalities', points out that south Wales experienced relatively high levels of infant mortality during the late nineteenth and early twentieth centuries; see also Woods, Watterson and Woodward, 'Causes of rapid infant mortality decline Part I', 353–7; I. M. Buchanan, 'Infant mortality in British coal mining communities, 1880–1911' (unpubl. University of London Ph.D. thesis, 1983), esp. 32; for further information on regional variations in infant mortality during the interwar period, see the *Registrar-General's Decennial Supplement, England and Wales 1931, Part IIa. Occupational Mortality*, pp. 168–9, 386–90, 399–404.

8.1 demonstrates, the infant mortality rates for the major administrative areas of south Wales were consistently higher in the interwar period than the aggregate rate for England and Wales.

Table 8.1. Quinquennial infant mortality averages, south Wales and England and Wales, 1920–39 (infant deaths per 1,000 live births)

	1920–4	1925–9	1930–4	1935–9
Cardiff CB	82.2	78.6	75.2	56.6
Merthyr CB	88.4	96.8	86.5	78.8
Swansea CB	79.2	74.4	67.4	56.4
Newport CB	70.8	72.0	76.8	62.3
Glamorgan AC	85.0	80.0	72.4	62.4
Monmouthshire AC	82.3	75.4	66.7	60.8
England and Wales	76.8	70.8	62.8	55.4

It is clear from this table that infant mortality in south Wales decreased in common with other areas of England and Wales in the interwar period and that the decline over the twenty years was, with the exception of Newport and Merthyr Tydfil, considerable. In fact, Newport experienced a rise in infant mortality in the late 1920s and early 1930s and only experienced a decline in mortality during the late 1930s.

It is also evident that the fall in infant mortality was not as great in south Wales as it was in other parts of England and Wales, with the result that regional inequality was growing in the fifteen years before the mid 1930s. It was only in the late 1930s that infant mortality in south Wales began to close the gap with England and Wales, although in Merthyr Tydfil the infant mortality rate continued to fall more slowly than the England and Wales average. Adopting a longer term perspective, many historians have noted that the rate of decrease in infant mortality in the first half of the twentieth century for Britain as a whole was at its lowest in the 1930s and that this is evidence that economic crisis was an important factor in the level of infant mortality.[10] That a depressed region such as south Wales experienced a slower rate of improvement in infant mortality than England and Wales as a whole suggests that unemployment and poverty were indeed important factors in the level of infant mortality.

By further disaggregating the infant mortality rates in south

[10] Lee, 'Regional inequalities'; Webster, 'Healthy or hungry thirties?', 123–4; Mitchell, 'Effects of unemployment on women and children', 107.

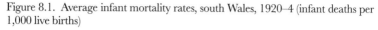

Figure 8.1. Average infant mortality rates, south Wales, 1920–4 (infant deaths per 1,000 live births)

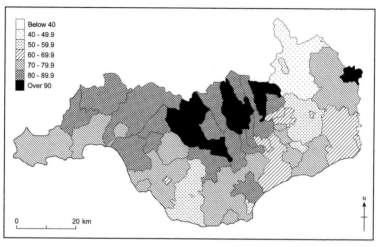

Below 40
40 - 49.9
50 - 59.9
60 - 69.9
70 - 79.9
80 - 89.9
Over 90

0   20 km

N

Note: For administrative districts, see Map 1, p. vx.

Wales it is possible to observe regional variations.[11] Infant mortality rates in the quinquennium 1920–4 are represented in Figure 8.1. It is evident from this figure and the material in Appendices 8.1 and 8.2 that the coalmining districts of south Wales experienced higher levels of infant mortality than the England and Wales aggregate, yet were experiencing a decline in the level of mortality during the interwar period. However, as was noted above, mortality levels did not decrease to the same extent as the England and Wales rate. Indeed, in districts such as Bedwas and Machen, Mynyddislwyn, Nantyglo and Blaina, Caerphilly, Maesteg, and Ogmore and Garw, the difference between the local rate and the national average increased during the course of the interwar period. In other districts, such as Glyncorrwg, Neath, Ogmore and Garw, Port Talbot, Rhondda, Pontardawe, Bedwellty, Pontypool and Rhymney, infant mortality increased or remained at about the same rate from 1920–4 to 1930–4 and only fell in the late 1930s.[12] As

---

[11]   See Appendices 8.1 and 8.2.
[12]   See Appendix 8.2; even in many of these districts the excess mortality over the England and Wales average was greater at the end of the interwar period than in the early 1920s.

might be expected, more rural districts, such as Cowbridge, Gower, Abergavenny, Chepstow, Magor and St Mellons, Monmouth and Pontypool, consistently experienced lower levels of mortality than the industrialized, urban areas of south Wales and, indeed, the England and Wales average. Similarly, small municipal boroughs such as Usk and Cowbridge and the coastal resort of Porthcawl experienced low levels of infant mortality, reflecting both the small number of births and the more salubrious sanitary conditions of such areas.

An investigation of the age-specific nature of infant mortality in south Wales allows further useful insights.[13] Neonatal mortality (that is, mortality in the first thirty days of life) has been used by historical demographers to reveal pre-natal causes of infant mortality and mortality due to the birth process. These 'endogenous' causes of infant mortality include developmental problems experienced in the womb, injury at birth, prematurity and other congenital causes of death, and stem primarily from maternal nutritional and health status. Post-neonatal mortality (that is, infant mortality after the first month of life but within twelve months), on the other hand, usually resulted from exogenous causes of death such as diarrhoeal, respiratory or common infections, accidents or other environmental factors. This type of infant mortality serves as an indicator of the quality of maternal care, the effectiveness of infant welfare services and the sanitary environment. Due to developments in modern medical science that prolong infant life for some time after the neonatal period, and the existence of some neonatal deaths due to exogenous factors, neonatal and post-neonatal mortality can no longer be assumed to be caused by endogenous and exogenous causes respectively, but the distinction remains valid for a study of infant mortality in the interwar period.

In common with most societies, infant mortality in south Wales was greatest immediately following birth and declined as age increased. Infant mortality was, with few exceptions, higher at all ages in south Wales than the England and Wales aggregate rate. As has been pointed out, neonatal mortality reflects the nutritional and health status of pregnant women. Poor or deteriorating maternal nutritional status increases neonatal mortality through increased likelihood of developmental problems in the womb, greater

[13]   See Appendix 8.3.

Figure 8.2. Neonatal mortality rates for selected areas of south Wales and England and Wales, 1920–39

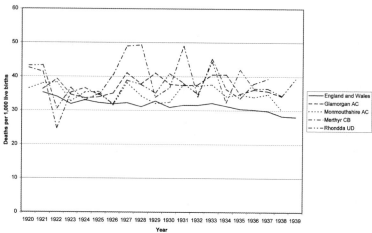

prematurity, an increased likelihood of difficult labour and lower birth weights.[14] It is evident that neonatal mortality was consistently higher in south Wales than the England and Wales average and also that, in common with the rest of England and Wales, neonatal rates in south Wales were more resistant to improvement than death rates for infants over the age of one month.

The quinquennial neonatal mortality averages show that the decrease in this rate in England and Wales was very small during the interwar period (33.6 deaths per 1,000 live births in 1921–4 to 29.4 in 1935–9).[15] The neonatal mortality rates for the boroughs of Cardiff and Swansea similarly fell during the same period but the decreases were even smaller. However, increases in neonatal mortality were experienced outside these more prosperous county boroughs. Figure 8.2 demonstrates that, following the high mortality of the hot

[14]   R. Lee, 'Infant, child and maternal mortality in Western Europe: a critique', in Brändström and Tedebrand, *Society, Health and Population during the Demographic Transition*, pp. 15–16.

[15]   See Appendix 8.3.

[16]   These hot summers produced an increase in mortality from diarrhoeal causes and while these causes of death are usually associated with the deaths of infants aged over three months, it seems that in years of epidemic diarrhoea younger infants also suffered high mortality rates from this cause; see for example Buchanan, 'Infant mortality in British coal mining communities', 110.

summers of 1920 and 1921,[16] neonatal mortality rates in south Wales closely approximated to, or marginally exceeded, the England and Wales rate during the early to mid 1920s. During the later 1920s, neonatal mortality in south Wales began to increase and to exceed the England and Wales rate by a larger margin. The rise in neonatal mortality rates in south Wales in Figure 8.2 is most clearly demonstrated in the cases of the administrative counties of Glamorgan and Monmouthshire where sufficiently large numbers of deaths produced a smoother trend line. It can be seen that neonatal mortality rates rose during the late 1920s, peaked during the early 1930s and declined thereafter. Merthyr, Newport and the Rhondda experienced small increases from the early 1920s to the late 1930s (and even larger increases from the early 1920s to the early 1930s). Therefore, levels of neonatal mortality in south Wales during the interwar period closely reflected the economic fortunes of the region as levels of unemployment and poverty also increased during the late 1920s, peaked during the early 1930s and decreased during the mid to late 1930s.

The increases in neonatal mortality are even more evident in smaller districts such as Abertillery, Mountain Ash and Penybont.[17] The neonatal mortality rate for the Abertillery Urban District increased from 38.2 deaths per 1,000 live births in 1920–4 to 42.3 in 1935–8 while the comparable rates for Mountain Ash were 28.4 and 40.5, and for Penybont 36.5 and 38.6.[18] In the cases of Penybont and Mountain Ash these increases occurred despite the highly developed and energetic nature of the infant welfare services in these localities.[19] The neonatal mortality rate is a particularly sensitive indicator of the nutritional status and health of expectant mothers, and it is significant that neonatal mortality rates increased in districts that experienced high levels of unemployment and poverty in the interwar period. Moreover, it is evident that south Wales's trend departed from that of England and Wales as a whole.

[17] See Appendix 8.3. The infant mortality rates are 'real' rates based upon 'definite' statistics and not estimates as in the case of total death rates. Penybont was mainly a rural district but its population was largely concentrated in the northern part of the district and primarily engaged in industrial activities – the census of 1921 enumerated 42 per cent of the males aged over 12 as employed in the coal industry, 7.2 per cent in agricultural occupations, 5 per cent in transport and 3.9 per cent as builders; Census of England and Wales 1921, Glamorgan, p. 66.

[18] See Appendix 8.3.

[19] See Penybont RD, RMOH (1920–39); Mountain Ash UD, RMOH (1920–39); the nature of these services is discussed below.

The pattern of neonatal mortality in south Wales had many of the same characteristics as the pattern for stillbirth mortality. As Nicky Hart has pointed out, stillbirths were a significant aspect of 'reproductive mortality' and yet they have not received the same attention from historical demographers as infant mortality.[20] While neonatal mortality is a useful indicator of the nutritional and health status of expectant and nursing mothers, the stillbirth rate highlights even more starkly the health status of childbearing women in interwar south Wales. As Hart comments:

> Stillbirth is . . . a valuable health status indicator . . . Where death occurs in utero the external environment is mediated by the mother's body, which is the foetal lifeline and a means of environmental insulation. The female body is the instrument of human procreation, and stillbirth is a good indicator of its capacity, its vitality. Since female physique reflects material conditions and the distribution of subsistence between the sexes, stillbirth is also an important potential indicator of inequality between them.[21]

Stillbirths and neonatal deaths share many of the same determinants. Both are primarily determined by the nature of the foetal environment in the period two to nine months after conception. It was recognized during the interwar period that the causes of deaths in the first week of life were the same as those causing stillbirths and that both were sensitive indicators of maternal health.[22] The stillbirth mortality rate for England and Wales decreased from about 40 deaths per 1,000 total births in the late 1920s to about 37 by the end of the 1930s.[23] The rates for south Wales were consistently, and often considerably, higher than the England and Wales aggregate.[24] Merthyr, in particular, experienced one of the highest stillbirth

[20]   Nicky Hart, 'Beyond infant mortality: gender and stillbirth in reproductive mortality before the twentieth century', *Population Studies*, 52, 2 (1998), 215–29.
[21]   Ibid., 227; a point also made by David Graham, 'Female employment and infant mortality: some evidence from British towns, 1911, 1931, 1951', *Continuity and Change*, 9, 2 (1994), 315.
[22]   See for example Swansea CB, RMOH (1925), p. 15. Out of 233 infant deaths in Swansea that year, 107 occurred within one week of age. If this is added to the number of stillbirths, the total number of perinatal deaths (288), as these deaths are described, was more than double the number of post-neonatal deaths (126).
[23]   See Appendix 8.4.
[24]   Ministry of Health, *Report on Maternal Mortality in Wales*, pp. 16–17, demonstrates that high stillbirth mortality was a characteristic of the whole of Wales; see also Winter, 'Unemployment, nutrition and infant mortality in Britain, 1920–50', 239.
[25]   Graham, 'Female employment and infant mortality', 315.

Figure 8.3. Stillbirth rates for large administrative areas of south Wales and England and Wales, 1928–39

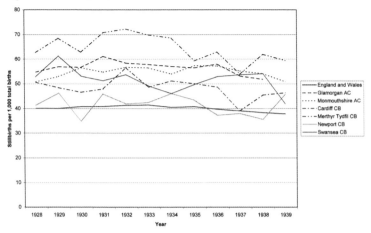

Source: Registrar-General's Statistical Review, 1928–39.

mortality rates in the whole of England and Wales during the 1930s.[25]

The greater levels of stillbirth mortality in south Wales are demonstrated in Figure 8.3. Stillbirths were made notifiable from 1 July 1927 and so reliable figures for the period before 1928 are not available for these areas. Nevertheless, some local medical officers in south Wales recorded the numbers of stillbirths in their annual reports.[26]

Figure 8.4 demonstrates that stillbirth rates in these districts increased during the course of the interwar period. This increase might have been due to the more precise registration of these deaths. The stillbirth figures for the Rhondda in the 1920s, for example, were supplied to the medical officer by the sextons of the three local cemeteries and since newspapers were full of reports of stillborn infants being found in rivers, canals and other places, it seems likely that figures for the 1920s underestimate the true extent of stillbirth mortality in south Wales.[27] Countering this to some extent is the fact that, prior to 1927, in cases where infants died soon after birth, doctors or midwives often counted them as stillbirths so

[26] See Appendix 8.4.
[27] See also Baker, *'Yan Boogie'*, pp. 49–50.

Figure 8.4. Stillbirths in selected districts of south Wales, 1920–39

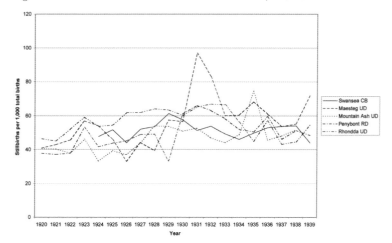

as to avoid the formalities of registration, thereby exaggerating the true extent of stillbirth mortality, although whether this would have changed over time to produce the trends shown seems unlikely.[28] Nevertheless, from 1928 onwards the statistics are more reliable and they show an excess of stillbirths in south Wales beyond the England and Wales average and a rise in stillbirths in south Wales in the early 1930s.

A further insight is gained by taking a longer term view of stillbirths in south Wales. Stillbirth rates for the Rhondda are available from 1901 and for Swansea borough from 1910 and these are shown in Figure 8.5. The figures for the Rhondda are the more complete and the resulting trend line is the more instructive. It shows that the stillbirth rate decreased in the decade before the First World War and continued to do so until 1920 when it reached 44.8 stillbirths per 1,000 total births. Thereafter, the stillbirth rate increased through the 1920s and reached a peak of 66.5 in 1933, after which a decline set in. The stillbirth rate for Swansea borough was similarly higher in the late 1920s and early 1930s relative to its level in the pre-First World War period. This pattern of high stillbirth rates in the late 1920s and early 1930s relative to the period

<hr />

[28]   Rhondda UD, RMOH (1923), pp. 28–9.

Figure 8.5. Stillbirth rates for the Rhondda Urban District and Swansea County Borough, 1901–39

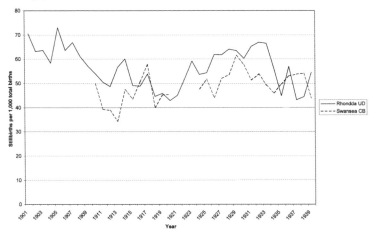

Source: Rhondda UD, RMOH (1920), pp. 19–20; Swansea CB, RMOH (1920), p. 23.

before the First World War might be explained by the more effective registration of stillbirths from July 1927, but it still fails to account for the increase in stillbirth mortality in the two districts before 1928. This is most marked in the Rhondda which, of course, experienced industrial depression throughout the 1920s. The method of counting stillbirths seems to have remained the same in the Rhondda for the period 1901 to 1927 and so the pattern of stillbirth mortality in the period before 1927 cannot be attributed to changes in the method of counting. Long-term changes in customs and attitudes toward stillbirths and burials might have affected the observed pattern but they cannot be accurately assessed.

For these reasons, it would seem that economic factors were important in determining the changing stillbirth rate for Swansea borough and the Rhondda valleys in the period 1901–39 and that the economic depression of the interwar years was instrumental in lowering the nutritional status of expectant mothers and increasing stillbirth mortality. The higher level of stillbirth mortality in the Rhondda reflects the greater level of unemployment and poverty experienced there. Developments in scientific medicine and improvements in the public environment failed to make a significant impact on neonatal mortality and, for the same reasons, made little difference to levels of stillbirth mortality. Expectant mothers, who were at the mercy of economic conditions that determined their nutritional status and a culture that ensured that a household's resources were devoted to the male 'breadwinners', paid a heavy price during the interwar depression as a large proportion of pregnancies resulted in stillbirths. Nicky Hart's assertion that neonatal and stillbirth mortality did not change appreciably during the economic depression of the 1930s, based as it is on the aggregate England and Wales rates, probably reflects the improvements experienced in more affluent areas of Britain rather than the effects of economic depression in the depressed areas.[29] In south Wales, neonatal and stillbirth mortality clearly increased and the same might be found in other depressed regions.

Mortality rates for infants over the age of one month experienced a greater decrease than neonatal mortality rates during the interwar period, with decreases of between a third and a half in most districts.[30] Once more, Merthyr lagged behind the other districts of south Wales both in terms of the absolute level of post-natal mortality and in the degree of improvement. Newport experienced the smallest decline in mortality but this was because of the relatively low rates in the early 1920s from which the decline in mortality began. It is evident that the decreases in post-neonatal mortality in Newport were not as great as for England and Wales as a whole and that from a favourable level of post-neonatal mortality Newport had, by the late 1930s, become a borough with a less favourable level of mortality relative to England and Wales. Interestingly, in those districts that experienced rising neonatal mortality rates, levels of mortality for older infants nevertheless decreased, often rapidly. The mortality rates for infants aged 9–12 months in Abertillery, for example, decreased from 11.0 deaths per 1,000 live births in 1920–4 to 3.7 in 1935–8 while in Mountain Ash comparable rates fell from 9.8 to 3.9 in the same period.

The worsened health status of women was further demonstrated by the increases in maternal mortality which occurred. Of the various forms of 'reproductive mortality', it is perhaps the issue of maternal mortality that received most attention during the interwar

---

[29] Hart, 'Beyond infant mortality', 227; Figure 8.3, however, suggests that the England and Wales stillbirth rate experienced a small increase from the late 1920s to the early 1930s.

[30] See Appendix 8.3.

[31] See for example Stevenson and Cook, *The Slump*, pp. 19–21, 38–46, 78–81; Winter,

period and has figured most prominently in the historiographical debates on unemployment and standards of health.[31] However, it is important to note that various investigations into maternal mortality carried out before the interwar depression found that mortality rates were significantly higher in Wales than in other parts of Britain.[32] This was as true of the rural areas of Wales as it was of the industrial valleys of the south. Therefore, the fact that maternal mortality was high in interwar south Wales relative to other parts of Britain is insufficient as evidence of the demographic impact of the Depression.

The more 'pessimistic' interpretations of health in interwar Britain argue that maternal mortality in the depressed areas increased and suggest that this increase was a direct result of economic depression and unemployment.[33] These assertions are, surprisingly, supported by an official source. The Ministry of Health's investigation into maternal mortality in Wales, published in 1937, found that puerperal mortality increased in south Wales in the period from 1924–8 to 1929–33.[34] Puerperal mortality in the Special Areas of south Wales increased from 5.16 deaths per 1,000 live births in the period 1924–8 to 6.50 deaths in 1929–33.[35] The report concluded that, while puerperal mortality rates had decreased or remained stationary for the rest of Wales, mortality rates for the Special Areas had increased 'considerably'.

The significance of these findings is contentious. Winter, for example, has argued that south Wales was exceptional and that

'Infant mortality, maternal mortality and public health'; Webster, 'Healthy or hungry thirties?', 117–18, 122–3; Mitchell, 'Effects of unemployment on women and children', 111, 115–16, 119.

[32] W. Williams, 'Puerperal mortality', *Transactions of the Epidemiological Society of London* (1895–96), 100–33; *Forty-Fourth Annual Report of the Local Government Board, 1914–15, Supplement Containing a Report on Maternal Mortality* [Cd. 8085], 1914–16, XXV, pp. 32–3, 36, 40; Ministry of Health, *Reports on Public Health and Medical Subjects*, 25: Janet M. Campbell, *Maternal Mortality* (London, 1924); Ministry of Health, *Reports on Public Health and Medical Subjects*, 68: Dame Janet Campbell, Isabella D. Cameron and Dilys M. Jones, *High Maternal Mortality in Certain Areas* (London, 1932).

[33] Webster, 'Healthy or hungry thirties?', 117; Mitchell, 'Effects of unemployment on women and children', 111, 115–16; a notable aspect of many of the 'pessimistic' interpretations of maternal mortality in interwar Britain is reference to the feeding experiments of the National Birthday Trust Fund in the Rhondda valleys but, as Williams, *Women and Childbirth in the Twentieth Century*, pp. 81, 90–1, 98, demonstrates, these experiments were methodologically flawed and cannot be used as evidence of low maternal nutritional status with the confidence that has hitherto been placed upon them.

[34] Ministry of Health, *Report on Maternal Mortality in Wales*, pp. 16–18, 25, 88–92, 114.

[35] Ibid., p. 88.

[36] Winter, 'Unemployment, nutrition and infant mortality', 243; Winter, 'Infant mortality, maternal mortality and public health', 454–5.

maternal mortality decreased in other parts of Britain during the period.[36] This is, of course, a legitimate and reasonable argument. More relevant is the work of Irvine Loudon. Loudon places less importance on socio-economic factors in maternal mortality and, instead, emphasizes the quality of obstetrical care, the virulence of streptococcal infection and increased levels of abortion.[37] Loudon dismisses the high and increasing puerperal mortality rates in the depressed areas of south Wales as, in the words of the Ministry of Health report, 'the cumulative result of a variety of unfavourable factors working in association' rather than the effects of malnutrition alone.[38] Moreover, if improved nutritional status was the crucial factor in the decrease in maternal mortality after 1935, Loudon argues, the decrease would have been more marked in relation to accidents of childbirth as opposed to puerperal sepsis. That the decrease in maternal mortality was primarily due to a decrease in puerperal sepsis, Loudon contends, demonstrates that it was the quality of obstetrical care that was the crucial factor.[39]

However, Loudon does not satisfactorily explain the increase in puerperal mortality in the depressed areas of south Wales, and his assertion that the migration of healthy young women from south Wales increased mortality rates is tenuous.[40] It seems unlikely that the quality of obstetrical services in Wales deteriorated in this particular period and in the Special Areas alone. This is confirmed by the fact that while mortality from puerperal sepsis in Wales exceeded the rates for England and Wales, excess mortality from 'other puerperal causes', which Loudon associates with social and economic factors, was much greater. Moreover, whereas mortality from puerperal sepsis increased slightly for England and Wales as a whole in the period 1924–35, mortality from 'other' puerperal causes decreased slightly. In contrast, Wales experienced increases in both puerperal sepsis mortality and 'other' puerperal mortality.[41] As Loudon argues, poor maternal health leads to greater levels of mortality from these 'other' causes whereas levels of puerperal

[37]   Irvine Loudon, *Death in Childbirth: An International Study of Maternal Care and Maternal Mortality, 1800–1950* (Oxford, 1992), pp. 243–4, 251; see also *idem*, 'On maternal and infant mortality, 1900–1960', *Social History of Medicine*, 4, 1 (1991), 29–73.

[38]   Irvine Loudon, 'Maternal mortality: 1880–1950. Some regional and international comparisons', *Social History of Medicine*, 1, 2 (1988), 197.

[39]   Ibid., 197–8.

[40]   Ibid., 197.

[41]   Ministry of Health, *Report on Maternal Mortality in Wales*, p. 14.

sepsis are primarily attributable to standards of obstetrical care. Therefore, south Wales experienced an increase in those forms of maternal mortality that Loudon associates with social and economic determinants.

Although unemployment and poverty affected the health of expectant mothers in depressed areas and resulted in increases in neonatal, stillbirth and maternal mortality rates, environmental improvements, improved childrearing techniques of mothers and the development of infant welfare services led to a decrease in the levels of mortality of older infants. This emphasizes once again that it was the women of south Wales who bore the brunt of the economic difficulties faced by families during the interwar depression. Women's inability to meet the demands placed on their bodies by pregnancy, exacerbated by the consequences of economic conditions for their nutritional intake, was reflected in the higher levels of stillbirth, neonatal and maternal mortality.

An examination of the causes of infant deaths sheds further light on infant mortality in interwar south Wales. However, the evidence for such an examination is sparse. The annual reports of the medical officers of the major administrative areas of south Wales provide the necessary information only in some cases, while in the smaller urban or rural districts the number of deaths in each cause-specific category was too few to calculate meaningful death rates. Nevertheless, enough evidence exists to calculate cause-specific infant mortality rates for a number of districts and to make a number of useful points.[42] These cause-specific infant mortality rates confirm a number of the assertions already made.

First, mortality from endogenous causes of mortality, usually occurring in the first month of life, was responsible for a significant proportion of infant mortality and experienced little improvement during the interwar period. This merely confirms the pattern revealed by the age-specific infant mortality rates. Death rates from constitutional and non-infective diseases remained roughly stationary during the interwar period and accounted for a growing proportion of infant deaths as deaths from other causes decreased. These endogenous causes accounted for between a third and a half of all infant deaths in the early 1920s but about half of all infant deaths by the late 1930s.

[42] For cause-specific infant mortality rates see Thompson, 'Social history of health', 489–94.

Secondly, deaths from exogenous causes, usually associated with the post-neonatal period, decreased significantly during the interwar period, both in absolute terms and as a proportion of total infant deaths. Changing patterns of infant deaths from infectious, diarrhoeal and respiratory diseases can be used to gauge the changing nature of the environment and developments in infant care. Deaths from infectious diseases, though displaying annual fluctuations, decreased markedly during the interwar period even though such deaths accounted only for a small proportion of total infant mortality at the beginning of the interwar period. The infant death rate from this cause stood at 5.4 deaths per 1,000 live births in Monmouthshire in the period 1920–4, and 4.1 in Swansea and 4.6 in the Rhondda in the same period. These rates decreased to 2.9, 2.5 and 1.6 respectively in the years 1935–9. Improvements in the efficiency of public health authorities in dealing with cases of infectious disease, through greater identification of cases and the isolation of carriers, and the smaller number of children in each family meant that the reservoir of infections grew smaller and the number of potential contacts decreased. Infants faced fewer risks of contracting an infectious disease during the course of the interwar period.[43]

Deaths from diarrhoeal diseases (diarrhoea, enteritis and gastritis) provide a sensitive indicator of the sanitary standards of a locality and the feeding methods practised by parents. The most notable aspect of the trend in diarrhoeal infant death rates was the great increase in mortality in 1921. The hot summer of that year produced a characteristic increase in diarrhoeal deaths. This 'sanitary test' posed by a hot summer was met with varying success in south Wales. In Monmouthshire the diarrhoeal death rate increased from 6.7 to 17.3 deaths per 1,000 live births. In Swansea the comparable rates were 9.8 and 14.2 and for the Rhondda they were 13.9 and 23.9. Colliery districts such as the Rhondda experienced higher levels of diarrhoeal mortality than districts like Swansea which possessed better sanitary infrastructure, such as efficient sewerage systems, plentiful supplies of clean water and a generally more hygienic public environment.

Nevertheless, it is evident that infant mortality from diarrhoeal or intestinal causes decreased to a significant extent in interwar south

---

[43] Sonalde Desai, 'When are children from large families disadvantaged? Evidence from cross-national analyses', *Population Studies*, 49, 2 (1995), 198.

Wales in most districts. Cardiff, Swansea, Rhondda and Pontypridd all experienced considerable decreases so that infant mortality from these causes accounted for only about 1–4 deaths per 1,000 live births by the late 1930s. For the administrative county of Monmouthshire, however, mortality from these causes seems to have remained stationary (with the exception of 1921) during the interwar period. This is rather unexpected when the improvements in water supply following the completion of the Grwyne Fawr and Taf Fechan reservoirs, both in 1928, are taken into account.

The last of these major exogenous causes of death, respiratory disease, accounted for a larger proportion of infant deaths than infectious and diarrhoeal diseases, but the interwar period saw a decrease in infant death rates from respiratory causes. Infant mortality rates from respiratory diseases fluctuated from one year to the next, partly reflecting the nature of these diseases and partly because of weather conditions.

Medical officers were of the opinion that infant deaths from respiratory disease were due to maternal neglect. A survey of infant deaths in Cardiff concluded that mothers took medical advice only after an infant had experienced a 'chesty cough' for two or three days, by which time it was too late for a doctor to prevent death. It was noted that in these cases the mother was also ill and the medical officer concluded that 'These mothers themselves were too ill to care'.[44] The Mountain Ash medical officer linked ignorance with housing conditions to explain deaths from respiratory causes. The fear of cold draughts and of 'catching colds' meant that people blocked fire-grates and flues and packed the crevices around windows with paper to prevent draughts. This, he claimed, prevented the circulation of fresh air and predisposed people to respiratory ailments.[45] Undoubtedly, housing conditions in interwar south Wales had an impact on infant respiratory mortality. The damp, poorly ventilated conditions experienced by such a large proportion of the population had a strong influence on respiratory mortality, especially during autumn and winter.[46] More importantly, infant mortality from respiratory disease has been associated with atmospheric pollution[47] and, as has been shown in Chapter 5, the

[44] Cardiff CB, RMOH (1935), pp. xxi, 16.
[45] Mountain Ash UD, RMOH (1925), p. 7.
[46] Lee, 'Infant, child and maternal mortality in Western Europe', p. 17.
[47] Buchanan, 'Infant mortality in British coal mining communities', 74–5.

atmosphere of south Wales was badly polluted by the various metal industries and the coal industry. Furthermore, the environment of the home was often ill-ventilated and polluted by coal fires that burned every day throughout the year. The large proportion of infant deaths in south Wales that was caused by respiratory diseases was partly a result of the atmospheric pollution that was endemic.

The causes of infant deaths, and their changing pattern over time, reveal a great deal about the social and sanitary conditions of interwar south Wales. They emphasize the points made earlier that while infant mortality from exogenous causes was declining in the interwar period, infant mortality from endogenous causes experienced no such dramatic decrease but instead either remained stationary or even, in some cases, increased. Nevertheless, despite the greater volume of infant mortality in south Wales relative to other parts of England and Wales, and despite the increase in regional inequalities, infant mortality declined considerably in south Wales during the interwar period. Explaining this decrease is not easy but a number of factors need to be considered. The nature of the environment in south Wales has been examined in Chapter 5 and it seems likely that improvements in water quality, sewerage systems, scavenging and the public environment had a beneficial impact on levels of infant mortality. The decrease in deaths from diarrhoeal causes supports this assertion. The effect of health education initiatives and maternal and child welfare care on falling levels of infant mortality are harder to evaluate.

Certainly, many medical officers and public health officials were convinced of the difference that such services could make to the level of infant mortality. Typical was the comment of the Rhondda medical officer:

> It may be confidently asserted . . . that the most important factor immediately affecting the preservation of infant life is the nature of the maternal care and attention given to the baby and it is in fostering and guiding this vital influence for good that the intensive and individual attention which can be given by the trained staff of a welfare department offers the most hopeful possibilities as a preventive of infantile deaths.[48]

The nature and scale of maternity and child welfare services varied from one district to another but efforts were made even in the most depressed districts to extend services during the interwar period. The

---

[48] Rhondda UD, RMOH (1925), pp. 37–8.

Maternity and Child Welfare Act of 1918 placed an obligation on local authorities to provide such services and, whereas services were relatively underdeveloped during the early 1920s, steady progress was made from the mid 1920s. There were 71 maternity and child welfare centres in Glamorgan by 1920 and 39 in Monmouthshire by June 1922, although the provision varied within the counties themselves. The urban district of Gelligaer, for example, with over 40,000 inhabitants, had established seven such centres by 1920, while Pontypridd, with a population of almost 50,000, had not established a single centre by that date. Rhondda, with over 180,000 people, possessed only two welfare centres by 1920.[49] The provision of welfare centres in scattered rural districts was especially problematic.[50] Despite the economic difficulties that faced local authorities, welfare services were extended during the interwar period. By 1938 Monmouthshire had 41 centres and Glamorgan had 97 by 1930.[51] Grants distributed by the Special Areas Commissioner in the 1930s were used to build dedicated premises for welfare clinics, replacing the often unsuitable buildings previously used.[52]

Antenatal services, however, were less developed in south Wales and progress in their provision was slow. The report into maternal mortality in Wales found that there were only eight antenatal clinics in the whole of Wales by 1924, two in Glamorgan, one each in the boroughs of Cardiff, Merthyr and Newport, and two in Swansea. By 1934, of the 87 clinics in Wales, 78 were in Glamorgan and Monmouthshire. There were 55 in Glamorgan, of which 5 were in the Cardiff County Borough, 4 in Merthyr and 3 in Swansea. There were 23 in Monmouthshire and 7 of these were in the borough of Newport. Attendance of expectant mothers at these clinics was still relatively low by 1934. Only between 30 per cent and 45 per cent of expectant mothers attended, although the figure for Merthyr was 60 per cent (the England and Wales average was 42.1 per cent).[53] The antenatal clinics in different districts of south Wales varied in their attitudes to nutritional supplementation.

[49]   Glamorgan CC, RMOH (1920), pp. 20–3; Monmouthshire CC, *Report upon Maternity and Child Welfare for the year 1921*, p. 11.

[50]   Glamorgan CC, RMOH (1927), p. 18.

[51]   Monmouthshire CC, *Report upon Maternity and Child Welfare for the year 1938*, p. 18; Glamorgan CC, RMOH (1930), p. 29.

[52]   Glamorgan CC, RMOH (1937–9).

[53]   Ministry of Health, *Report on Maternal Mortality in Wales*, pp. 27–8. Monmouthshire County Council had extended its antenatal services to 19 clinics by 1938; Monmouthshire County Council, *Report upon Maternity and Child Welfare for the year 1938*, p. 17.

Rhondda Urban District Council spent £112 per 1,000 population
in 1935, Mountain Ash Urban District £64, Merthyr County
Borough £41 and Monmouthshire County Council £5.[54]

Despite the fact that the number of centres in south Wales
increased and welfare services were extended, financial considerations hindered developments. Elizabeth Peretz examined the
maternity and child welfare services provided by Merthyr Tydfil
County Borough Council during the interwar period and found
that, in comparison with certain councils in England, it offered a
restricted service despite being controlled by a Labour majority for
much of the period.[55] In 1920 there were four infant welfare clinics
in the borough and a minor ailments clinic. By 1937 welfare services had been extended to include clinics for dental and orthopaedic
care, a maternity wing at a local authority hospital, midwives, an
artificial sunlight clinic and antenatal clinics. Cod liver oil and milk
were distributed free by the council to infants and expectant
mothers in need and various charitable bodies distributed other
foodstuffs, though this was on a much less comprehensive basis.
Peretz argues that the relatively poor service offered by Merthyr
council was partly attributable to its lack of financial resources and
partly because councillors preferred to give more money to families
rather than to develop welfare services. Such services were viewed
as the patronizing methods of Liberals and Conservatives.
Working-class women in Merthyr were skilled in household
management and childrearing and had no need for the patronizing
advice of meddling professional officials.[56]

The reasons for the development of welfare services in a district
were numerous and cannot be attributed to the political complexion
of the local council alone. In Cardiff it was clearly the size of the
borough and the financial resources at the disposal of the council
that were crucial. In 1920 the borough had already established five

[54]   Webster, 'Health, welfare and unemployment during the Depression', 223.
[55]   It is ironic that H. R. S. Phillpott, in his examination of Labour-controlled councils
throughout Britain, focused on Merthyr's maternity and child welfare services as evidence
of the success of Labour councils in extending essential public health services; see
H. R. S. Phillpott, *Where Labour Rules: A Tour Through Towns and Counties* (London, 1934), pp.
87–9.
[56]   Elizabeth Peretz, 'The costs of modern motherhood to low income families in
interwar Britain', in Valerie Fildes, Lara Marks and Hilary Marland (eds), *Women and Children
First: International Maternal and Infant Welfare, 1870–1945* (London, 1992), pp. 257–80. This
interpretation is contradicted to some extent by the relatively high levels of attendance at
antenatal clinics in Merthyr noted above.

infant welfare and two antenatal clinics, employed ten health visitors and supplied milk to expectant and nursing mothers and infants under the age of 5 free or at less than cost price subject to a means test. The borough council also arranged for the Cardiff Royal Infirmary to take difficult pregnancies. An artificial light treatment clinic was opened in 1928, dental clinics for expectant mothers were established, and even a post-natal clinic was added in 1934. This was indeed a rarity in interwar south Wales. The number of infant welfare clinics had increased to eleven by 1938.[57] Swansea similarly utilized its considerable financial capabilities to develop relatively comprehensive maternity and child welfare services.[58]

Financial ability was not the only determinant of welfare services. The efficiency and energy of the council seems to have been important, as the example of Penybont Rural District demonstrates. Its council had established five infant welfare clinics and an antenatal clinic by 1920 (the only other antenatal clinic in Glamorgan in 1920 was in Margam). Four more infant welfare services were opened in 1926, one in 1927, one in 1928 and three others in 1935 so that there were fourteen centres by the late 1930s.[59]

On numerous occasions, public health officials made the point that they faced, and had to overcome, the ignorance and inertia of mothers in their efforts to disseminate information on maternal health and on the most appropriate methods of child raising. The effort to persuade expectant and nursing mothers to attend antenatal and child welfare clinics was a constant battle that had to be fought with each generation of women. A typical comment in this vein was that of the Mountain Ash medical officer, who stated:

> One of the difficulties we have to overcome is to convince women of the value of ante-natal supervision as most women desire as little examination as possible and do not realise how great a safeguard it may be, particularly if they have passed successfully through previous confinements without physical examination.[60]

As historians have pointed out on numerous occasions, such criticism undoubtedly reflected the arrogance of professional public health officials and their ignorance of working-class values and

[57] Cardiff CB, RMOH (1920), pp. 49–50; (1924), p. 38; (1929), p. 59; (1934), p. 69; (1938), p. 67.
[58] Swansea CB, RMOH (1920–39).
[59] Glamorgan CC, RMOH (1920), pp. 22–3; Penybont RD, RMOH (1939), p. 39.
[60] Mountain Ash UD, RMOH (1927), p. 54.

patterns of behaviour.[61] Public health officials who made these statements seem to have had no conception of the difficulties faced by working-class women in attending clinics. Long and expensive journeys faced many women, while the care of other children and the innumerable daily household tasks they faced were further disincentives. In any case, as the Aberdare medical officer found, general practitioners were themselves apathetic, and even anti-pathetic, in their attitudes towards antenatal clinics and had to be educated as to the benefits they could bring to expectant mothers.[62]

Furthermore, Margery Spring Rice's study of working-class women noted that the hopefulness and optimism that characterized the outlook of young wives and mothers in their twenties were eroded by the unremitting toil of everyday life, so that by their thirties working-class women were fatalistic and resigned to their lives of drudgery. Younger wives made real efforts to learn as much as possible about taking care of themselves and their families and were eager to obtain information from welfare centres or district nurses.[63] This is borne out by the observations of public health officials that it was the younger mothers who attended the clinics and who were keen to receive any advice that was given.[64] Behaviour that was criticized by public health officials was, therefore, partly a result of the massive pressures on working-class women rather than ignorance or fecklessness. It was perhaps also the case that women learned childrearing techniques when they first became mothers at younger ages and saw no reason to attend clinics during subsequent pregnancies.

The efforts made by medical officers and other public health officials to extend their influence into the lives of ordinary people were gradually successful. Annual reports constantly pointed to improved attendance figures for the antenatal and welfare clinics during the interwar period.[65] By 1938 the Mountain Ash medical officer could claim of infant welfare centres in his district that 'We have the

---

[61]   Eilidh Garrett and Andrew Wear, 'Suffer the little children: mortality, mothers and the state', *Continuity and Change*, 9, 2 (1994), 181.

[62]   Aberdare UD, RMOH (1924), p. 75.

[63]   Spring Rice, *Working Class Wives*, pp. 77–8, 82–3.

[64]   Geoffrey Chamberlain and A. Susan Williams, 'Antenatal care in south Wales, 1934–1962', *Social History of Medicine*, 8, 3 (1995), 481, notes that 70 per cent of the women attending antenatal clinics in the Rhondda in the period 1934–46 were below the age of 29.

[65]   See for example Mountain Ash UD, RMOH (1928), p. 60; (1930), p. 72; (1933), p. 27; (1934), p. 26.

impression that mothers attend now freely, no matter what their financial position.'[66] However, only 40 per cent of expectant mothers in Cardiff attended antenatal clinics during the early 1930s although this had increased to about 50 per cent by the end of the decade. Although there seems to have been an increase in attendance at antenatal clinics in the 1930s it was slight and half the expectant mothers of Cardiff continued to give birth without attending antenatal clinics.[67]

Those women who did visit clinics or who received home visits from health visitors[68] were informed about the most effective methods of feeding and caring for their infants and appropriate standards of domestic hygiene.[69] Margery Spring Rice's study suggested that working-class women learnt a great deal about childrearing, health and domestic sanitation in this way. While general practitioners were called only 'in an emergency', when the focus of attention was on the sick member of the family, the more informal nature of health visits and clinic attendances meant that working-class women were able to discuss relevant matters and learn approved methods of childrearing and domestic sanitation. Male doctors merely treated illness without discussing in any detail questions of a more general concern. 'The function of a doctor in these circumstances is merely therapeutic', concluded Spring Rice, 'that of the Welfare Centre prophylactic.'[70] Furthermore, the huge range of media through which prophylactic knowledge was disseminated, from handbills and posters to films shown at the local cinemas and lectures held in local halls, and to women's columns and commercial advertisements in the local newspapers, meant that working-class women were increasingly well-informed during the interwar period.

While it is difficult to ascertain the extent to which working-class

[66] Mountain Ash UD, RMOH (1938), p. 25.

[67] Cardiff CB, RMOH (1932–7).

[68] Newborn babies were visited as soon as possible after ten days of age and subsequently every four weeks until the child reached three months of age. Thereafter, the child was visited every three months until it was five years of age. This was in cases where the progress of the child was considered to be satisfactory. More frequent visits were made if it was thought necessary.

[69] See Maesteg UD, RMOH (1936), p. 16; for official interpretations of the importance of these educational efforts see Rhondda UD, RMOH (1925), pp. 37–8; Pontardawe RD, RMOH (1931), p. 7; for criticism of this emphasis on individual behaviour, lifestyle choices and personal responsibility see Jones, *Health and Society*, pp. 76, 78.

[70] Spring Rice, *Working Class Wives*, pp. 47–8.

women acted on the advice given to them or how far childrearing practices changed during the interwar period, it seems reasonable to suggest that the advice disseminated by public health authorities was increasingly internalized by working-class mothers and acted upon. As Pat Thane has argued, genuinely valuable advice was disseminated by health visitors and clinic nurses and 'At very low levels of knowledge, health and living standards, even small accretions of knowledge could have major effects.'[71] Thus, the gradual extension of welfare services and the increasing use made of them by women in south Wales suggests that greater knowledge was indeed a factor in the fall in infant mortality.

More subtly, medical officers believed that there had been a transformation in attitudes toward infant life and a corresponding improvement in childrearing techniques by the interwar period. The Glamorgan medical officer was of the opinion that there had occurred in the years after the First World War a 'revolution' in the attitude of society towards childhood. He argued that the decrease in the birth rate and the tendency towards smaller families fostered 'maternal pride' and inspired greater efforts to improve the quality of life of the fewer children in each family. 'When children are fewer', he maintained, 'they are more treasured possessions than when there is a superabundance, and with small families the amount of attention it is possible to give each child is correspondingly increased.'[72] Similarly, the Pontardawe medical officer commented in 1920 that:

> Publicity has arrested the attention of mothers to the importance of their functions as mothers, and has made them feel that the Community does not regard children as superfluities and a nuisance but as its most promising and most plastic element, and therefore demanding the utmost care. My experience is that although there may not be more maternal affection, there is greater anxiety shewn when a child is out of sorts than used to be, and springs from a less fatalistic outlook. Health visiting and Infant Welfare

---

[71]   Pat Thane, 'Visions of gender in the making of the British welfare state: the case of women in the British Labour Party and social policy, 1906–45', in Gisela Bock and Pat Thane (eds), *Maternity and Gender Politics: Women and the Rise of European Welfare States, 1880s-1950s* (London, 1991), p. 103.

[72]   Glamorgan CC, RMOH (1930), p. 21; see also (1929), p. 10; (1938), p. 31.

[73]   Pontardawe RD, RMOH (1920), p. 6; see also Penybont RD, RMOH (1924), p. 5.

Centres undoubtedly foster and nourish this brighter hope and increased confidence.[73]

These observations echo the more recent assertion of David Reher that as fewer children were born to each family and as fewer died, and those who did, did so at an earlier age (as in interwar south Wales), the total amount of time a mother was able to devote to the upbringing and care of an individual child increased. Since the amount of parental time dedicated to the child is a significant factor in child health and survival, it served to lessen infant mortality and morbidity.[74] Therefore, decreases in the birth rate and smaller family sizes in interwar south Wales tended to increase the parental investment in a child's upbringing and served to increase infant survival chances. Although this is impossible to measure, anecdotal evidence suggests that this was the case.

It is evident that despite the economic vicissitudes experienced by south Wales during the interwar period, all districts of the region shared in the decrease in infant mortality that occurred throughout Britain. This decrease seems to have been a result partly of the declining fertility rates, partly of the environmental improvements made during the interwar period and, more especially perhaps, the extension of maternity and infant welfare services and the consequent improvements in childrearing techniques. The large decreases in post-neonatal mortality support the last two of these three factors. However, it also needs to be recognized that the decline in mortality in south Wales did not occur to the same extent as the decrease in mortality for England and Wales as a whole. Regional inequalities increased during this period. The precise causes of this slower decline, whether economic, social or medical, are hard to discern. A clue may be offered by Elizabeth Peretz's study. Although the number of infant welfare centres increased and the services they offered broadened during the interwar period, it seems that the development of services in interwar south Wales lagged behind those in other regions of Britain. Since the nature and extent of health services have been found to be especially significant for infant standards of health and levels of mortality,[75] the

---

[74] David Reher, 'Wasted investments: some economic implications of childhood mortality patterns', *Population Studies*, 49, 3 (1995), 519–36, esp. 536.

[75] Stockwell, 'Infant mortality'.

retarded growth of services in interwar south Wales might have widened infant mortality differentials between the region and the rest of England and Wales. This was another way in which the interwar economic depression influenced levels of mortality.

Furthermore, the overall improvement in levels of infant mortality needs to be qualified by a recognition that stillbirth and neonatal mortality did not decrease to the same extent as the mortality of older infants and, in the more depressed communities of south Wales, actually increased during the depths of the economic depression in the late 1920s and early 1930s. It was here that poverty had its most obvious effect on infant mortality, as poor and deteriorating maternal nutritional and health status resulted in increasing stillbirth and neonatal mortality rates.

CONCLUSION

The demographic history of the interwar years, along with the impact of the economic depression on standards of health and levels of mortality, was complex and subtle. Undoubtedly, there were improvements in mortality rates in interwar south Wales, but the period was also characterized by the intensification of regional and class inequalities and even increases in mortality levels for certain sections of the population. This complexity needs to be recognized. First, some improvements can be discerned in the general mortality rates. Standardized death rates remained roughly stationary in the two administrative counties of Glamorgan and Monmouthshire and in Merthyr Tydfil but other districts in south Wales, most noticeably the county boroughs of Cardiff, Swansea and Newport, shared in the decline in mortality that occurred more generally.

Improvements in levels of infant mortality were even more marked. Infant mortality rates for the major administrative units of south Wales fell by between 25 per cent and 30 per cent during the course of the interwar period.[1] Since infant mortality is commonly considered 'the most sensitive indicator of the overall health status of any population group', the decrease in infant mortality during the interwar period is highly significant.[2] It suggests that improvements in the material conditions of the lives of infants continued to be made despite the economic depression of the period. However, as with mortality rates more generally, the more depressed areas of south Wales did not share in the same high rate of decrease in mortality experienced in England and Wales as a whole and by the more prosperous parts of south Wales. Many districts in the depressed mining valleys saw only very small levels of improvement in infant mortality rates and much of this improvement occurred in the mid to late 1930s. Similarly, inequalities in the heights and weights of children intensified during the interwar period as

---

[1]   The infant mortality rate for Newport CB fell from a low rate in the early 1920s and so its fall was only about 10 per cent; see Chapter 8.

[2]   Stockwell, 'Infant mortality', in Kiple, *Cambridge World History of Human Disease*, p. 224.

children in south Wales increased in stature at a slower rate than
children in more prosperous parts of England and Wales.

The increase in regional inequalities in mortality levels was as
important an aspect of the demographic history of interwar Britain
as the generally improving levels of mortality that government officials of the period chose to emphasize. This, it might be argued, was
one way in which the influence of economic depression registered
in standards of health. Unemployment and poverty served to retard
improvements in mortality rates in economically depressed regions
of Britain. Not only did regional inequalities intensify in a British
context but inequalities also intensified within south Wales. Cardiff,
Swansea and Newport shared in the improvements that other parts
of England and Wales experienced during the period whereas the
communities of the mining valleys did not. It was during the
interwar period that these two parts of south Wales fell increasingly
out of step with each other in demographic terms. Gwyn Williams's
assertion that in the interwar period 'Whole areas of Wales became
and have remained problem areas' is, to some extent, borne out by
this evidence.[3]

Certainly there were improvements in the mortality levels of the
population of south Wales and these improvements were highly
significant. Similarly, the fact that certain areas of south Wales did
not experience improvements in mortality levels to the same extent
as England and Wales as a whole is also significant. But it is important, too, to note the increases in mortality from particular causes or
for particular groups of the population and the part played by
economic depression in these trends. Mortality from tuberculosis,
for example, often considered a sensitive indicator of standards of
living, increased in the Rhondda and other valley communities.
Similarly, neonatal mortality decreased by only a small ratio in the
more prosperous areas of south Wales but increased in areas such as
Merthyr, the Rhondda, Abertillery and Mountain Ash which
suffered the highest levels of unemployment and poverty. Increases
in stillbirth mortality were also notable in these deprived communities. This timing was significant. Increases in these forms of
'reproductive mortality' took place during the late 1920s and early
1930s during the trough of the Depression when unemployment
and poverty were the experience of a significant proportion of the

[3]   Williams, *When was Wales?*, p. 253.

population. Even over the interwar period as a whole, there was little or no improvement in levels of 'reproductive mortality' in the depressed valley districts.

Increases in these forms of mortality suggest that it was the women of south Wales who suffered disproportionately the effects of economic depression. This conclusion is supported by the fact that the increase in tuberculosis mortality in Merthyr during the interwar period, while evident for males, was more marked for females. The inferior status of women in mining communities and the specific nature of their everyday lives in the insanitary conditions of such communities meant that females suffered higher levels of mortality than their counterparts in other communities. While mortality levels in south Wales exceeded those for England and Wales as a whole, it is evident that female death rates in the industrial valleys exceeded corresponding rates for England and Wales as a whole to a greater extent than did male death rates.

Webster concluded that the health problems of the 1930s were 'rooted in economic disadvantage'.[4] This detailed investigation of south Wales, focusing on the material circumstances of working-class life and the detailed patterns of mortality, suggests that mortality was indeed rooted in economic disadvantage but that this economic disadvantage was in turn partly rooted in the specific nature of the industrial communities of south Wales. Patterns of mortality were the product of a specific social, economic and ecological environment as much as of the economic depression of the period. The high death rates of adult women in Edwardian south Wales support this assertion. This is not to underestimate the effects of the Depression, which clearly had implications for levels of mortality in south Wales, not least in the increases in adult female mortality, but it is to recognize the specific social and economic characteristics of individual communities. Specificities of space as well as of time are important and the mortality landscape of interwar south Wales was as much a product of the peculiar characteristics of Welsh society as it was of the economic conditions of the interwar period. Those who enter the debate over the 'healthy or hungry' nature of the interwar period would do well to remember the importance of these specific environmental factors, and analyses of mortality in the 1920s and 1930s must be anchored in

---

[4]   Webster, 'Healthy or hungry thirties?', 125.

the realities of lived experience. This is one way in which Landers's conceptualization of the 'vital regime' can inform contributions to the 'healthy or hungry' debate by its recognition of the specific social, economic and political environment of demographic phenomena.

Income was one of the most important factors that influenced the levels and trends of mortality. Most mortality indicators displayed sharp disparities according to income. However, establishing a causal link between unemployment and mortality is problematic. Examination of the material aspects of working-class life demonstrates why it is impossible to view unemployment as an independent variable and health and mortality as dependent variables. The effects of unemployment were mediated through, and complicated by, a host of social and environmental factors, and Winter's assertion that unemployment 'must be seen as part of a network of economic relations, support systems and social attitudes' is demonstrated by this study of health in interwar south Wales.[5]

When examining the mortality statistics of local authority districts, it must be remembered that the unemployed did not constitute the total population in a district and so the influence of their mortality patterns on those of the district as a whole was complicated by the existence of families which did not suffer the effects of unemployment. While unemployment did reach levels approaching 80 per cent and even 90 per cent in south Wales, this occurred in certain particularly depressed districts and only in the depths of the Depression in the early 1930s. On the whole, the unemployed generally made up a minority of the population at any one time in most districts of south Wales. Furthermore, it is evident that there was no neat and clear difference between the incomes of 'employed' and 'unemployed' families. On the whole, unemployment caused a decrease in income for a family but there were enormous variations in incomes and needs. It was a common observation, for example, that workers experiencing short-time working were worse off than those who were wholly unemployed.

These circumstances were further complicated by the efficacy of the strategies utilized by families to ameliorate the reduction in income that unemployment usually entailed. It is impossible accurately to assess the benefits that survival strategies brought to families

---

[5] Winter, 'Unemployment, nutrition and infant mortality in Britain, 1920–50', 252.

but it is obvious that they made some difference. As Paul Johnson argues, working-class families did not waste money on types of saving or borrowing week after week if they derived little or no advantage from them, and similarly they would not have continually utilized survival strategies if the family obtained no benefit.[6] The strategies saved, or made available, only very small amounts of money in real terms, but at the low levels of income at which the poor and the unemployed existed, the money was significant in proportional terms and helped mitigate the worst effects of poverty. These strategies, therefore, acted as 'shock absorbers' against the worst effects of unemployment and poverty, and served to lessen mortality and health inequalities even though they could not eradicate them.

This is not to argue that unemployment and poverty were without consequences for health and mortality patterns. It remains the case that, despite the many factors that complicated the relationship between income and mortality, there was nevertheless a strong correlation between income and levels of mortality. For most families, unemployment in interwar south Wales entailed a significant decrease in income and, if the spell of unemployment was prolonged, a corresponding deterioration in dietary standards. Contemporaries were agreed that the unemployed existed on diets inferior to those enjoyed by the rest of the population. Unfortunately, the level of analysis cannot be more detailed than local authority districts and the effects of unemployment can be perceived only through the distorting influence of a range of mediating factors. Nevertheless, increases in certain forms of mortality among the most vulnerable members of the community at times when unemployment was at its most severe demonstrate that unemployment did have an adverse effect on mortality.

Standards of health and levels of mortality were more favourable in the interwar period than in the Edwardian or Victorian periods, but it seems difficult to reconcile these improvements in mortality in interwar south Wales with the popular perception of the period as a time of ill health and premature mortality.[7] E. P. Thompson, in his contribution to the 'standard of living' debate, challenged the

---

[6] Johnson, *Saving and Spending*, pp. 5–6.

[7] However, Aneurin Bevan's argument that people do not live in the past but in the present must also be remembered – 'Discontent arises from a knowledge of the possible, as contrasted with the actual'; Bevan, *In Place of Fear*, p. 22.

assumption that there exists a simple correlation between the standard of living, as indicated by statistical indices, and the quality of
life, either objectively or as it is subjectively perceived and experienced. As an example, Thompson pointed to the rise in wages in
the coalmining industry in the period 1790–1840 which coincided
with 'intensified exploitation, greater insecurity, and increasing
human misery'.[8] He commented that 'by 1840 most people were
"better off" than their forerunners had been fifty years before, but
they had suffered and continued to suffer this slight improvement as
a catastrophic shock'. A similar argument might be posited in relation to the interwar period. Despite the decreases in certain
mortality indicators and the improvements in real wages and
benefit levels since the Victorian and Edwardian periods, popular
perceptions of the interwar period were, and continue to be,
pessimistic ones. By the interwar period, most people were 'better
off' than their counterparts had been twenty or thirty years previously but many of them experienced this improvement, if not as a
'catastrophic shock', at least as a deterioration in the subjective
quality of life.

This was because large numbers of families experienced unemployment and poverty, or else witnessed them in their
communities, and attributed the large amount of ill health and
premature death to that unemployment and poverty. It was in the
interwar period, of course, that health and mortality became politicized to a significant extent and came to figure in public debates
about the effectiveness of welfare provision and the role of central
government in the welfare of the population. The issue of health
came to occupy a central position in the bitter political disagreements of the 1920s and, more especially, the 1930s and has
remained an important aspect of popular memories of the period.

The precise effects of the economic depression on patterns of
mortality were more complex than is recognized in the popular
perception, or indeed the historiography, of the period. Unemployment and poverty influenced patterns of mortality in interwar
south Wales in many complex and subtle ways. It is not adequate to
point out that areas that experienced high levels of unemployment
were also characterized by high levels of morbidity or mortality, as

---

[8]   H. J. Kaye, *British Marxist Historians: An Introductory Analysis* (Oxford, 1984), pp. 184–5;
E. P. Thompson, *The Making of the English Working Class* (London, 1963), p. 231.

many studies do. Broader perspectives need to be adopted that recognize the continuities with the Victorian and Edwardian periods, the interdependent nature of the determinants of health and mortality, and the specific nature of working-class communities in different parts of Britain.

APPENDICES

Appendix 1.1. Unemployment percentages at employment exchanges in south Wales, 1927–39

	Aberdare	Aberkenfig	Bargoed	Barry	Bridgend	Caerphilly	Cardiff
1927	27.0	24.0	14.2	20.2	17.5	7.5	14.0
1928	35.7	24.2	17.7	23.9	22.5	25.6	17.8
1929	23.6	24.3	12.1ᵃ	23.7	23.3	16.2	18.6
1930	23.9	23.2	18.5	29.7	22.5	24.9	23.9
1931	28.6	28.9	25.7	37.6	33.9	44.1	29.7
1932	40.1	34.3	37.7	38.5	30.5	50.8	29.6
1933	40.2	31.7	42.5	37.4	29.9	46.3	29.4
1934	42.8	29.8	41.8	36.4	27.3	42.3	27.2
1935	47.5	31.6	32.2	35.1	32.7	40.0	26.8
1936	45.6	29.0	32.6	33.2	31.6	37.6	25.2
1937	25.7	22.8	18.5	28.6	22.3	26.3	18.8
1938	26.3	16.5	19.3	24.3	16.8	26.1	18.4
1939	26.3	–	16.6	22.7	11.9	22.9	14.8

	Clydach	Cymmer	Dowlais	Ferndale	Gorseinon	Maesteg	Merthyr Tydfil
1927	17.3	31.2	37.2	41.4	20.8	25.6	47.6
1928	19.0	41.2	40.0	37.9	18.5	39.0	66.4
1929	11.6	25.4	26.6	32.9	16.6	24.5	44.7
1930	20.4	31.1	38.7	34.4	21.9	28.2	55.3
1931	36.8	40.8	52.5ᵇ	56.4	28.1	53.1	61.0
1932	40.5	42.0	–	67.2	28.9	64.6	60.9
1933	27.2	28.8	–	67.7	21.9	58.7	58.5
1934	21.7	26.9	–	62.2	21.9	54.7	59.2
1935	24.5	22.3	–	67.6	26.4	50.2	55.5
1936	16.4	25.4	–	67.1	24.2	55.2	52.9
1937	10.3	15.5	–	48.1	16.2	30.6	41.6
1938	20.3	17.9	–	48.9	30.2	36.5ᶜ	41.8
1939	9.6	21.7	–	43.1	18.1	–	25.8

	Morriston	Mountain Ash	Neath	Ogmore Vale	Pontardawe	Pontar-dulais	Pont-lottyn
1927	21.8	29.7	17.4	17.9	14.7	18.1	31.1
1928	14.5	25.4	27.7	17.1	17.5	16.2	42.3
1929	15.5	18.1	22.2	17.2	20.1	12.9	30.8[d]
1930	23.9	23.4	31.0	24.8	28.5	19.0	–
1931	36.0	30.9	39.6	47.2	39.2	19.1	47.9
1932	36.2	37.2	36.8	48.8	36.2	26.0	57.4
1933	29.5[e]	38.9	29.5	49.3	29.7	26.2	58.9
1934	–	44.3	32.1	41.6	33.7	27.8	64.9
1935	–	37.7	32.1	36.1	35.2	28.9	55.3
1936	–	42.4	29.0	41.8	24.2	26.2	56.8
1937	–	22.0	15.6	19.2	14.4	13.4	39.8
1938	–	30.9	23.4	43.6	37.5	35.3	40.6
1939	–	13.9	14.8	13.5	16.1	18.1	35.6

	Pontyclun	Pont-ycymmer	Pontypridd	Porth	Porthcawl	Port Talbot	Resolven
1927	18.9	28.3	34.3	20.5	6.7	34.3	4.9
1928	16.6	38.2	26.5	19.4	8.8	35.8	18.0
1929	14.8	31.4	30.9	14.3	8.1	31.0	11.1
1930	29.0	38.1	40.5	24.7	10.4	37.9	8.6
1931	36.5	43.6	49.1	32.8	13.7	52.0	11.6
1932	42.8	49.5	60.5	41.0	17.1	48.9	14.7
1933	36.9	51.8	52.4	36.4	15.2	42.4	13.9
1934	32.6	48.4	54.7	37.4	12.9	30.4	18.8[f]
1935	33.2	43.8	52.8	41.6	–	32.5[g]	10.7
1936	24.4	43.0	52.1	44.2	–	31.5	10.0
1937	16.4	26.8	37.4	30.0	–	19.9	4.5
1938	19.0	42.0	34.9	32.3	–	28.7	4.5
1939	13.9	18.3	33.1	31.3	–	19.1	4.25

	Swansea	Taffs Well	Tonypandy	Tonyrefail	Treharris	Treorchy	Ystaly-fera
1927	18.7	22.7	32.3	21.1	10.5	18.8	27.2
1928	20.7	29.8	26.9	21.3	5.6	18.3	32.4
1929	22.8	39.3	38.8	16.5	3.9	15.6	13.4
1930	29.3	40.1	50.6	24.8	25.4	26.5	19.8
1931	39.0	57.7	56.3	24.0	16.4[h]	30.0	20.9
1932	37.5	80.2	57.5	40.3	–	33.6	27.7
1933	33.8	51.6	59.5	38.5	–	32.4	18.8

	Swansea	Taffs Well	Tonypandy	Tonyrefail	Treharris	Treorchy	Ystaly-fera
1934	30.6	38.3	50.2	34.0	–	36.8	25.6
1935	34.1	37.8	51.2	33.2	–	35.2	31.9
1936	32.2	33.1	54.3	29.1	–	35.3	29.2
1937	23.5	21.6	37.2	22.8	–	22.3	24.3
1938	28.7	18.9	38.3	26.4	–	25.2	25.4
1939	23.1	17.4	36.0	20.9	–	25.9	25.3

	Aber-gavenny	Aber-tillery	Blackwood	Blaenavon	Blaina	Crumlin	Ebbw Vale
1927	8.7	28.0	13.7	33.9	46.0	25.3	20.5
1928	10.3	31.5	13.8	36.9	55.3	19.7	14.1
1929	12.1	21.5	13.8	31.4	50.1	20.8	12.6
1930	16.3	28.2	14.5	–	42.3	19.3	32.0
1931	22.0	32.8	20.6	32.2	47.5	23.9	35.3
1932	28.0	54.4	33.6	40.2	93.0	36.3	38.6
1933	26.3	61.5	33.3	36.7	75.6	37.0	40.3
1934	28.9	53.9	34.1	29.3	75.5	28.9	36.1
1935	29.6	48.9	33.2	37.0	60.0	20.2	35.3
1936	28.6	41.9	32.6	34.5	60.8	27.4	32.8
1937	22.1	23.7	22.4	25.1	40.0	12.0	15.1
1938	22.1	26.8	21.4	23.0	57.2	14.4	14.2
1939	16.5	25.3	19.2	17.5	–	14.0	11.2

	Newport	Pontnewydd	Pontypool	Risca	Tredegar
1927	15.2	31.5	24.6	31.4[i]	8.0
1928	20.6	36.0	27.8	25.8	16.2
1929	22.7	32.4	25.0	32.7	18.2
1930	31.1	–	37.7	24.2	17.7
1931	38.1	54.9	36.6	37.4	22.7
1932	37.4	59.8	47.7	47.3	31.7
1933	34.6	63.2	41.2	45.4	33.7
1934	29.0	53.7	38.1	43.8	28.8
1935	27.7	51.0	36.1	39.6	29.6
1936	25.9	45.6	32.7	43.4	32.2
1937	19.7	35.0	24.4	22.2	20.2
1938	23.7	47.6	27.4	33.5	21.6
1939	17.6	27.7	17.4	22.4	19.4

	Glamorgan	Monmouthshire
1927	21.7	21.3
1928	24.5	22.9
1929	21.3	22.5
1930	28.1	28.8
1931	36.8	33.8
1932	40.4	42.0
1933	37.9	40.2
1934	36.9	36.0
1935	36.4	33.5
1936	34.9	32.7
1937	23.7	21.1
1938	26.4	23.6
1939	21.0	18.0

Source: Ministry of Labour, *Local Unemployment Index* (1927–39). Percentage of insured workers registered as unemployed. Monthly figures have been used to calculate annual averages.

[a] From September Pontlottyn figures were included in the Bargoed exchange.

[b] January to June only. Included in Merthyr exchange thereafter.

[c] Maesteg figures included with Cymmer exchange from 1939.

[d] January to August only. Figures included in Bargoed exchange until December 1930.

[e] Presumably included with Swansea exchange from 1934.

[f] Figures for 1934 and 1935 include men from elsewhere attending Training Centres.

[g] Includes juveniles from other areas.

[h] January to June only. Figures included in Merthyr exchange from July 1931.

[i] The figure for November is illegible and the average has been calculated from the eleven monthly percentages.

Appendix 1.2. Average weekly unemployment insurance benefits, 1920–39 (shillings)

	Single adult man	Single adult woman	Man, wife and 2 children
1920	11.7	11.2	11.7
1921	16.7	13.3	17.8
1922	15.0	12.0	22.0
1923	15.0	12.0	22.0
1924	16.3	13.3	24.1
1925	18.0	15.0	27.0
1926	18.0	15.0	27.0
1927	18.0	15.0	27.0
1928	17.3	15.0	27.7
1929	17.0	15.0	28.0
1930	17.0	15.0	29.7
1931	16.6	14.6	29.3
1932	15.3	13.5	27.3

	Single adult man	Single adult woman	Man, wife and 2 children
1933	15.3	13.5	27.3
1934	16.1	14.3	28.6
1935	17.0	15.0	30.3
1936	17.0	15.0	32.0
1937	17.0	15.0	32.0
1938	17.0	15.0	32.8
1939	17.0	15.0	33.0

Sources: Final Report of the Royal Commission on Unemployment Insurance [Cmd. 4185], 1932, xiii, p. 20; Ministry of Labour, *Twenty-Second Abstract of Labour Statistics of the United Kingdom* (1922–36) [Cmd. 5556], 1937, xxvi, pp. 68–71; Ministry of Labour, Annual Report (1938), p. 54. Monthly averages have been used to calculate annual averages.

Appendix 1.3. Unemployment benefits index and real benefits index, 1920–39

	Single adult man	Single adult woman	Man, wife and 2 children
1920	68.8	74.7	39.4
1921	98.2	88.7	59.9
1922	88.2	80.0	74.1
1923	88.2	80.0	74.1
1924	95.9	88.7	81.1
1925	105.9	100.0	90.9
1926	105.9	100.0	90.9
1927	105.9	100.0	90.9
1928	101.8	100.0	93.3
1929	100.0	100.0	94.3
1930	100.0	100.0	100.0
1931	97.6	97.3	98.7
1932	90.0	90.0	91.9
1933	90.0	90.0	91.9
1934	94.7	95.3	96.3
1935	100.0	100.0	102.0
1936	100.0	100.0	107.7
1937	100.0	100.0	107.7
1938	100.0	100.0	110.4
1939	100.0	100.0	111.1

Real Unemployment Benefits Index

	Single adult man	Single adult woman	Man, wife and 2 children
1920	43.7	47.4	25.0
1921	68.7	62.0	41.9
1922	76.2	69.1	64.0
1923	80.1	72.7	67.3
1924	86.6	80.1	73.2
1925	95.1	89.8	81.6
1926	97.2	91.8	83.5
1927	99.9	94.3	85.8
1928	96.9	95.1	88.8
1929	96.3	96.3	90.8
1930	100.0	100.0	100.0
1931	104.5	104.2	105.7
1932	98.8	98.8	100.9
1933	101.6	101.6	103.7
1934	106.2	106.8	107.6
1935	110.5	110.5	112.7
1936	107.5	107.5	115.8
1937	102.6	102.6	110.5
1938	101.3	101.3	111.9
1939	–	–	–

Sources: Final Report of the Royal Commission on Unemployment Insurance [Cmd. 4185], 1932, xiii, p. 20; Ministry of Labour, *Twenty-Second Abstract of Labour Statistics of the United Kingdom* (1922–36) [Cmd. 5556], 1937, xxvi, pp. 68–71; Ministry of Labour, *Annual Report* (1938), 54; B. R. Mitchell and P. Deane, *Abstract of British Historical Statistics* (Cambridge, 1962). 1930=100. Real rates have been calculated using the Ministry of Labour Cost of Living Index.

Appendix 4.1. Houses built by local authorities in south Wales, 1920–38

District	Houses built 1920–38	Rate per 1,000 population (1939)	Houses built as % of 1921 housing stock
Abercarn UD	201	10.96	5.53
Abergavenny UD	168	21.45	8.62
Abertillery UD	160	5.73	2.40
Bedwas and Machen UD	386	46.47	23.44
Bedwellty UD	762	27.09	14.00
Blaenavon UD	150	15.43	6.08
Caerleon UD	46	13.47	11.47
Chepstow UD	50	12.39	4.75
Cwmbran UD	272	24.89	11.73
Ebbw Vale UD	563[a]	18.94	9.32

District	Houses built 1920–38	Rate per 1,000 population (1939)	Houses built as % of 1921 housing stock
Monmouth MB	179	37.37	19.04
Mynyddislwyn UD	395	30.15	14.91
Nantyglo and Blaina UD	192	16.62	6.49
Pontypool UD	1,120	27.79	12.96
Rhymney UD	60	6.48	2.72
Risca UD	357	24.40	11.04
Tredegar UD	360[b]	17.46	8.09
Usk UD	0	0	0
Abergavenny RD	48	5.80	2.66
Chepstow RD	110	12.63	5.98
Magor and St Mellons RD	212	18.37	6.51
Monmouth RD	36	6.17	2.30
Pontypool RD	36	6.59	3.09
Monmouthshire AC	5863	19.30	8.76
Aberdare UD	547	12.83	5.11
Barry UD	818	22.57	12.25
Bridgend UD	144	12.8	8.13
Caerphilly UD	741	23.16	11.32
Cowbridge MB	13	12.75	5.18
Gelligaer UD	642	17.66	8.31
Glyncorrwg UD	300	31.67	16.71
Llwchwr UD	688	27.04	15.08
Maesteg UD	182	8.21	3.69
Mountain Ash UD	268	8.10	3.52
Neath MB	777	24.80	21.75
Ogmore and Garw UD	208	8.84	3.95
Penarth UD	152	9.48	4.94
Pontypridd UD	571	14.93	6.88
Porthcawl UD	0	0	0
Port Talbot MB	1,278	31.62	16.65
Rhondda UD	297[c]	2.48	1.06
Cardiff RD	388	11.99	4.73
Cowbridge RD	372	25.92	20.63
Gower RD	20	1.90	1.06
Llantrisant and Llantwit Fardre RD	860	35.77	19.07
Neath RD	672	16.60	7.51
Penybont RD	1,087	38.57	23.01
Pontardawe RD	916	27.12	13.39
Glamorgan AC	11,941	16.83	8.14
Cardiff CB[d]	6,722	29.80	20.80
Merthyr CB	794	12.92	5.02

Swansea CB	5,058	31.39	17.48
Newport CB	1,259	13.13	8.28

Sources: Annual reports of the Medical Officers of Health of Glamorgan CC, Monmouthshire CC, 1920–39; Census of England and Wales, 1921, Glamorgan, Monmouthshire; *National Register, United Kingdom and the Isle of Man, Statistics of Population on 29 September 1939* (London, 1944). Authorities are as constituted in 1939.

ᵃ Does not include 45 hut dwellings erected in 1920–1 which housed 2 families each.

ᵇ Does not include 24 wooden bungalows erected in 1920–1.

ᶜ Does not include 16 huts erected in 1920–2.

ᵈ Figure derived from M. C. Bourne, 'A study of council building activity in post-war Cardiff', unpublished UWIST M.Sc. thesis (1981); figure includes houses built in 1939.

Appendix 7.1. Crude death rates, major administrative areas, 1920-39 (deaths per 1,000 population)

	England and Wales	Glam. AC	Mon. AC	Cardiff CB	Merthyr CB	Swansea CB	Newport CB
1920	12.4	11.9	11.9	11.3	14.1	12.6	12.4
1921	12.1	11.2	11.3	11.6	12.7	11.9	11.1
1922	12.7	12.1	11.4	13.2	14.2	13.5	12.6
1923	11.6	10.5	10.4	12.0	12.1	12.2	10.7
1924	12.2	10.9	10.6	12.1	12.3	12.6	11.3
1925	12.1	11.2	10.6	12.8	12.7	12.4	11.9
1926	11.6	10.5	9.4	10.8	12.0	11.8	10.5
1927	12.3	11.1	11.0	12.6	12.9	13.5	12.5
1928	11.7	11.5	10.9	11.7	12.6	12.6	11.2
1929	13.4	11.0	11.3	12.9	14.2	13.5	12.6
1930	11.4	10.7	10.2	11.4	12.5	12.8	11.0
1931	12.3	12.1	12.0	12.8	14.2	12.6	13.1
1932	12.0	11.9	11.1	12.5	13.7	13.2	11.9
1933	12.3	12.7	11.5	13.5	13.9	14.5	13.2
1934	11.8	11.7	11.7	12.3	13.9	12.9	12.1
1935	11.7	12.0	11.5	12.3	14.7	12.9	12.4
1936	12.1	12.2	12.2	12.6	13.9	14.1	12.1
1937	12.4	12.9	12.6	12.6	14.3	13.9	12.8
1938	11.6	12.6	12.1	11.9	15.7	13.2	12.1
1939	12.1	13.1	12.8	13.7	14.5	12.4	12.9

Sources: Annual reports of the Medical Officers of Health for Glamorgan CC, Monmouthshire CC, and the county boroughs of Cardiff, Merthyr Tydfil, Newport and Swansea, 1920–39; *Registrar-General's Statistical Review of England and Wales*, 1920–39.

Appendix 7.2. Quinquennial crude death rate averages, all administrative districts, 1920–39 (deaths per 1,000 population)

	1920–4	1925–9	1930–4	1935–9
Abercarn UD	10.6	9.6	10.9	11.5
Abergavenny MB	13.1	13.3	13.6	15.5
Abersychan UD	10.2	9.8	10.2	–
Abertillery UD	9.8	9.5	10.6	12.2
Bedwas and Machen UD	12.1	10.7	12.1	11.4
Bedwellty UD	11.0	10.1	11.9	11.6
Blaenavon UD	14.2	12.2	13.5	15.1
Caerleon UD	10.5	9.2	10.6	10.6
Chepstow UD	12.8	12.6	15.4	13.2
Cwmbran UD	–	–	–	12.1
Ebbw Vale UD	11.3	10.9	11.6	12.4
Llanfrechfa Upper UD	10.8	11.0	10.9	–
Llantarnam	11.6	10.4	10.8	–
Monmouth MB	14.9	15.9	14.4	14.6
Mynyddislwyn UD	9.7	9.5	9.9	10.9
Nantyglo and Blaina UD	10.7	10.4	11.7	13.7
Panteg UD	10.5	11.6	11.1	–
Pontypool UD	12.6	11.4	11.6	–
Rhymney UD	12.7	12.0	12.4	13.5
Risca UD	9.9	9.9	10.7	12.0
Tredegar UD	11.4	10.9	11.3	12.0
Usk UD	9.9	11.6	16.3	15.7
Abergavenny RD	11.5	10.0	10.8	11.6
Chepstow RD	10.8	12.1	10.7	11.6
Magor RD	11.2	10.7	10.4	–
Magor and St Mellons RD	–	–	–	11.7
Monmouth RD	14.0	12.2	13.6	12.7
Pontypool RD	12.0	11.8	11.7	11.3
St Mellons RD	10.4	9.9	9.9	–
Aberdare UD	12.1	12.1	13.0	14.5
Barry UD	10.6	10.9	11.9	12.6
Bridgend UD	11.4	10.8	10.4	12.8
Caerphilly UD	11.3	11.1	12.0	13.0
Cowbridge MB	13.3	13.6	16.3	13.3
Gelligaer UD	11.1	11.0	11.5	12.3
Glyncorrwg UD	11.2	11.1	10.7	10.8
Llwchwr UD	–	–	10.1	11.1
Maesteg UD	11.5	11.0	12.1	13.2
Mountain Ash UD	11.6	11.4	12.3	13.5
Neath MB	12.4	11.3	12.0	12.5
Ogmore and Garw UD	10.5	10.6	11.0	12.2
Penarth UD	10.3	10.1	10.8	12.1

	1920–4	1925–9	1930–4	1935–9
Pontypridd UD	12.4	11.8	12.3	13.6
Porthcawl UD	11.6	11.1	12.8	12.7
Port Talbot UD	11.4	10.9	12.0	12.1
Rhondda UD	11.8	11.7	12.5	13.6
Cardiff RD	10.0	9.5	10.5	10.5
Cowbridge RD	11.0	10.9	10.6	11.2
Gower RD	11.0	10.9	11.7	11.2
Llantrisant and Llantwit				
Fardre RD	10.8	11.2	11.2	11.9
Neath RD	11.0	10.3	11.2	11.3
Penybont RD	10.5	9.2	10.6	11.4
Pontardawe RD	11.2	10.7	11.6	12.0
Swansea RD	10.4	10.2	–	–
Glamorgan AC	11.3	11.1	11.8	12.6
Monmouthshire AC	11.1	10.6	11.3	12.2
Cardiff CB	12.0	12.2	12.5	12.6
Merthyr CB	13.1	12.9	13.6	14.6
Swansea CB	12.6	12.8	13.2	13.3
Newport CB	11.6	11.7	12.3	12.5
England and Wales	12.2	12.2	12.0	12.0

Sources: Annual reports of the Medical Officers of Health for Glamorgan CC, Monmouthshire CC, and the county boroughs of Cardiff, Merthyr Tydfil, Newport and Swansea, 1920–39; *Registrar-General's Statistical Review of England and Wales*, 1920–39.

Appendix 7.3. Standardized death rates (by direct method), major administrative districts, 1920–39 (deaths per 1,000 population)

	England and Wales	Glam. AC	Mon. AC	Cardiff CB	Merthyr CB	Swansea CB	Newport CB
1920	–	12.6	–	–	–	–	–
1921	11.3	11.8	11.3	12.4	13.1	11.4	11.4
1922	11.8	13.0	11.8	13.4	14.8	12.9	12.8
1923	10.6	11.2	10.9	12.1	12.5	11.7	10.9
1924	11.1	11.6	10.9	11.7	12.6	11.7	11.7
1925	11.1	11.9	10.9	13.0	13.2	11.5	12.3
1926	10.5	11.3	9.6	10.6	12.5	11.1	10.8
1927	11.0	11.9	11.5	12.6	13.3	12.4	12.7
1928	10.4	11.9	11.3	11.7	13.1	11.4	11.3
1929	11.9	12.4	11.7	13.0	14.7	12.4	12.9
1930	10.1	11.6	10.6	11.2	12.9	11.5	11.2
1931	10.1	11.5	11.1	11.3	13.5	10.5	11.9
1932	9.8	11.2	10.3	11.0	12.3	10.7	10.5
1933	9.9	12.0	10.5	11.8	13.1	11.8	11.9

	England and Wales	Glam. AC	Mon. AC	Cardiff CB	Merthyr CB	Swansea CB	Newport CB
1934	9.5	11.0	10.7	10.7	12.8	10.3	10.7
1935	9.3	12.2	10.4	10.4	13.2	10.4	10.5
1936	9.6	11.2	10.9	10.5	12.5	10.8	10.4
1937	9.7	11.9	11.2	10.6	12.6	11.2	10.8
1938	9.1	11.6	10.7	9.8	14.0	10.4	10.5
1939	9.2	12.0	11.4	10.7	12.9	10.7	10.8

Sources: Census of England and Wales, 1901; Annual reports of the Medical Officers of Health for Glamorgan CC, Monmouthshire CC, and the county boroughs of Cardiff, Merthyr Tydfil, Newport and Swansea, 1920–39; *Registrar-General's Statistical Review of England and Wales,* 1920–39.

Appendix 7.4. Standardized death rates (indirect method), all administrative districts, 1920-39 (England and Wales = 100)

	1920–4	1925–9	1930–4	1935–9
Aberdare UD	111.2	116.2	123.3	136.1
Barry UD	102.1	105.1	107.0	112.1
Bridgend UD	100.0	91.2	86.3	106.3
Caerphilly UD	113.2	114.7	120.9	130.6
Cowbridge MB	100.1	93.9	113.1	89.8
Gelligaer UD	107.8	115.8	122.7	134.5
Glyncorrwg UD	113.2	120.8	118.4	122.8
Llwchwr UD	–	–	103.8	115.2
Maesteg UD	111.8	122.0	124.5	138.5
Mountain Ash UD	111.6	115.6	122.4	133.3
Neath MB	112.9	103.5	119.8	128.8
Ogmore and Garw UD	101.9	112.3	113.3	126.0
Penarth UD	92.7	90.3	93.0	105.5
Pontypridd UD	112.5	113.2	116.9	130.0
Porthcawl UD	91.2	89.7	98.0	95.9
Port Talbot UD	–	–	120.4	125.1
Rhondda UD	114.7	119.3	125.1	135.1
Cardiff RD	–	–	91.0	90.2
Cowbridge RD	90.6	92.9	95.2	101.1
Gower RD	83.0	85.1	97.6	93.2
Llantrisant and Llantwit Fardre RD	106.9	114.4	114.0	123.1
Neath RD	103.2	101.2	115.7	120.2
Penybont RD	86.0	80.9	98.6	107.6
Pontardawe RD	102.0	102.6	117.2	124.1
Swansea RD	99.1	100.3	–	–
Glamorgan AC	106.4	108.3	114.9	123.1

	1920–24	1925–29	1930–34	1935–39
Cardiff CB	112.0	111.0	112.1	111.3
Merthyr CB	118.2	121.1	129.8	136.4
Swansea CB	106.8	107.7	116.5	115.0
Newport CB	105.2	109.7	111.7	112.2
Abercarn UD	101.8	96.3	110.9	118.7
Abergavenny UD	98.5	98.3	102.4	116.6
Abersychan UD	98.2	98.0	100.1	–
Abertillery UD	98.9	103.9	108.8	125.2
Bedwas and Machen UD	121.0	107.3	123.4	119.3
Bedwellty UD	113.8	109.0	129.8	130.1
Blaenavon UD	123.4	111.0	123.4	137.9
Caerleon UD	79.0	71.0	70.5	65.4
Chepstow UD	90.4	103.4	118.7	100.3
Ebbw Vale UD	105.6	109.1	116.5	126.5
Llanfrechfa Upper UD	96.7	100.2	102.2	–
Llantarnam UD	98.9	94.6	95.9	–
Monmouth MB	99.8	103.5	98.1	99.5
Mynyddislwyn UD	99.4	102.2	111.4	126.5
Nantyglo and Blaina UD	97.0	104.2	112.0	129.6
Panteg UD	90.6	99.8	97.6	–
Pontypool UD	112.2	107.6	112.7	–
Rhymney UD	115.6	117.4	125.5	138.8
Risca UD	93.1	97.8	102.2	119.2
Tredegar UD	100.2	102.0	109.2	116.9
Usk UD	77.3	82.4	107.7	101.7
Abergavenny RD	77.4	68.8	74.4	77.7
Chepstow RD	84.5	95.7	84.5	96.8
Magor RD	85.3	80.7	87.0	–
Monmouth RD	96.0	84.5	101.1	94.7
Pontypool RD	82.5	85.8	90.5	87.0
St Mellons RD	89.7	86.4	92.3	–
Monmouthshire AC	100.0	99.8	106.7	116.4

Sources: Annual reports of the Medical Officers of Health for Glamorgan CC, Monmouthshire CC, and the county boroughs of Cardiff, Merthyr Tydfil, Newport and Swansea, 1920–39; *Registrar-General's Statistical Review of England and Wales*, 1920–39.

Appendix 8.1. Infant mortality rates, all administrative districts, 1920–39 (deaths of infants under one year of age per 1,000 live births)

	England and Wales	Glam. AC	Mon. AC	Cardiff CB	Merthyr CB	Swansea CB	Newport CB
1920	80	90	88	84	84	88	–
1921	83	93	92	94	90	70	82

	England and Wales	Glam. AC	Mon. AC	Cardiff CB	Merthyr CB	Swansea CB	Newport CB
1922	77	90	83	81	102	82	63
1923	69	75	73	74	86	76	65
1924	75	77	76	78	80	80	73
1925	75	83	84	92	99	70	89
1926	70	76	66	60	83	80	64
1927	69	86	87	80	103	83	67
1928	65	75	72	77	93	61	70
1929	74	80	68	84	107	78	70
1930	60	69	65	72	91	63	55
1931	66	77	72	77	105	69	79
1932	65	72	68	76	73	69	77
1933	64	79	72	77	90	74	94
1934	59	65	57	74	74	62	80
1935	57	64	61	59	74	59	70
1936	59	63	62	55	79	57	64
1937	58	65	64	64	79	56	62
1938	53	60	56	52	77	50	62
1939	50	60	61	53	86	60	54

Sources: Annual reports of the Medical Officers of Health for Glamorgan CC, Monmouthshire CC, and the county boroughs of Cardiff, Merthyr Tydfil, Newport and Swansea, 1920–39; *Registrar-General's Statistical Review of England and Wales,* 1920–39.

Appendix 8.2. Quinquennial infant mortality averages, all administrative districts, 1920–39 (deaths of infants under one year of age per 1,000 births)

	1920–4	1925–9	1930–4	1935–9
Aberdare UD	94.8	89.4	74.0	61.8
Barry UD	72.6	71.0	56.0	45.0
Bridgend UD	68.6	64.6	52.2	47.8
Caerphilly UD	86.2	97.0	78.8	71.0
Cowbridge MB	25.8	25.2	23.0	29.6
Gelligaer UD	91.0	91.4	78.4	65.0
Glyncorrwg UD	83.2	71.2	76.4	58.8
Llwchwr UD	—	—	75.2	55.8
Maesteg UD	89.8	90.2	81.2	78.2
Mountain Ash UD	80.8	80.8	73.4	73.6
Neath MB	75.4	83.2	72.4	54.6
Ogmore and Garw UD	79.2	83.0	80.2	65.8
Penarth UD	58.6	63.2	47.0	56.2
Pontypridd UD	95.6	79.8	72.2	67.4
Porthcawl UD	71.4	46.2	33.4	36.2
Port Talbot UD	84.3	72.8	75.6	65.6
Rhondda UD	91.6	82.6	78.2	66.8

	1920–4	1925–9	1930–4	1935–9
Cardiff RD[a]	73.2	61.8	56.4	50.4
Cowbridge RD	55.8	75.4	55.0	56.2
Gower RD	71.4	62.4	56.0	51.0
Llantrisant and Llantwit Fardre RD	87.2	76.0	75.6	60.6
Neath RD	82.8	84.6	69.2	64.2
Penybont RD	74.4	70.8	67.8	61.0
Pontardawe RD	84.0	70.6	68.2	58.8
Swansea RD[b]	89.2	70.6	–	–
Glamorgan AC	85.0	80.0	72.4	62.4
Cardiff CB	82.2	78.6	75.2	56.6
Merthyr CB	88.4	96.8	86.5	78.8
Swansea CB	79.2	74.4	67.4	56.4
Newport CB	70.8[c]	72.0	76.8	62.3
Abercarn UD	84.6	67.9	59.9	63.6
Abergavenny UD	56.1	55.6	57.2	50.0
Abersychan UD	83.5	78.1	55.2	–
Abertillery UD	92.6	73.3	70.9	68.3
Bedwas and Machen UD	83.3	90.1	69.3	64.8
Bedwellty UD	90.0	87.3	81.1	65.5
Blaenavon UD	112.6	82.1	77.7	73.8
Caerleon UD	53.6	16.7	64.1	65.2
Chepstow UD	67.4	49.2	48.7	36.9
Cwmbran UD	–	–	–	73.1
Ebbw Vale UD	85.8	81.9	69.2	66.5
Llanfrechfa Upper UD	70.6	103.9	79.4	–
Llantarnam UD	75.3	67.1	66.0	–
Monmouth MB	96.0	71.1	75.4	33.8
Mynyddislwyn UD	80.3	85.3	68.6	66.7
Nantyglo and Blaina UD	95.0	78.9	83.0	74.5
Panteg UD	67.8	84.7	59.6	–
Pontypool UD	67.4	73.3	75.3	58.0[d]
Rhymney UD	91.4	84.5	75.8	57.0
Risca UD	66.2	68.4	55.9	52.2
Tredegar UD	82.8	73.9	75.9	63.4
Usk UD	61.0	52.9	85.4	16.7
Abergavenny RD	44.6	53.9	56.4	48.3
Chepstow RD	66.3	55.9	45.7	57.3
Magor RD	60.8	62.8	52.7	–
Magor and St Mellons RD	–	–	–	43.6
Monmouth RD	70.2	63.1	71.5	42.6
Pontypool RD	59.9	65.0	49.9	45.6
St Mellons RD	72.7	67.1	43.9	–
Monmouthshire AC	82.3	75.4	66.7	60.8
England and Wales	76.8	70.8	62.8	55.4

Sources: Annual reports of the Medical Officers of Health for Glamorgan CC, Monmouthshire CC, and the county boroughs of Cardiff, Merthyr Tydfil, Newport and Swansea, 1920–39; *Registrar-General's Statistical Review of England and Wales*, 1920–39.
[a] Cardiff RD was created by boundary changes in 1922 but the local authority in this area previously had been Llandaff and Dinas Powys RD.
[b] This local authority became Llwchwr UD in 1931.
[c] 1921 to 1924 only.
[d] Boundary changes during 1935.

Appendix 8.3. Quinquennial age-specific infant mortality averages, 1920–39 (infant deaths per 1,000 live births)

	Under 1 month	1–3 months	3–6 months	6–9 months	9–12 months
England and Wales					
1921–4	33.6	12.8	11.5	9.5	8.7
1925–9	32.1	11.4	10.3	8.8	8.3
1930–4	31.5	10.0	8.5	6.7	5.9
1935–9	29.4	8.8	7.7	5.3	4.1
Glamorgan AC					
1921–4	36.0	14.7	13.2	10.5	9.3
1925–9	37.8	12.8	10.4	9.8	9.2
1930–4	38.8	10.8	8.5	7.4	6.8
1935–8	35.3	9.5	8.0	5.9	4.8
Monmouthshire AC					
1920–4	36.2	13.8	10.6	10.5	10.3
1925–9	34.4	11.3	10.2	9.7	8.8
1930–4	35.8	9.9	7.1	6.8	6.4
1935–8	33.4	9.9	6.6	5.9	4.4
Cardiff CB					
1920–4	32.2	15.4	13.9	10.9	10.2
1925–9	34.0	12.4	13.5	10.3	8.7
1930–4	37.9	13.1	10.0	7.7	6.5
1935–9	31.1	8.9	7.3	4.8	4.6
Merthyr Tydfil CB					
1921–4	36.0	15.7	16.9	10.3	11.8
1925–9	42.0	16.2	13.4	12.0	14.0
1930–4	39.8	14.4	15.3	9.7	7.8
1935–8	36.8	15.1	11.4	8.1	6.5
Swansea CB					
1920–4	35.3	13.6	12.1	9.4	9.1
1925–9	37.2	11.2	10.0	9.3	7.0
1930–4	33.5	12.1	8.1	7.2	6.8
1935–9	32.8	8.7	7.1	4.4	3.8
Newport CB					
1921–4	32.3	11.8	10.3	9.5	7.3
1925–9	33.9	10.5	10.5	7.9	9.1

	Under 1 month	1–3 months	3–6 months	6–9 months	9–12 months
1930–4	42.3	11.3	9.5	6.5	7.7
1935–8	32.8	9.4	9.6	8.0	4.9
Abertillery UD					
1920–4	38.2	15.2	12.4	16.9	11.0
1925–9	36.8	11.4	10.1	9.8	4.3
1930–4	42.1	11.1	5.6	6.5	5.6
1935–8	42.3	11.3	7.0	8.1	3.7
Mountain Ash UD					
1920–4	28.4	16.6	13.6	10.8	9.8
1925–9	35.3	11.3	10.8	12.2	11.1
1930–4	33.9	13.0	9.5	8.5	8.4
1935–8	40.5	9.4	12.1	5.1	3.9
Penybont RD					
1920–4	36.5	12.1	9.2	10.1	7.6
1925–9	34.2	10.7	9.6	7.3	8.3
1930–4	36.7	9.5	6.6	7.0	7.8
1935–9	38.6	7.1	6.1	4.9	5.3
Pontypridd UD					
1920–4	–	–	–	–	–
1925–9	37.5	12.2	11.2	9.3	8.9
1930–4	42.9	11.6	5.9	6.5	5.3
1935–9	35.3	10.9	9.2	6.9	5.3
Rhondda UD					
1920–4	37.3	14.7	14.9	11.4	10.5
1925–9	35.7	11.6	11.5	10.2	10.9
1930–4	38.1	11.8	9.5	6.6	7.9
1935–9	37.7	7.2	8.2	5.4	3.2

Sources: Annual reports of the Medical Officers of Health for Glamorgan CC, Monmouthshire CC, and the county boroughs of Cardiff, Merthyr Tydfil, Newport and Swansea, 1920–39; *Registrar-General's Statistical Review of England and Wales*, 1920–39.

Appendix 8.4. Stillbirths per 1,000 total births, 1920–39

	England and Wales	Glam. AC	Mon. AC	Cardiff CB	Merthyr CB	Newport CB	Swansea CB
1928	40.1	54.8	50.8	50.6	62.7	41.3	52.9
1929	40.0	57.0	53.0	48.5	68.5	46.2	61.3
1930	40.8	56.6	56.5	46.6	62.8	35.0	53.1
1931	40.9	61.1	54.8	48.0	70.8	45.9	51.3
1932	41.3	58.4	56.7	56.6	72.3	41.9	53.8
1933	41.4	57.8	56.5	48.6	69.9	42.5	49.2
1934	40.5	57.1	54.0	51.2	68.6	46.1	46.0
1935	40.7	56.5	57.4	50.1	59.3	43.5	49.7

	England and Wales	Glam. AC	Mon. AC	Cardiff CB	Merthyr CB	Newport CB	Swansea CB
1936	39.7	58.0	57.3	48.7	62.9	37.2	52.9
1937	39.0	53.1	55.2	39.0	53.9	37.9	53.7
1938	38.3	51.8	54.1	45.5	61.9	35.6	54.1
1939	37.8	–	50.8	46.4	59.4	45.7	41.9

Source: Registrar-General's Statistical Review of England and Wales, 1928–39. Figures calculated from birth statistics found in the annual reports of the local medical officer of health.

	Swansea CB	Maesteg UD	Mountain Ash UD	Penybont RD	Rhondda UD
1920	43.4	40.9	40.5	37.7	46.3
1921	–	42.8	40.3	37.1	45.0
1922	–	45.6	37.7	37.8	52.0
1923	–	57.0	46.0	52.9	59.2
1924	47.6	53.8	33.2	41.6	53.6
1925	51.6	45.8	39.3	43.7	54.3
1926	44.0	33.1	36.8	45.1	61.8
1927	52.0	44.2	44.0	48.8	61.8
1928	53.5	39.3	54.0	48.9	64.0
1929	61.3	57.5	53.7	33.1	63.4
1930	57.6	56.5	50.7	61.2	60.2
1931	51.3	96.9	52.7	66.0	65.2
1932	53.8	83.1	46.8	63.1	66.8
1933	49.2	59.9	44.0	58.3	66.5
1934	46.0	60.4	48.8	51.8	56.2
1935	49.7	68.3	74.6	50.5	44.9
1936	52.9	61.1	45.5	59.4	56.9
1937	53.7	53.6	48.1	46.1	43.1
1938	54.1	55.2	51.8	51.3	44.5
1939	43.8	72.0	–	48.4	54.5

Source: Annual Reports of the relevant Medical Officers of Health, 1920–39.

BIBLIOGRAPHY

1. MANUSCRIPTS

Glamorgan Record Office, Cardiff
Cardiff CBC, Housing, Town Planning, etc., Committee minutes.
Glamorgan CC, *Summary Report of the Medical Officer of Health for the years 1914–19* (1921).
Rhondda UDC, Correspondence and papers relating to air pollution.

Gwent Record Office, Cwmbran
Monmouthshire CC, *Annual Report of the Medical Officer of Health*, 1919.
Monmouthshire Education Committee, *Annual Report of the Medical Inspection Department* (1920–39).
Nantyglo and Blaina UDC, Sanitary Inspector's Report Book.
Tredegar Workingmen's Medical Aid Society records.

Museum of Welsh Life, St Fagans (Sound Archive).
Janet Davies, 26 July and 2 August 1984 (Tapes 7089 and 7090).
Lorna Rubbery, Rhyd-y-Car (Tape 7224).

National Archives, Kew
Board of Education records (ED 50).
Ministry of Health records (HLG 30, MH55, MH57, MH 79, MH96).

National Library of Wales, Aberystwyth
E. L. Chappell papers.
T. Alban Davies papers.
Thomas Jones C.H. papers.
Welsh Board of Health collection.
NLW, MS 306B, T. D. Gwernogle Evans, 'Llysieuwyr (Herbalists) Hen, a Newydd, Yng Nghymru', Eisteddfod Genedlaethol Llanelly, 1930.

South Wales Coalfield Collection, University of Wales Swansea
Bedlinog Medical Committee minutes.
Maesteg Medical Fund minutes.
Mardy Distress Committee Records.
Mountain Ash and Penrhiwceiber Hospital records.
New Tredegar, Tirphil and District Central Relief Committee statement.
Phillip Abraham papers.
Stan Nind papers.

South Wales Miners' Library, University of Wales Swansea
Recordings and transcripts of interviews:
    William Rosser Jones, 4 July 1973 (AUD/180).
    Henry Lewis, 4 December 1972 (AUD/201).

West Glamorgan Record Office, Swansea
Neath RDC, Housing and Town Planning Committee minutes.
Neath RDC, Report upon the Sanitary Conditions of District by the Medical Officer of
    Health and the Surveyors, April 1920.
Port Talbot MB, Highways and Housing Committee minutes.
Port Talbot MB, Housing and Town Planning Committee minutes.
Port Talbot MB, Letting Committee minutes.
Swansea CB, Engineer's Department, Housing Returns.
Swansea CB, Housing Sub-Committee minutes.
Swansea CB, Housing of the Working Classes Committee minutes.
Swansea CB, Joint report of the Borough Treasurer, Borough Architect and Borough Estate
    Agent, 1927.

2. OFFICIAL PUBLICATIONS (IN CHRONOLOGICAL ORDER)

Census of England and Wales, 1901.
Report as to the Practice of Medicine and Surgery by Unqualified Persons in the United Kingdom
    [Cd. 5422], 1910, xliii.
Forty-Second Annual Report of the Local Government Board, Part III [Cd. 6982], 1912–13, LXVII.
Forty-Fourth Annual Report of the Local Government Board, 1914–15, Supplement Containing a Report on
    Maternal Mortality [Cd. 8085], 1914–16, XXV.
Report of the Commission appointed to inquire into Industrial Unrest [Cd. 8662], 1917–18, xv.
Commission of Enquiry into the Coal Industry [Cmd. 360], 1919, xii.
Ministry of Health, *Manual on Unfit Houses and Unhealthy Areas* (London, 1919).
Census of England and Wales, 1921.
Ministry of Health, *Report of the South Wales Regional Survey Committee* (London, 1921).
Ministry of Health, Reports on Public Health and Medical Subjects, 25: Janet M. Campbell,
    Maternal Mortality (London, 1924).
Ministry of Labour, *Local Unemployment Index* (1927–39).
The Registrar-General's Decennial Supplement of England and Wales, 1921: Part II. Occupational
    Mortality, Fertility and Infant Mortality (London, 1927).
Ministry of Health, *Report on Investigation in the Coalfield of South Wales and Monmouthshire*
    [Cmd. 3272], 1928–9, viii.
Census of England and Wales, 1931.
Ministry of Health, Reports on Public Health and Medical Subjects, 68: Dame Janet
    Campbell, Isabella D. Cameron and Dilys M. Jones, *High Maternal Mortality in Certain Areas*
    (London, 1932).
Board of Trade, *An Industrial Survey of South Wales* (London, 1932).
Final Report of the Royal Commission on Unemployment Insurance [Cmd. 4185], 1932, xiii.
Ministry of Labour, *Reports of the Investigation into the Industrial Conditions in certain Depressed Areas,*
    III: South Wales and Monmouthshire [Cmd. 4728], 1933–4, xiii.
Particulars of the Slum Clearance Programmes Furnished by Local Authorities [Cmd. 4535], 1933–4,
    xxi.
Ministry of Health, *Housing. House Production, Slum Clearance, etc. England and Wales, 1935–39.*
Second Report of the Commissioner for the Special Areas [Cmd. 5090], 1935–6, xiii.
Annual Report of the Unemployment Assistance Board [Cmd. 5177], 1935–6, xiii.
Ministry of Health, *Report on the Overcrowding Survey of England and Wales* (London, 1936).
Return of the Number of Payments Made at Local Offices of the Ministry of Labour, 26 June 1936
    [Cmd. 5240], 1935–6, xvii.
Ministry of Labour, *Twenty-Second Abstract of Labour Statistics of the United Kingdom (1922–1936)*
    [Cmd. 5556], 1936–7, xxvi.
Ministry of Health, *Report on Maternal Mortality in Wales* [Cmd. 5423], 1936–7, xi.

Third Report of the Commissioner for the Special Areas [Cmd. 5303], 1936–7, xii.

Ministry of Health, Reports on Public Health and Medical Subjects, 86: E. Lewis-Faning, *A Study of the Trend of Mortality Rates in Urban Communities of England and Wales, with Special Reference to 'Distressed Areas'* (London, 1938).

The Registrar-General's Decennial Supplement of England and Wales, 1931: Part IIa. Occupational Mortality (London, 1938).

Ministry of Health, *Report of the Committee of Inquiry into the Anti-Tuberculosis Service in Wales and Monmouthshire* (London, 1939).

National Register, United Kingdom and the Isle of Man, Statistics of Population on 29 September 1939 (London, 1944).

Ministry of Fuel and Power, *South Wales Coalfield Regional Survey Report* (London, 1946).

Welsh Office, *Better Health – Better Wales* (London, 1998).

3. NEWSPAPERS AND PERIODICALS

Newspapers

Aberdare Leader
Abergavenny Chronicle
Barry Herald
Caerphilly Journal
Cardiff Times and South Wales Weekly News
Daily Herald
Free Press of Monmouthshire
Glamorgan Gazette
Guardian
Llais Llafur
Llanelly Mercury
Llanelly Star
Merthyr Express
Neath Guardian
New York Times
Rhondda Leader
Rhondda Vanguard
South Wales Daily News
South Wales Echo
South Wales Evening Express
South Wales Evening Post
South Wales Gazette
South Wales Weekly Argus
The Times
Western Mail

Periodicals

Better Health
British Medical Journal
Co-operative Congress Reports
Friend
Labour Woman
Lancet
Maternity and Child Welfare
Medical Herbalist
Medical Officer
Miner
Ministry of Labour Gazette
Planning
Public Health
Welsh Housing and Development Association Yearbook
Welsh Journal of Agriculture
Welsh Outlook
World's Children

4. WORKS OF REFERENCE AND REPORTS

Works of reference

Cule, John, *Wales and Medicine* (Aberystwyth, 1980).

Jones, Beti, *Newsplan Cymru/Wales* (London, 1994).

Kendall, M. G. (ed.), *The Sources and Nature of the Statistics of the United Kingdom* (London, 1952).

Miller-Keane Encyclopedia and Dictionary of Medicine, Nursing, and Allied Health, 6th edn (London, 1997).

Mitchell, B. R. and Deane, Phyllis, *Abstract of British Historical Statistics* (Cambridge, 1962).

Williams, John, *Digest of Welsh Historical Statistics* (Pontypool, 1985), 2 vols.

Reports
Annual reports by the following:
Chief Medical Officer
Chief Medical Officer of the Board of Education
Co-operative Congress
Miners' Welfare Fund
Ministry of Health
Registrar General's Statistical Review of England and Wales
Welsh Housing and Development Association
Welsh National Memorial Association

5. MEDICAL OFFICER OF HEALTH REPORTS

Annual reports of the medical officers of the following districts in the period 1920–39 have
been used. A large proportion of these reports is held in the Welsh Board of Health
Collection at the National Library of Wales.

Glamorgan

Aberavon Municipal Borough
Aberdare Urban District
Barry Urban District
Bridgend Urban District
Briton Ferry Urban District
Caerphilly Urban District
Cardiff County Borough
Cardiff Rural District
Cowbridge Municipal Borough
Cowbridge Rural District
Gelligaer Urban District
Glamorgan Administrative County
Glyncorrwg Urban District
Gower Rural District
Llandaff and Dinas Powys Rural District
Llantrisant and Llantwit Fardre Rural
    District

Llwchwr Urban District
Maesteg Urban District
Margam Urban District
Merthyr Tydfil County Borough
Mountain Ash Urban District
Neath Municipal Borough
Neath Rural District
Ogmore and Garw Urban District
Penarth Urban District
Penybont Rural District
Pontardawe Rural District
Pontypridd Urban District
Porthcawl Urban District
Port Talbot Municipal Borough
Rhondda Urban District
Swansea County Borough
Swansea Rural District

Monmouthshire

Abercarn Urban District
Abergavenny Municipal Borough
Abergavenny Rural District
Abersychan Urban District
Abertillery Urban District
Bedwas and Machen Urban District
Bedwellty Urban District
Blaenavon Urban District
Caerleon Urban District
Chepstow Rural District
Chepstow Urban District
Cwmbran Urban District
Ebbw Vale Urban District
Llanfrechfa Upper Urban District
Llantarnam Urban District

Magor Rural District
Magor and St Mellons Rural District
Monmouth Municipal Borough
Monmouthshire Administrative County
Mynyddislwyn Urban District
Nantyglo and Blaina Urban District
Newport County Borough
Panteg Urban District
Pontypool Urban District
Rhymney Urban District
Risca Urban District
St Mellons Rural District
Tredegar Urban District
Usk Urban District

Annual reports of the school medical officers for the following local education authorities have also been used. These were often bound with the corresponding annual medical officer of health reports.

Aberdare Urban District

Monmouthshire County Council

Abertillery Urban District

Mountain Ash Urban District

Barry Urban District

Pontypridd Urban District

Cardiff County Borough

Rhondda Urban District

Ebbw Vale Urban District

6. CONTEMPORARY WORKS

An Industrial Survey of South Wales: Made for the Board of Trade by University College of South Wales and Monmouthshire (London, 1932).

Armitage, C. Phyllis, *Health Visiting: The New Profession. A Handbook for Health Visitors and School Nurses* (London, 1927).

Astor, J. J. et al., *The Third Winter of Unemployment: The Report of an Enquiry Undertaken in the Autumn of 1922* (London, 1923).

Beales, H. L., and R. S. Lambert (eds), *Memoirs of the Unemployed* (London, 1934).

Booth, Charles, *Life and Labour* (London, 1892).

British Waterworks Association, *British Waterworks Year Book and Directory* (1926).

Burns, John, and W. Halliday Welsh, *Everybody's Book on Tuberculosis* (Cardiff, 1914).

Cassie, E., *Maternity and Child Welfare: A Text-Book for Public Health Workers* (London, 1929).

Cathcart, E. P., and A. M. T. Murray, *An Inquiry into the Diet of Families in Cardiff and Reading*, MRC Special Report Series, 165, (London, 1932).

Chappell, Edgar L., *Gwalia's Homes: 50 Points for Housing Reform* (Ystalyfera, 1911).

Communist Party, *TB: The White Scourge in Wales* (Cardiff, c.1939).

Cox, J. Glyn, *Report of an Investigation into the Incidence of Tuberculosis in the County of Anglesey and the Urban District of Barry* (Cardiff, 1937).

Cronin, A. J., *The Citadel* (London, 1937).

Davies, Miles, 'The Rhondda Valley', *Geographical Magazine*, 2, 5 (1936), 372–86.

Davies, Rhys, *My Wales* (London, 1937).

—— 'From my Notebook (III)', *Wales*, 22 (1946), 13–19.

Edwards, H. W. J., *The Good Patch* (London, 1938).

Evans, Thomas Gwernogle, *The Cup of Health* (Cardiff, 1922).

Fenner Brockway, A., *Hungry England* (London, 1932).

Ginzberg, Eli, *A World Without Work* (London, 1942).

Glover, J. A., 'The place of the Public health department in relation to council housing estates', *Journal of the Royal Sanitary Institute*, 59, 1 (1938), 64–70.

Griffiths, James, *The Price Wales Pays for Poverty* (c.1939).

Hannington, Wal, *The Problem of the Distressed Areas* (London, 1937).

Hanley, James, *Grey Children: A Study in Humbug and Misery* (London, 1937).

Hastings, S., *A National Physiological Minimum* (London, 1934).

Harris, Oliver, *Poor Law Administration: A Report on the Investigation into Poor Law Relief Cases in the Bedwellty Union* (c.1929).

Harrison, G., and F. C. Mitchell, *The Home Market: A Handbook of Statistics* (London, c.1936).

Harry, E. Ll., 'Consumption of milk in a distressed area of south Wales', *Welsh Journal of Agriculture*, 11 (1935), 23–48.

—— 'Meat consumption in the Rhondda Valley', *Welsh Journal of Agriculture*, 12 (1936), 69–86.

—— 'The consumption of milkstuffs and meatstuffs in the Rhondda Valley', *Welsh Journal of Agriculture*, 13 (1937), 69–81.

—— and J. R. E. Phillips, 'Household budgets in the Rhondda Valley', *Welsh Journal of Agriculture*, 12 (1937), 81–93.

—— 'Expenditure of unemployed and employed households', *Welsh Journal of Agriculture*, 14 (1938), 91–108.

Hazell, W., *The Gleaming Vision, being the History of the Ynysybwl Co-operative Society Ltd, 1889–1954*.

Herbert, S. Mervyn, *Britain's Health* (Harmondsworth, 1939).

Housing Committee of the County Borough of Swansea, *Municipal Housing in Swansea* (Gloucester, 1940).

Hutt, Allen, *The Condition of the Working Class in Britain* (London, 1933).

Jennings, Hilda, *Brynmawr: A Study of a Distressed Area* (London, 1934).

Jones, T. A., 'The Royal Gwent Hospital (Workmen's Fund)', in *Newport Encyclopedia. Coronation Year and Royal Visit Souvenir* (Newport, 1937).

Jones, W. H., and W. J. Cowie, 'The consumption of milk in Cardiff', *Welsh Journal of Agriculture*, 10 (1934), 83–107.

Kelly's Directory of Monmouthshire and South Wales.

Labour Party, *Reports on Nutrition and Food Supplies and Women in Offices* (London, 1936).

Labour Party Committee of Inquiry, *The Distress in South Wales: Health of Babies and Mothers Imperilled* (London, 1928).

Lewes, Mary L., *The Queer Side of Things* (London, 1923).

Massey, P., *Portrait of a Mining Town, Fact*, 8 (1937).

McNally, C. E., *Public Ill Health* (London, 1935).

Meara, Gwynne, *Unemployment in Merthyr Tydfil: A Survey Made at the Request of the Merthyr Settlement* (Newtown, 1935).

Men Without Work: A Report made to the Pilgrim Trust (Cambridge, 1938).

M'Gonigle, G. C. M., and J. Kirby, *Poverty and Public Health* (London, 1936).

Morton, H. V., *In Search of Wales* (London, 1945 edn).

National Housing and Town Planning Council, *Programme of Housing and Town Planning Conference for Wales and Monmouthshire*, 8–9 July 1921 at Llandrindod Wells.

Orr, John Boyd, *Food, Health and Income* (London, 1936).

Phillips, J. R. E., 'Some further studies of household budgets in the Rhondda Valley', *Welsh Journal of Agriculture*, 15 (1939), 29–40.

Phillpott, H. R. S., *Where Labour Rules: A Tour Through Towns and Counties* (London, 1934).

Political and Economic Planning (PEP), *The Problem of South Wales, Planning*, 94, 9 (March 1937).

—— *Report on the British Health Services* (London, 1937).

Powys Greenwood, H., *Employment and the Depressed Areas* (London, 1936).

Save the Children Fund, *Unemployment and the Child* (London, 1933).

Singer, H. W., *Unemployment and the Unemployed* (London, 1940).

Spring Rice, Margery, *Working Class Wives: Their Health and Conditions* (Harmondsworth, 1939).

Swansea County Borough, *Souvenir of the Opening of the Guildhall* (Swansea, 1934).

The Second Industrial Survey of South Wales (Cardiff, 1937).

Trevelyan, M., *Folk-lore and Folk-Stories of Wales* (London, 1909).

'Unemployment: The Wider Problem', *Round Table*, 103 (June 1936), 546–9.

Walters, R. C. S., *The Nation's Water Supply* (London, 1936).

Williams, Lady, 'Modern theories of nutrition in relation to Welsh migration', *Public Health in Wales*, Addresses delivered to the Welsh School of Social Services, Llandrindod Wells, 10–13 August 1936.

—— 'Malnutrition as a cause of maternal mortality', *Public Health*, 1, vol. 50 (October, 1936), pp. 11–19.

Williams, W., 'Puerperal mortality', *Transactions of the Epidemiological Society of London* (1895–96).

Zweig, F., *Men in the Pits* (London, 1948).

7. AUTOBIOGRAPHIES

Ackerman, John, *Up the Lamb* (Bridgend, 1998).
Baker, Eileen, *'Yan Boogie'. The Autobiography of a Swansea Valley Girl* (Pretoria, 1992).
Beales, H. L., and R. S. Lambert, *Memoirs of the Unemployed* (Wakefield, 1973).
Berry, Ron, *History is What You Live* (Llandysul, 1998).
Butler, Marian, *Everything I Hold Sacred: A Biography of a Spiritual Healer* (London, 1994).
Coombes, B. L., *I am a Miner, Fact*, 23 (London, 1939).
—— *These Poor Hands* (London, 1939).
—— *Those Clouded Hills* (London, 1944).
—— *Miners Day* (London, 1945).
Courtney, Edith, *A Mouse Ran up my Nightie* (Llandysul, 1974).
Cronin, A. J., *Adventures in Two Worlds* (London, 1952).
Davies, Edith S., *The Innocent Years: The Story of My Childhood in Ynysybwl* (Creigiau, 1995).
Davies, Rosina, *The Story of My Life* (Llandysul, 1942).
Davies, Rhys, *Print of a Hare's Foot* (London, 1969).
Davies, Walter Haydn, *The Right Place – The Right Time: Memories of Boyhood Days in a Welsh Mining Community* (Llandybie, 1972).
—— *Ups and Downs* (Swansea, 1975).
—— *Blithe Ones* (Port Talbot, 1979).
Eckley, Simon, and Don Bearcroft (eds), *Voices of Abertillery, Aberbeeg and Llanhilleth* (Stroud, 1996).
Edwards, C. B., '"It was like this": personal recollections of Garndiffaith in the 1930s', part I, *Gwent Local History*, 76 (1994), 21–34; part II, *Gwent Local History*, 77 (1994), 37–46.
Edwards, Ifan, *No Gold on my Shovel* (London, 1947).
Evans, Gwyneth E., 'Reminiscences of the 1920s and early 1930s', Afon Tâf Research Group, *Recollections of Merthyr's Past* (Newport, 1979), pp. 55–61.
Eyles, Anne, and Con O'Sullivan, *In the Shadow of the Steelworks: Reminiscences of a Splott Childhood in the 1930s* (Cardiff, 1992).
—— *In the Shadow of the Steelworks II* (Cardiff, 1992).
Finch, Harold, *Memoirs of a Bedwellty MP* (Newport, 1972).
Grenfell-Hill, J. (ed.), *Growing up in Wales 1895–1939* (Llandysul, 1996).
Hardy, Barbara, *Swansea Girl: A Memoir* (London, 1994).
Healy, Kathleen, *Growing up in a Welsh Valley* (Ilfracombe, 1999).
Horner, Arthur, *Incorrigible Rebel* (London, 1960).
John, Jean, *Grey Trees: Childhood Memories of Llwydcoed* (Bristol, 1996).
Jones, Thomas, *Rhymney Memories* (Newtown, 1938).
Lee, R. L., *The Town that Died* (London, 1975).
Llewelyn Davies, M. (ed.), *Life as we have Known it* (London, 1931).
Luxton, Brian, *In our own Words, in our own Pictures, People's History to Commemorate the Barry Docks Centenary* (Barry, 1989).
Menadue, Clive, *The Foxglove Sun: Moments from Childhood Recalled* (Blaengarw, 1996).
Morgan, Elaine, *Mad Morgan: Child of the Forest, Man of the Mines. The Autobiography of Reginald Victor Morgan* (Bradford, 1995).
Morgan, Robert, *My Lamp Still Burns* (Llandysul, 1981).
Mor-O'Brien, Anthony (ed.), *The Autobiography of Edmund Stonelake* (Cardiff, 1981)
Mullin, James, *The Story of a Toiler's Life* (London, 1921).
Nicholson, Mavis, *Martha Jane and Me: A Girlhood in Wales* (London, 1991).
O'Sullivan, Florance, *Return to Wales* (Tenby, 1974).
Parnell, Mary Davies, *Block Salt and Candles: A Rhondda Childhood* (Bridgend, 1991).
Paynter, Will, *My Generation* (London, 1972).
Phillips, Bill, *A Kid from Splott* (Cardiff, 1985).
Prothero, Cliff, *Recount* (Ormskirk, 1982).

Pryce Jones, Maggie, *Kingfisher of Hope* (Llandysul, 1993).

Radcliffe, Grafton, *Back to Blaengarw* (Blaengarw, 1994).

Smith, Francis Maylett, *The Surgery at Aberffrwd: Some Encounters of a Colliery Doctor Seventy Years Ago* (Hythe, Kent, 1981).

Thomas, Chris, *My Early Struggles* (Swansea, 1997).

Thomas, Gwyn, *A Few Selected Exits* (London, 1968).

Twamley, Bill, *Cardiff and Me – Sixty Years Ago: Growing up in the Twenties and Thirties* (Cardiff, 1984).

Watkins, Percy, *A Welshman Remembers* (Cardiff, 1944).

Webb, Rachael Ann, *From Caerau to the Southern Cross* (Port Talbot, 1987).

—— *Sirens over the Valley* (Port Talbot, 1988).

8. SECONDARY BOOKS

Aldcroft, Derek H., *The Inter-War Economy: Britain, 1919–1939* (London, 1970).

Andrews, Elizabeth, *A Woman's Work is Never Done* (Ystrad, Rhondda, 1957).

Beddoe, Deirdre, *Back to Home and Duty: Women between the Wars, 1918–1939* (London, 1989).

—— *Out of the Shadows: A History of Women in Twentieth-Century Wales* (Cardiff, 2000).

Benjamin, Bernard, *Population Statistics: A Review of UK Sources* (Aldershot, 1989).

Benson, John, *The Penny Capitalists: A Study of Nineteenth-Century Working-Class Entrepreneurs* (Dublin, 1983).

—— *Entrepreneurism in Canada: A History of 'Penny Capitalists'* (Lampeter, 1990).

Berridge, Virginia, *Health and Society since 1939* (Cambridge, 1999).

Bevan, Aneurin, *In Place of Fear* (London, 1961).

Bideau, A., B. Desjardins and H. Pérez-Brignoli (eds), *Infant and Child Mortality in the Past* (Oxford, 1997).

Bourke, Joanna, *Working-Class Cultures in Britain, 1890–1960: Gender, Class and Ethnicity* (London, 1994).

Bowley, Marian, *Housing and the State, 1919–1945* (London, 1945).

Brändström, A., and L.-G. Tedebrand (eds), *Society, Health and Population during the Demographic Transition* (Stockholm, 1988).

Bridges, E. M., *Healing the Scars; Derelict Land in Wales* (Llandysul, 1988).

Bryder, Linda, *Below the Magic Mountain: A Social History of Tuberculosis in Twentieth Century Britain* (Oxford, 1988).

Burnett, John, *A History of the Cost of Living* (Harmondsworth, 1969).

—— *A Social History of Housing, 1815–1970* (London, 1986).

—— *Plenty and Want. A Social History of Diet in England* (London, 1989).

—— *Idle Hands: The Experience of Unemployment, 1790–1990* (London, 1994).

Bynum, W. F., and Roy Porter (eds), *Living and Dying in London, Medical History Supplement*, 11 (London, 1991).

—— (eds), *Companion Encyclopedia of the History of Medicine* (London, 1993).

Calder, Angus, and Dorothy Sheridan (eds), *Speak for Yourself: A Mass-Observation Anthology, 1927–49* (London, 1984).

Chapman, A. L., and R. Knight, *Wages and Salaries in the United Kingdom, 1920–1938* (Cambridge, 1953).

Chapman, S. D., *The History of Working-Class Housing: A Symposium* (Newton Abbot, 1971).

Cherry, Steven, *Medical Services and the Hospitals in Britain, 1860–1939* (Cambridge, 1996).

Clapp, B. W., *An Environmental History of Britain since the Industrial Revolution* (London, 1994).

Cole, G. D. H., *The British Co-operative Movement in a Socialist Society* (London, 1951).

Coleman, D. A., and John Salt, *The British Population: Patterns, Trends, and Processes* (Oxford, 1992).

Constantine, Stephen, *Unemployment in Britain between the Wars* (London, 1980).

Cooter, Roger (ed.), *Studies in the History of Alternative Medicine* (London, 1988).

Corsini, C. A., and P. P. Viazzo (eds), *The Decline of Infant Mortality and Child Mortality: The European Experience, 1750–1990* (The Hague, 1997).

Cross, Gary S., *Time and Money: The Making of Consumer Culture* (London, 1993).

Crowther, Anne, *Social Policy in Britain, 1914–1939* (London, 1988).

Daunton, Martin J., *Coal Metropolis: Cardiff, 1870–1914* (Leicester, 1977).

—— *House and Home in the Victorian City: Working-Class Housing, 1850–1914* (London, 1983).

—— (ed.), *Councillors and Tenants: Local Authority Housing in English Cities, 1919–1939* (Leicester, 1984).

Davies, John, *A History of Wales* (Harmondsworth, 1994).

Davies, T. G., *Deeds Not Words: A History of the Swansea General and Eye Hospital, 1817–1948* (Cardiff, 1988).

Davin, Anna, *Growing up Poor: Home, School and Street in London, 1870–1914* (London, 1996).

Deacon, Alan, *In Search of the Scrounger: The Administration of Unemployment Insurance in Britain, 1920–1931* (London, 1976).

—— and Jonathan Bradshaw, *Reserved for the Poor: The Means Test in British Social Policy*, (Oxford, 1983).

Dewey, Peter, *War and Progress: Britain, 1914–1945* (London, 1997).

Dobson, Mary J., *Contours of Death and Disease in Early Modern England* (Cambridge, 1997).

Douglas, Mary and Baron Isherwood, *The World of Goods: Towards an Anthropology of Consumption* (Harmondsworth, 1980 edn).

Duncombe, L., D. Page, D. Stokes and S. Wilcox (eds), *Under the Doctor* (Pontypool, 1995).

Ellis, E. L., *T. J.: A Life of Dr Thomas Jones C.H.* (Cardiff, 1992).

Evans, D. Gareth, *A History of Wales, 1906–2000* (Cardiff, 2000).

Evans, Richard J., *Death in Hamburg: Society and Politics in the Cholera Years, 1830–1910* (Oxford, 1987).

Eveleth, Phyllis B., and J. M. Tanner, *Worldwide Variation in Human Growth* (Cambridge, 1976).

Fildes, Valerie, *Breasts, Babies and Bottles: A History of Infant Feeding* (Edinburgh, 1986).

Finlayson, Geoffrey, *Citizen, State, and Social Welfare in Britain, 1830–1990* (Oxford, 1994).

Fisk, M. J., *Home Truths. Issues for Housing in Wales* (Llandysul, 1996).

—— *Housing in the Rhondda, 1800–1940* (Cardiff, 1996).

Floud, Roderick, Kenneth W. Wachter and Annabel Gregory, *Height, Health and History: Nutritional Status in the United Kingdom, 1750–1980* (Cambridge, 1990).

Foot, Michael, *Aneurin Bevan: A Biography* (London, 1963).

Francis, Hywel, and Dai Smith, *The Fed: A History of the South Wales Miners in the Twentieth Century* (London, 1980).

Fraser Brockington, C., *Public Health in the Nineteenth Century* (London, 1965).

Frazer, W. M., *A History of English Public Health, 1834–1939* (London, 1950).

Garcia, J., R. Kilpatrick and M. Richards (eds), *The Politics of Maternity Care: Services for Childbearing Women in the Twentieth Century Britain* (Oxford, 1990).

Garside, W., *The Measurement of Unemployment: Methods and Sources in Great Britain, 1850–1979* (Oxford, 1980).

Gauldie, E., *Cruel Habitations: A History of Working-Class Housing, 1780–1918* (London, 1974).

Gazeley, Ian, *Poverty in Britain, 1900–1965* (Basingstoke, 2003).

Gilbert, B. B., *British Social Policy, 1914–39* (London, 1970).

Gladstone, David, *The Twentieth-Century Welfare State* (London, 1999).

Glynn, Sean, and John Oxborrow, *Interwar Britain: A Social and Economic History* (London, 1976).

—— and Alan Booth, *Modern Britain: An Economic and Social History* (London, 1996).

Gray, Nigel, *The Worst of Times: An Oral History of the Great Depression in Britain* (Aldershot, 1985).

Gray-Jones, A., *A History of Ebbw Vale* (Risca, 1970).

Green, David G., *Working-Class Patients and the Medical Establishment: Self Help in Britain from the Mid-Nineteenth Century to 1948* (Aldershot, 1985).

Greenhalgh, Susan (ed.), *Situating Fertility: Anthropology and Demographic Inquiry* (Cambridge, 1995)

Gurney, Peter, *Co-operative Culture and the Politics of Consumption in England, 1870–1930* (Manchester, 1996).

Gwyther, Cyril E., *The Valley shall be Exalted* (London, 1949).

Hardy, Anne, *The Epidemic Streets: Infectious Disease and the Rise of Preventive Medicine, 1856–1900* (Oxford, 1993).

Harris, Bernard, *The Health of the Schoolchild: A History of the School Medical Service in England and Wales* (Buckingham, 1995).

—— *The Origins of the British Welfare State: Social Welfare in England and Wales, 1800–1945* (Basingstoke, 2004).

Hazelgrove, Jennifer, *Spiritualism and British Society between the Wars* (Manchester, 2000).

Helman, Cecil, *Culture, Health and Illness* (Oxford, 1984).

Herbert, Trevor, and Gareth Elwyn Jones (eds), *Wales between the Wars* (Cardiff, 1988).

Hole, W. V., and M. T. Pountney, *Trends in Population, Housing and Occupancy Rates, 1861–1961* (London, 1971).

John, Arthur H., and Glanmor Williams (eds), *Glamorgan County History*, vol. 5, *Industrial Glamorgan* (Cardiff, 1980).

John, Angela V. (ed.), *Our Mothers' Land: Chapters in Welsh Women's History, 1830–1939* (Cardiff, 1991).

Johnes, Martin, *Soccer and Society: South Wales, 1900–1939* (Cardiff, 2002).

Johnson, Paul, *Saving and Spending: The Working Class Economy in Britain, 1870–1939* (Oxford, 1985).

Jones, Helen, *Health and Society in Twentieth-Century Britain* (London, 1994).

Jones, Philip N., *Colliery Settlement in the South Wales Coalfield, 1850 to 1926* (Hull, 1969).

Jones, R. Merfyn, *Cymru 2000: Hanes Cymru yn yr Ugeinfed Ganrif* (Caerdydd, 1999).

Jones T. B., and W. J. T. Collins, *History of the Royal Gwent Hospital* (Newport, 1948).

Jones, W. R. D., *Maesycwmmer: The Hidden Landscape (1826–1939)* (Newport, 1989).

Kaye, H. J., *British Marxist Historians: An Introductory Analysis* (Oxford, 1984).

Kiple, Kenneth (ed.), *The Cambridge World History of Human Disease* (Cambridge, 1993).

Kleinman, Arthur K., *Patients and Healers in the Context of Culture* (London, 1980).

Landers, John, *Death and the Metropolis: Studies in the Demographic History of London, 1670–1830* (Cambridge, 1993).

Landy, David (ed.), *Culture, Disease and Healing: Studies in Medical Anthropology* (London, 1977).

Lawrence, Chris, *Medicine in the Making of Modern Britain, 1700–1920* (London, 1994).

Lewis, Jane, *The Politics of Motherhood: Child and Maternal Welfare in England, 1900–1939* (London, 1980).

—— *What Price Community Medicine? The Philosophy, Practice and Politics of Public Health since 1919* (Brighton, 1986).

—— (ed.), *Labour and Love: Women's Experience of Home and Family, 1850–1940* (Oxford, 1989 edn).

Loudon, Irvine, *Death in Childbirth: An International Study of Maternal Care and Maternal Mortality, 1800–1950* (Oxford, 1992).

—— (ed.), *Western Medicine* (Oxford, 1997).

Lupton, Deborah, *Medicine as Culture: Illness, Disease and the Body in Western Societies* (London, 1994).

Mabbitt, J. H. L., *The Health Services of Glamorgan* (Cowbridge, 1977).

McKeown, Thomas, *The Modern Rise of Population* (London, 1976).

—— *The Role of Medicine: Dream, Mirage or Nemesis?* (Princeton, 1979).

McKibbin, Ross, *The Ideologies of Class: Social Relations in Britain, 1880–1950* (Oxford, 1994).

Mackintosh, J. M., *Trends of Opinion about the Public Health, 1901–51* (London, 1953).

Marsh, D. C., *National Insurance and Assistance in Great Britain* (London, 1950).

Mercer, A. J., *Disease, Mortality and Population in Transition* (Leicester, 1990).

Minchinton, W. E., *The British Tinplate Industry: A History* (Oxford, 1957).

Morgan, J. E., *A Village Workers' Council and what it Accomplished, Being A Short History of the Lady Windsor Lodge, South Wales Miners' Federation* (Pontypridd, 1956).

Morgan, K. O., *Rebirth of a Nation: Wales, 1880–1980* (Oxford, 1981).

Morgan, Prys (ed.), *Glamorgan County History*, vol. 6, *Glamorgan Society, 1780–1980* (Cardiff, 1988).

Mowat, Charles L., *Britain between the Wars, 1918–40* (London, 1955).

Naylor, B., *Quakers in the Rhondda 1926–1986* (Chepstow, 1986).

Nicholas, K., *The Social Effects of Unemployment in Teesside* (Manchester, 1986).

Oddy, D. J., and D. Miller (eds), *The Making of the Modern British Diet* (London, 1975).

Perry, Matt, *Bread and Work: Social Policy and the Experience of Unemployment, 1918–39* (2000).

Phillips, Gordon, and Noel Whiteside, *Casual Labour: The Unemployment Question in the Port Transport Industry, 1880–1970* (Oxford, 1985).

Pollard, A. H., F. Yusuf and G. N. Pollard, *Demographic Techniques* (Oxford, 1981).

Pooley, Colin G. (ed.), *Housing Strategies in Europe, 1880–1930* (Leicester, 1992).

—— and Jean Turnbull, *Migration and Mobility in Britain since the Eighteenth Century* (London, 1998).

Porter, Dorothy (ed.), *The History of Health and the Modern State* (Amsterdam, 1994).

—— *Health, Civilization and the State: A History of Public Health from Ancient to Modern Times* (London, 1999).

Porter, Roy (ed.), *Patients and Practitioners: Lay Perceptions of Medicine in Pre-Industrial Society* (Cambridge, 1985).

—— (ed.), *The Cambridge Illustrated History of Medicine* (Cambridge, 1996).

—— *The Greatest Benefit to Mankind: A Medical History of Humanity from Antiquity to the Present* (London, 1997).

Pressat, Roland, *Demographic Analysis: Methods, Results, Applications* (London, 1972).

Ramsey, Matthew, *Professional and Popular Medicine in France, 1770–1830* (Cambridge, 1988).

Riley, James C., *Sickness, Recovery and Death: A History and Forecast of Ill Health* (London, 1989).

—— *Sick, Not Dead: The Health of British Workingmen during the Mortality Decline* (Baltimore, 1997).

Roberts, Elizabeth, *A Woman's Place: An Oral History of Working-Class Women, 1890–1940* (Oxford, 1984).

Robins, N. A., *Homes for Heroes: Early Twentieth-Century Council Housing in the County Borough of Swansea* (Swansea, 1992).

Routh, Guy, *Occupation and Pay in Great Britain, 1906–79* (London, 1980).

Schofield, R., D. Reher and A. Bideau (eds), *The Decline of Mortality in Europe* (Oxford, 1991).

Shorter, Edward, *A History of Women's Bodies* (London, 1983).

Smith, F. B., *The People's Health, 1830–1910* (London, 1979).

—— *The Retreat of Tuberculosis, 1850–1950* (London, 1988).

Stedman Jones, Gareth, *Outcast London* (London, 1971).

Stevenson, John, *British Society, 1914–45* (Harmondsworth, 1984).

—— and Chris Cook, *The Slump* (London, 1977), revised as *Britain in the Depression: Society and Politics, 1929–39* (Harlow, 1994).

Swenarton, Mark, *Homes Fit for Heroes: The Politics and Architecture of Early State Housing in Britain* (London, 1981).

Tanner, Duncan, Chris Williams and Deian Hopkin (eds), *The Labour Party in Wales, 1900–2000* (Cardiff, 2000).

Taylor, A. J. (ed.), *The Standard of Living in the Industrial Revolution* (London, 1975).

Tebbutt, Melanie, *Making Ends Meet: Pawnbroking and Working-Class Credit* (London, 1984).

Thane, Pat, *Foundations of the Welfare State* (London, 1996).

Thomas, Gwyn, *Where did I Put my Pity? Folk Tales from the Modern Welsh* (London, 1946).

—— *A Point of Order* (London, 1956).

—— *A Welsh Eye* (London, 1964).

—— *Sorrow for Thy Sons* (London, 1986).

Thomas, Keith, *Religion and the Decline of Magic* (Harmondsworth, 1973).

Thompson, E. P., *The Making of the English Working Class* (London, 1963).

Thorpe, Andrew, *Britain in the 1930s* (Oxford, 1992).

Tranter, Neil L., *British Population in the Twentieth Century* (London, 1996).

Treble, J. H., *Urban Poverty in Britain, 1830–1914* (London, 1979).

Vincent, David, *Poor Citizens: The State and the Poor in Twentieth Century Britain* (Harlow, 1991).

Ward, Stephen V., *The Geography of Interwar Britain: The State and Uneven Development* (London, 1988).

Wear, Andrew (ed.), *Medicine in Society: Historical Essays* (Cambridge, 1992).

White, Carol, and Sian Rhiannon Williams (eds), *Struggle or Starve: Women's Lives in the South Wales Valleys between the Two World Wars* (Dinas Powys, 1998).

Williams, A. Susan, *Women and Childbirth in the Twentieth Century: A History of the National Birthday Trust Fund, 1928–93* (Stroud, 1997).

Williams, Chris, *Capitalism, Community and Conflict: The South Wales Coalfield, 1898–1947* (Cardiff, 1998).

Williams, Gwyn A., *The Welsh in their History* (London, 1982).

—— *When was Wales?* (London, 1985).

Winter, J. M., *The Great War and the British People* (London, 1986).

Wohl, Anthony, *Endangered Lives: Public Health in Victorian Britain* (London, 1983).

Woods, Robert, and John Hugh Woodward (eds), *Urban Disease and Mortality in Nineteenth-Century England* (London, 1984).

9. SECONDARY ARTICLES AND ESSAYS

Anderson, Michael, 'The social implications of demographic change', in F. M. L. Thompson (ed.), *The Cambridge Social History of Britain, 1750–1950*, vol. 2, *People and their Environment* (Cambridge, 1990), pp. 1–70.

Armstrong, W. A., 'The trend of mortality in Carlisle between the 1780s and the 1840s: a demographic contribution to the standard of living debate', *Economic History Review*, 34, 1 (1981), 94–114.

Baber, Colin and Dennis Thomas, 'The Glamorgan economy, 1914–1945', in Arthur H. John and Glanmor Williams (eds), *Glamorgan County History*, vol. 5, *Industrial Glamorgan from 1700–1970* (Cardiff, 1980), pp. 519–79.

Beddoe, Deirdre, 'Munitionettes, maids and mams: women in Wales, 1914–1939', in Angela V. John (ed.), *Our Mothers' Land: Chapters in Welsh Women's History, 1830–1939* (Cardiff, 1991), pp. 189–209.

Benson, Susan Porter, 'Gender, generation, and consumption in the United States: working-class families in the interwar period', in Susan Strasser, Charles McGovern and Matthias Judt (eds), *Getting and Spending: European and American Consumer Societies in the Twentieth Century* (Cambridge, 1998), pp. 223–40.

Berger, S., 'The uses of the traditional sector in Italy', in F. Bechhofer and B. Elliott (eds), *The Petite Bourgeoisie: Comparative Studies of the Uneasy Stratum* (London, 1981), pp. 71–89.

Berridge, Virginia, 'Health and medicine', in F. M. L. Thompson (ed.), *The Cambridge Social History of Britain, 1750–1950*, vol. 3, *Social Agencies and Institutions* (Cambridge, 1990), pp. 171–242.

Brieger, Gert, 'The historiography of medicine', in W. F. Bynum and Roy Porter (eds), *Companion Encyclopedia of the History of Medicine* (London, 1993), vol. 1, pp. 24–44.

Brown, P. S., 'The vicissitudes of herbalism in late nineteenth- and early twentieth-century Britain', *Medical History*, 29, 1 (1985), 71–92.

Bryder, Linda, 'The First World War: healthy or hungry?', *History Workshop Journal*, 24 (1987), 141–57.

Burke, Peter 'Res et verba: conspicuous consumption in the early modern world', in John Brewer and Roy Porter (eds), *Consumption and the World of Goods* (London, 1993), pp. 148–61.

Cage, R. A., 'Infant mortality rates and housing: twentieth century Glasgow', *Scottish Economic and Social History*, 14 (1994), 72–92.

Chamberlain, Geoffrey, and A. Susan Williams, 'Antenatal care in south Wales, 1934–1962', *Social History of Medicine*, 8, 3 (1995), 480–8.

Chandler, Andy, '"The black death on wheels"; unemployment and migration – the experience of inter-war south Wales', in Tim Williams (ed.), *Papers in Modern Welsh History*, 1 (Cardiff, 1982), pp. 1–15.

Cherry, Steven, 'Beyond national health insurance: the voluntary hospitals and hospital contributory schemes: a regional study', *Social History of Medicine*, 5, 3 (1992), 455–82.

Cooter, Roger, 'Bones of contention? Orthodox medicine and the mystery of the bonesetters craft', in W. F. Bynum and Roy Porter (eds), *Medical Fringe and Medical Orthodoxy, 1750–1850* (London, 1987), pp. 158–73.

Crafts, N. F. R., 'Long-term unemployment in Britain in the 1930s', *Economic History Review*, 40, 3 (1987), 418–32.

Croll, Andy, 'Writing the insanitary town: G. T. Clark, slums and sanitary reform', in Brian L. James (ed.), *G. T. Clark. Scholar Ironmaster in the Victorian Age* (Cardiff, 1998), pp. 24–47.

Cronjé, Gillian, 'Tuberculosis and mortality decline in England and Wales, 1851–1910', in Robert Woods and John Hugh Woodward (eds), *Urban Disease and Mortality in Nineteenth-Century England* (London, 1984), pp. 79–101.

Crook, Rosemary, '"Tidy women": women in the Rhondda between the wars', *Oral History*, 10, 2 (1982), 40–6.

Crosby, A. W., 'Influenza', in Kenneth Kiple (ed.), *The Cambridge World History of Human Disease* (Cambridge, 1993), pp. 807–11.

Cross, G., 'Consumer history and the dilemmas of working-class history', *Labour History Review*, 62, 3 (1997), 261–74.

Daunton, Martin J., 'Miners' houses: South Wales and the Great Northern Coalfield, 1880–1914', *International Review of Social History*, 25, 2 (1980), 143–75.

—— 'Housing', in F. M. L. Thompson (ed.), *The Cambridge Social History of Britain, 1750–1950*, vol. 2, *People and their Environment* (Cambridge, 1990), pp. 195–250.

Davies, John, 'The communal conscience in Wales in the inter-war years', *Transactions of the Honourable Society of the Cymmrodorion* (1998), 145–60.

Davies, Sam, '"Three on the hook and three on the book": dock labourers and unemployment insurance between the wars', *Labour History Review*, 59, 3 (1994), 34–43

Deacon, Alan, 'Systems of interwar unemployment relief', in Sean Glynn and Alan Booth (eds), *The Road to Full Employment*, (London, 1987), pp. 31–42.

Desai, Sonalde, 'When are children from large families disadvantaged? Evidence from cross-national analyses', *Population Studies*, 49, 2 (1995), 195–210.

Duffin, Jacalyn, 'Pneumonia', in Kenneth Kiple (ed.), *The Cambridge World History of Human Disease* (Cambridge, 1993), pp. 938–9.

Duffy, John, 'History of public health and sanitation in the West since 1700', in Kenneth Kiple (ed.), *The Cambridge World History of Human Disease* (Cambridge, 1993), pp. 200–6.

Earwicker, Ray, 'Miners' medical services before the First World War: The South Wales Coalfield', *Llafur*, 3, 2 (1981), 39–52.

Eichengreen, Barry, 'Unemployment in interwar Britain: new evidence from London', *Journal of Interdisciplinary History*, 17, 2 (1986), 335–58.

Eichegreen, B., and T. J. Hatton, 'Interwar unemployment in international perspective: an overview', in idem (eds), *Interwar Unemployment in International Perspective* (Dordrecht, 1988), 1–59.

Evans, Neil, '"South Wales has been roused as never before": marching against the means test, 1934–1936', in David W. Howell and Kenneth O. Morgan (eds), *Crime, Protest and Police in Modern British Society: Essays in Memory of David J. V. Jones* (Cardiff, 1999), pp. 176–206.

Evans, Neil, and Dot Jones, '"A blessing for the miner's wife": the campaign for pithead baths in the south Wales coalfield, 1908–1950', *Llafur*, 6, 3 (1994), 5–28.

Fildes, Valerie, 'Infant feeding practices and infant mortality in England, 1900–1919', *Continuity and Change*, 13, 2 (1998), 251–80.

Finlayson, Geoffrey, 'A moving frontier: voluntarism and the state in British social welfare, 1911–1949', *Twentieth Century British History*, 1, 2 (1990), 183–206.

Fontaine, Laurence, and Jürgen Schlumbohm, 'Household strategies for survival: an introduction', *International Review of Social History*, 45 (2000), supplement 8, 1–17.

Garrett, Eilidh, and Andrew Wear, 'Suffer the little children: mortality, mothers and the state', *Continuity and Change*, 9, 2 (1994), 179–84.

Graham, David, 'Female employment and infant mortality: some evidence from British towns, 1911, 1931 and 1951', *Continuity and Change*, 9, 2 (1994), 313–46.

Green, A. and M. MacKinnon, 'Unemployment and relief in Canada', in Eichengreen and Hatton, *Interwar Unemployment in International Perspective*, p. 388.

Greenhalgh, Susan, 'Anthropology theorizes reproduction: integrating practice, political economic, and feminist approaches', in eadem (ed.), *Situating Fertility: Anthropology and Demographic Inquiry* (Cambridge, 1995), pp. 3–28.

Griffin, Colin P., '"Three days down the pit and three days play": underemployment in the East Midland Coalfields between the wars', *International Review of Social History*, 38 (1993), 321–43.

Harris, Bernard, 'The height of schoolchildren in Britain, 1900–1950' in John Komlos (ed.), *Stature, Living Standards, and Economic Development: Essays in Anthropometric History* (London, 1994), pp. 25–38.

Hart, Nicky, 'Beyond infant mortality: gender and stillbirth in reproductive mortality before the twentieth century', *Population Studies*, 52, 2 (1998), 215–29.

Hopkin, Deian, 'Social reactions to economic change', in Trevor Herbert and Gareth Elwyn Jones (eds), *Wales between the Wars* (Cardiff, 1988), pp. 52–98.

Huck, P., 'Infant mortality and living standards of English workers during the Industrial Revolution', *Journal of Economic History*, 55, 3 (1995), 528–50.

Jenner, Mark S. R., review of John Landers, *Death and the Metropolis: Studies in the Demographic History of London, 1670–1830* (Cambridge, 1993), and J. A. I. Chapman (ed.), *Epidemic Disease in London* (London, 1993), in *Urban History*, 22, 2 (1995), 295–7.

Jennings, J. H., 'Geographical implications of the municipal housing programme in England and Wales, 1919–39', *Urban Studies*, 8, 2 (1971), 121–38.

Johansson, Sheila Ryan, 'Sex and death in Victorian England: an examination of age- and sex-specific death rates, 1840–1910', in Martha Vicinus (ed.), *A Widening Sphere: Changing Roles of Victorian Women* (London, 1977), pp. 163–82.

Johnson, Paul A., 'Credit and thrift and the British working class, 1870–1939', in J. M. Winter (ed.), *The Working Class in Modern British History* (Cambridge, 1983), pp. 147–70.

—— 'Conspicuous consumption and working-class culture in late-Victorian and Edwardian Britain', *Transactions of the Royal Historical Society*, 38 (1988), 27–42.

Johnston, W. D., 'Tuberculosis', in Kenneth Kiple (ed.), *The Cambridge World History of Human Disease* (Cambridge, 1993), pp. 1059–68.

Jones, Dot, 'Counting the cost of coal: women's lives in the Rhondda, 1881–1911', in Angela V. John (ed.), *Our Mothers' Land: Chapters in Welsh Women's History, 1830–1939* (Cardiff, 1991), pp. 109–33.

Jones, Ieuan Gwynedd, 'The people's health in mid-Victorian Wales', in idem, *Mid Victorian Wales: The Observer and the Observed* (Cardiff, 1992), pp. 24–53.

Kertzer, David, I., 'Political-economic and cultural explanations of demographic behaviour', in Susan Greenhalgh (ed.), *Situating Fertility: Anthropology and Demographic Inquiry* (Cambridge, 1995), pp. 29–52.

Lawrence, R. J., 'Domestic space and society: a cross cultural study', *Comparative Studies in Society and History*, 24 (1982), 104–30.

Lee, C. H., 'Regional inequalities in infant mortality in Britain, 1861–1971: patterns and hypotheses', *Population Studies*, 45, 1 (1991), 55–65.

Lee, R., 'Infant, child and maternal mortality in Western Europe: a critique', in A. Brändström and L.-G. Tedebrand (eds), *Society, Health and Population during the Demographic Transition* (Stockholm, 1988), pp. 9–21.

Lewis, Jane, 'Providers, "consumers", the state and the delivery of health-care services in twentieth-century Britain', in Andrew Wear (ed.), *Medicine in Society: Historical Essays* (Cambridge, 1992), pp. 317–45.

Loudon, Irvine, 'Maternal mortality: definition and secular trends in England and Wales, 1850–1970', in Kenneth Kiple (ed.), *The Cambridge World History of Human Disease* (Cambridge, 1995), pp. 214–24.

Loux, F., 'Popular culture and knowledge of the body: infancy and the medical anthropologist', in Roy Porter and Andrew Wear (eds), *Problems and Methods in the History of Medicine* (London, 1987), pp. 81–97.

Loux, Françoise, 'Folk medicine', in W. F. Bynum and Roy Porter (eds), *Companion Encyclopedia of the History of Medicine* (London, 1993), vol. 1, pp. 661–75.

Luckin, Bill, and Graham Mooney, 'Urban history and historical epidemiology: the case of London, 1860–1920', *Urban History*, 24, 2 (1997), 37–55.

McInnes, Angus, 'Surviving the slump: an oral history of Stoke-on-Trent between the wars', *Midland History*, 18 (1993), 121–40.

McKenna, Madeline, 'The suburbanization of the working-class population of Liverpool between the wars', *Social History*, 16, 2 (1991), 173–89.

Marshall, J. L., 'The pattern of housebuilding in the inter-war period in England and Wales', *Scottish Journal of Political Economy*, 15, 2 (1968), 184–205.

Mayhew, Madeleine, 'The 1930s nutrition controversy', *Journal of Contemporary History*, 23, 3 (1988), 445–64.

Miley, Ursula, and John V. Pickstone, 'Medical botany around 1850: American medicine in industrial Britain', in Roger Cooter (ed.), *Studies in the History of Alternative Medicine* (London, 1988), pp. 140–54.

Mitchell, Margaret, 'The effects of unemployment on the social conditions of women and children in the 1930s', *History Workshop Journal*, 19 (1985), 105–27.

Oddy, Derek J., 'The health of the people', in T. Barker and M. Drake (eds), *Population and Society in Britain 1850–1950* (London, 1982), pp. 121–41.

—— 'Food, drink and nutrition', in F. M. L. Thompson (ed.), *The Cambridge Social History of Britain, 1750–1950*, vol. 2, *People and their Environment* (Cambridge, 1990), pp. 251–78.

Page, S. J., 'The mobility of the poor: a case study of Edwardian Leicester', *Local Historian*, 21, 3 (1991), 109–19.

Pamuk, E. R., 'Social class inequality in mortality from 1921 to 1972 in England and Wales', *Population Studies*, 39 (1985), 17–31.

Pelling, Margaret, 'Unofficial and unorthodox medicine', in Irvine Loudon (ed.), *The Oxford Illustrated History of Western Medicine* (Oxford, 1997), pp. 264–76.

Peretz, Elizabeth, 'The costs of modern motherhood to low income families in interwar Britain', in Valerie Fildes, Lara Marks and Hilary Marland (eds), *Women and Children First: International Maternal and Infant Welfare, 1870–1945* (London, 1992), pp. 257–80.

Phillips, Gervase, 'An army of giants: height and medical characteristics of Welsh soldiers, 1914–1918', *Archives*, 22, 97 (1997), 141–6.

Pickstone, John V., 'Establishment and dissent in nineteenth-century medicine: an exploration of some correspondence and connections between religious and medical belief systems in early industrial England', in W. J. Sheils (ed.), *The Church and Healing* (Oxford, 1982), pp. 165–89.

Pickstone, John V., review of R. Porter and W. F. Bynum (eds), *Living and Dying in London* (London, 1991), *Social History of Medicine*, 7, 1 (1994), 147–8.

Pooley, Colin G., 'Introduction', in idem (ed.), *Housing Strategies in Europe, 1880–1930* (Leicester, 1992), pp. 1–10.

—— 'England and Wales', in idem (ed.), *Housing Strategies in Europe, 1880–1930* (Leicester, 1992), pp. 73–104.

Pooley, Colin G., and S. Irish, 'Access to housing on Merseyside, 1919–39', *Transactions of the Institute of British Geographers*, 12 (1987), 177–90.

Porter, Dorothy, 'Public health', in W. F. Bynum and R. Porter (eds), *Companion Encyclopedia of the History of Medicine* (London, 1993), vol. 2, pp. 1231–61.

Porter, Roy, 'The patient's view: doing medical history from below', *Theory and Society*, 14 (1985), 175–98.

—— '"I think ye both quacks": the controversy between Dr Theodor Myersbach and Dr John Coakley Lettsom', in W. F. Bynum and Roy Porter (eds), *Medical Fringe and Medical Orthodoxy, 1750–1850* (London, 1987), 56–78.

—— and Andrew Wear, 'Introduction', in idem (eds), *Problems and Methods in the History of Medicine* (London, 1987), pp. 1–11.

Powell, Martin, 'How adequate was hospital provision before the NHS? An examination of the 1945 South Wales Hospital Survey', *Local Population Studies*, 48 (1992), 22–32.

—— 'Hospital Provision before the National Health Service: a geographical study of the 1945 hospital surveys', *Social History of Medicine*, 5, 3 (1992), 483–504.

—— 'The geography of English hospital provision in the 1930s', *Journal of Historical Geography*, 18, 3 (1992), 307–16.

—— 'Did politics matter? Municipal public health expenditure in the 1930s', *Urban History*, 22, 3 (1995), 360–79.

Preston, Samuel H., 'Population studies of mortality', *Population Studies*, 50 (1996), 525–36.

Rather, L. J., 'The "six things non-natural": a note on the origins and fate of a doctrine and a phrase', *Clio Medica*, 3, 4 (1968), 337–47.

Rees, R., 'The south Wales copper-smoke dispute, 1833–95', *Welsh History Review*, 10, 4 (1981), 480–96.

Reher, David, 'Wasted investments: some economic implications of childhood mortality patterns', *Population Studies*, 49, 3 (1995), 519–36.

Richards, H., 'Investment in public health provision in the mining valleys of south Wales, 1860–1914', in Colin Baber and John Williams (eds), *Modern South Wales: Essays in Economic History* (Cardiff, 1986), pp. 128–39.

Riley, James C., 'Measuring morbidity and mortality', in Kenneth Kiple (ed.), *The Cambridge World History of Human Disease* (Cambridge, 1993), pp. 230–8.

Roberts, Elizabeth, 'Working-class standards of living in Barrow and Lancaster, 1890–1914', *Economic History Review*, 30, 2 (1977), 306–21.

—— 'Oral history investigations of disease and its management by the Lancashire working class, 1890–1939', in J. V. Pickstone (ed.), *Health, Disease and Medicine in Lancashire, 1750–1950: Four Papers on Sources, Problems and Methods* (Manchester, 1980), pp. 33–51.

—— 'Women's strategies, 1890–1940', in Jane Lewis (ed.), *Labour and Love: Women's Experience of Home and Family, 1850–1940* (Oxford, 1989), pp. 223–47.

Rosen, George, 'Social variables and health in an urban environment: the case of the Victorian city', *Clio Medica*, 8, 1 (1973), 1–17.

Ryder, R. 'Council house building in County Durham, 1900–39: the local implementation of national policy', in Martin J. Daunton (ed.), *Councillors and Tenants: Local Authority Housing in English Cities, 1919–1939* (Leicester, 1984).

Saito, Osamu, 'Historical demography: achievements and prospects', *Population Studies*, 50, 3 (1996), 537–53.

Scott, Peter, 'The state, internal migration, and growth of new industrial communities in inter-war Britain', *English Historical Review*, 115, 461 (2000), 329–53.

Sigsworth, Michael, and Michael Worboys, 'The public's view of public health in mid-Victorian Britain', *Urban History*, 21, 2 (1994), 237–50.

Stockwell, E. G., 'Infant mortality', in Kenneth Kiple (ed.), *The Cambridge World History of Human Disease* (Cambridge, 1993), pp. 224–30.

Stolnitz, George J., 'A century of international mortality trends: II', *Population Studies*, 10, 1 (1956–7), 17–42.

Swenarton, M., and S. Taylor, 'The scale and nature of the growth of owner-occupation in Britain between the wars', *Economic History Review*, 38, 3 (1985), 373–92.

Szreter, Simon, 'The importance of social intervention in Britain's mortality decline c.1850–1914: a reinterpretation of the role of public health', *Social History of Medicine*, 1 (1988), 1–37.

—— and Graham Mooney, 'Urbanisation, mortality and the standard of living debate: new estimates of the expectation of life at birth in nineteenth-century British cities', *Economic History Review*, 51 (1997), 84–112.

Taylor, Avram, '"You never told your man": women's management of household finances and credit during the inter-war period', *North East Labour History Society*, 30 (1996), 51–65.

Tebbutt, Melanie, 'Women's talk? Gossip and "women's words" in working-class communities, 1880–1939', in Andrew Davies and Steven Fielding (eds), *Workers' Worlds: Cultures and Communities in Manchester and Salford, 1880–1939* (Manchester, 1992), pp. 49–73.

Thane, Pat, 'Visions of gender in the making of the British welfare state: the case of women in the British Labour Party and social policy, 1906–45', in Gisela Bock and Pat Thane (eds), *Maternity and Gender Politics: Women and the Rise of European Welfare States 1880s-1950s* (London, 1991), pp. 93–118.

Thomas, Mark, 'Labour market structure and the nature of unemployment in interwar Britain', in B. Eichengreen and T. J. Hatton (eds), *Interwar Unemployment in International Perspective* (Dordrecht, 1988), pp. 97–148.

Thompson, Steven, 'Hospital provision, charity and public responsibility in Edwardian Pontypridd', *Llafur*, 8, 3 (2002), 53–65.

—— '"That beautiful summer of severe austerity": health, diet and the working-class domestic economy in south Wales in 1926', *Welsh History Review*, 21, 3 (2003), 552–74.

—— 'A proletarian public sphere: working-class self-provision of medical services and care in south Wales, *c.*1900–1948', in Anne Borsay (ed.), *Medicine in Wales, c.1800–2000: Public Service or Private Commodity?* (Cardiff, 2003), pp. 86–107.

—— 'To relieve the sufferings of humanity, irrespective of party, politics or creed: conflict, consensus and voluntary hospital provision in Edwardian south Wales', *Social History of Medicine*, 16, 2 (2003), 247–62.

—— '"Conservative bloom on Socialism's compost heap": working-class home ownership in South Wales, *c.*1890–1939', in R. R. Davies and Geraint H. Jenkins (eds) *From Medieval to Modern Wales: Historical Essays in Honour of Kenneth O. Morgan and Ralph A. Griffiths* (Cardiff, 2004), pp. 246–63.

Tudor Hart, J., 'The inverse care law', *The Lancet* (27 Feb. 1971), 405–12.

Webster, Charles, 'Healthy or hungry thirties?', *History Workshop Journal*, 13 (1982), 110–29.

—— 'Health, welfare and unemployment during the Depression', *Past and Present*, 109 (1985), 204–29.

Whiteside, Noel, 'The social consequences of interwar unemployment', in S. Glynn and A. Booth (eds), *The Road to Full Employment* (London, 1987), pp. 17–30.

—— 'Counting the cost: sickness and disability among working people in an era of industrial recession, 1920–1939', *Economic History Review*, 40, 2 (1987), 228–46.

Whiteside, Noel, and J. A. Gillespie, 'Deconstructing unemployment: developments in Britain in the interwar years', *Economic History Review*, 44, 4 (1991), 665–82.

Williams, A. Susan, 'Relief and research: the nutrition work of the National Birthday Trust Fund, 1935–9', in David F. Smith (ed.), *Nutrition in Britain: Science, Scientists and Politics in the Twentieth Century* (London, 1997), pp. 99–122.

Williams, Gareth, 'From grand slam to great slump: economy, society and rugby football in Wales during the Depression', in idem, *1905 and All That: Essays on Rugby Football, Sport and Welsh Society* (Llandysul, 1991), pp. 175–200

Williams, Mari A., 'Yr ymgyrch i "Achub y Mamau" yng nghymoedd diwydiannol de Cymru, 1918–1939', *Cof Cenedl*, 11 (Llandysul, 1996), 117–46.

—— '"In the wars": Wales 1914–1945', in Gareth Elwyn Jones and Dai Smith (eds), *The People of Wales* (Llandysul, 1999), pp.179–206.

Williams, Sian Rhiannon, 'The Bedwellty Board of Guardians and the Default Act of 1927', *Llafur*, 4, 2 (1979), 65–77.

Winter, Jay Murray, 'The impact of the First World War on civilian health in Britain', *Economic History Review*, 30, 3 (1977), 487–503.

—— 'Infant mortality, maternal mortality and public health in Britain in the 1930s', *Journal of European Economic History*, 8, 2 (1979), 439–62.

—— 'The decline of mortality in Britain, 1870–1950', in T. Barker and M. Drake (eds), *Population and Society in Britain, 1850–1950* (London, 1982), pp. 100–20.

—— 'Unemployment, nutrition and infant mortality in Britain, 1920–50', in idem (ed.), *The Working Class in Modern British History* (Cambridge, 1983), pp. 232–55.

—— *The Great War and the British People* (London, 1986).

—— 'Public health and the political economy of war: a reply to Linda Bryder', *History Workshop Journal*, 26 (1988), 163–73.

Woods, R. I., P. A. Watterson and J. H. Woodward, 'The causes of rapid infant mortality decline in England and Wales, 1861–1921 part I', *Population Studies*, 42, 3 (1988), 343–66.

—— 'The causes of rapid infant mortality decline in England and Wales, 1861–1921, part II', *Population Studies*, 43, 1 (1989), 113–32.

Woods, R., 'Public health and public hygiene: the urban environment in the late nineteenth and early twentieth centuries', in R. Schofield, D. Reher and A. Bideau (eds), *The Decline of Mortality in Europe* (Oxford, 1991), pp. 233–47.

—— 'Infant mortality in Britain: a survey of current knowledge on historical trends and variations', in A. Bideau, B. Desjardins and H. Pérez-Brignoli (eds), *Infant and Child Mortality in the Past* (Oxford, 1997), pp. 74–88.

Wrigley, E. A., 'The prospects for population history', *Journal of Interdisciplinary History*, 12, 2 (1981), 207–26.

10. Unpublished theses

Armbruster, G. H., 'The social determination of ideologies: being a study of a Welsh mining community', University of London Ph.D. (1940).

Bourne, M. C., 'A study of council house building activity in post-war Cardiff', UWIST M.Sc., (1981).

Buchanan, I. M., 'Infant mortality in British coal mining communities, 1880–1911', University of London Ph.D. (1983).

Chandler, A. J., 'The re-making of a working class: migration from the South Wales Coalfield to the new industry areas of the Midlands *c*.1920–1940', University of Wales Ph.D. (1989).

Grenfell-Hill, J. Du C., 'Mother and infants in South Wales, 1900–1930', University of Wales Ph.D. (1993).

Hadfield, J., 'Health in the industrial North-East 1919–39', University of Sheffield Ph.D. (1977).

Harris, B. J., 'Medical inspection and the nutrition of schoolchildren in Britain, 1900–1950', University of London Ph.D. (1989).

Keane, J. M., 'The impact of unemployment: a study of the effects of unemployment in a working-class district of Cardiff in the depression years, 1930–35', University of Wales M.Sc. (Econ.) (1983).

Leiper, N. J., 'Health and unemployment in Glamorgan, 1923–1938', University of Wales M.Sc. (1986).

Thompson, Steven, 'A social history of health in interwar South Wales', University of Wales Ph.D. (2001).

Tingle, A. J., 'The School Medical Service in Cardiff, 1902–44', University of Wales M. Ed. (1980).

Wright, J. F., 'The development of public water supplies in the Swansea area, 1837–1989', University of Wales Local History Diploma (1991).

INDEX

Note: page references followed by n, fig or t indicate material in footnotes, figures and tables respectively.

Theha - p119

https://unnail.glam.ac.uk
excheage

p 230
229